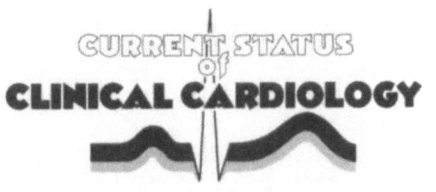

CURRENT STATUS
of
CLINICAL CARDIOLOGY

Series Editor J. P. Shillingford

CURRENT STATUS
OF CLINICAL
CARDIOLOGY 1990

CURRENT STATUS OF CLINICAL CARDIOLOGY

Series Editor J.P. Shillingford

All the chapters in this book, with the exception of Chapter 7, are revised and updated versions of chapters which were originally published in the volumes of the *Current Status of Clinical Cardiology* series, as follows:

Chapters 1, 4, 11: from Spry, C.J.F. (ed.) *Immunology and Molecular Biology of Cardiovascular Diseases* (1987)

Chapters 2, 3: from Camm, A.J. and Ward, D.E. (eds.) *Clinical Aspects of Cardiac Arrhythmias* (1988)

Chapter 5: from Goodwin, J.F. (ed.) *Heart Muscle Disease* (1985)

Chapter 6: from Macartney, F.J. (ed.) *Congenital Heart Disease* (1986)

Chapters 8, 9, 10: from Fox, K.M. (ed.) *Ischaemic Heart Disease* (1987)

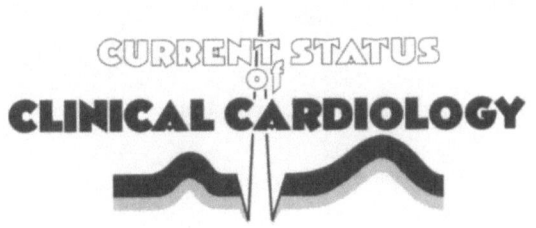

CURRENT STATUS
OF
CLINICAL CARDIOLOGY

Series Editor J.P. Shillingford

CURRENT STATUS OF CLINICAL CARDIOLOGY 1990

Edited by
D.G. Julian

Consultant Medical Director
British Heart Foundation;
Emeritus Professor of Cardiology
University of Newcastle upon Tyne

KLUWER ACADEMIC PUBLISHERS
DORDRECHT / BOSTON / LONDON

Distributors

for the United States and Canada: Kluwer Academic Publishers, PO Box 358, Accord Station, Hingham, MA 02018-0358, USA
for all other countries: Kluwer Academic Publishers Group, Distribution Center, PO Box 322, 3300 AH Dordrecht, The Netherlands

ISBN-13:978-94-010-6813-0   e-ISBN-13:978-94-009-0729-4
DOI: 10.1007/978-94-009-0729-4

Contents

List of Contributors

L D Allan
Department of Perinatal Cardiology
Guy's Hospital
15th floor, Guy's Tower
St Thomas Street
London SE1 9RT
UK

D J Betteridge
Department of Medicine
University College and Middlesex
    School of Medicine
The Rayne Institute
University Street
London WC1E 6JJ
UK

A Cheng
Department of Cardiology
Harefield Hospital
Harefield
Middlesex UB9 6JH
UK

P Chisholm
Immunology Section
Division of Biomolecular Sciences
Kings College
University of London
Camden Hill Road
London W8 7AH
UK

P A Crean
Regional Cardiology Unit
St James' Hospital
James Street
Dublin 8
Republic of Ireland

S E Humphries
Charing Cross Sunley Research
    Centre
1 Lurgan Avenue
Hammersmith
London W6 8LW
UK

C D J Ilsley
Department of Cardiology
Harefield Hospital
Harefield
Middlesex UB9 6JH
UK

D G Julian
Consultant Medical Director
British Heart Foundation
102 Gloucester Place
London W1H 4DH
UK

C M Oakley
Department of Medicine (Clinical
    Cardiology)
Hammersmith Hospital
Royal Postgraduate Medical School
Ducane Road
London W12 0NN
UK

E G J Olsen
Department of Histopathology
(Cardiovascular Division)
Brompton Hospital
Fulham Road
London SW3 6HP
UK

E J Perrins
Department of Cardiology
The General Infirmary at Leeds
Great George Street
Leeds LS1 3EX
UK

A A Quyyumi
National Heart, Lung and Blood
    Institute
National Institutes of Health,
    Building 10 7B15
Bethesda
MD 20892
USA

A Tybjærg-Hansen
Charing Cross Sunley Research
    Centre
1 Lurgan Avenue
Hammersmith
London W6 8LW
UK

D A Zideman
Department of Anaesthetics
Hammersmith Hospital
Royal Postgraduate Medical School
Ducane Road, London W12 0HS
UK

Foreword

D.G. JULIAN

Cardiology has been advancing on a broad front and in recent years we have learned much about the basic mechanisms underlying heart disease, and developed many new methods of diagnosis and treatment. This book discusses in depth some of the most important aspects of these.

One of the most exciting areas of research has been in molecular biology; Tybjærg-Hansen and Humphries describe how, following the pioneering Nobel prize-winning work of Goldstein and Brown, gene probes are being used to discover the genetic causes of coronary artery disease, especially in the hyperlipidaemias but also in thrombotic states. These developments, together with the introduction of powerful lipid-lowering agents has triggered interest in the primary hyperlipidaemias, which are frequently hereditary. Betteridge discusses their diagnosis and management. Quyyumi describes how a greater knowledge of the physiology and pathology of the coronary circulation has led to a better understanding of the causes of angina pectoris and of 'silent ischaemia'. Crean deals with the difficult topic of unstable angina, which has caused a lot of controversy in the past, but whose investigation and management is now broadly agreed.

Probably nowhere in medicine in recent years has there been a more exciting and important advance than the introduction of thrombolytic agents in acute myocardial infarction. This subject is dealt with in detail by Cheng and Ilsley, but they also consider the role of angioplasty and surgery in this context, as well as the place of drugs including aspirin and β-blockers. It is disappointing that 30 years after the introduction of modern cardiopulmonary resuscitation, so few patients in or out of hospital are saved from cardiac arrest, when the potential is so great. This is partly because many doctors do not know as much as they should about the procedures to be followed. Zideman outlines the modern management of cardiac arrest and cites the latest recommendations of the use of drugs in this situation. Cardiac pacing has become a highly specialised field, as pacemakers become more complex. This certainly has worked for the benefit of patients, but perhaps to the confusion of many doctors. The rate of pacemaker implantation in the United Kingdom is notoriously low and probably reflects both ignorance on the part of the medical profession and financial constraints. Perrins describes the various types of pacemaker available and the indications for their use.

Fetal echocardiography is a technique that is insufficiently well-known and one that deserves much wider application. Lindsey Allan, who is one of the leaders in this field, illustrates very clearly what can be achieved by this method. In the long term it should lead to a substantial reduction in the number of cases of severe congenital heart disease.

Amyloid heart disease is a relative rarity but, as Celia Oakley points out, one of considerable clinical interest.

Immunology has until recently had a relatively minor impact in cardiology, but, as Olsen shows, there are a large number of cardiac conditions from rheumatic disease to cardiomyopathy in which immune processes play an important role.

Heart transplantation is now an accepted form of treatment for advanced cardiac disease and the results today are very much better than they were only a few years ago. Nevertheless, there is still a long way to go in solving the problems of rejection; Chisholm discusses the various models which are being currently studied with the hope that a better understanding of the processes involved will lead to substantial improvements in survival and the quality of life of survivors.

The authorities who have contributed to this book have addressed their subjects in a comprehensible and stimulating way. Readers will certainly find much to interest them amongst the wide range of topics discussed.

1
Experimental cardiac transplantation

P. M. CHISHOLM

INTRODUCTION

Cardiac transplantation is not of course a cardiovascular disease, but the procedure is carried out as a consequence of disease. The immune response of the recipient animal to the histocompatibility differences between the donor and recipient of the graft also results in cardiac pathology, i.e. the destruction of cardiac tissue and loss of organ function. Experimental cardiac transplantation has as its raison d'etre the need to understand the fundamental nature of the immune response to organ or tissue allografts transplanted between different members of the same species, and the mechanisms by which these allografts are rejected. From this understanding strategies should develop for the diagnosis and prevention of graft rejection which will be applicable in man.

In the published proceedings of the last two International Congresses of the Transplantation Society, held in Helsinki, Finland in 1986[1] and in Sydney, Australia in 1988[2], almost all the papers presented in experimental transplantation described results obtained in rodent models and a substantial proportion of those used cardiac allograft models. This is primarily a reflection of the explosion over the past two decades in research in cellular immunology and immunogenetics using inbred strains of mice and rats, which has resulted both in a thorough understanding of the genetics and biology of the major histocompatibility complex (MHC), the gene complex which codes for the tissue antigens involved in transplant rejection, and in a comprehensive description of the cellular mechanisms responsible for the immunological rejection of organ allografts. It is also a reflection of the recognition that many features of the immune response to MHC-disparate grafts are universally applicable to grafts of different tissues in different species. Thus it has become clear that although the MHC is highly polymorphic, i.e. the extent of MHC-encoded antigenic variation between individuals of a species is very large, the number of effector mechanisms in graft rejection directed at those differences is strictly limited: differences in the fate of different organ grafts in the same or different species can be considered as variations on a single, although complex immunobiological theme.

1

This great increase in transplantation research has generated an enormous literature. In a number of recent reviews on the immunobiology of transplantation and the mechanisms of graft rejection[3,4] results obtained from experimental cardiac transplantation have made a significant contribution. It is my intention here not to review the field once more, but instead to simply highlight the key features of experimental cardiac transplantation which may be of interest to the non-immunological cardiologist or biologist, and which I believe are of most relevance to the practice and understanding of clinical heart transplantation. The first section comprises a brief consideration of those aspects of tissue immunogenicity which govern the fate of transplanted tissues, and a description of the types of immune mediated injury which occur during the process of transplant rejection. The second section describes the various models of rodent cardiac transplantation in common use. The final section describes the molecular and cellular events which take place within allogeneic cardiac tissue during uninterrupted graft rejection, and shows how these events can be modified by immunological intervention.

THE IMMUNOBIOLOGY OF GRAFT REJECTION

Tissue immunogenicity

The molecules which induce the immune response to organ allografts are the major and minor histocompatibility antigens of the species. The major antigens are coded for by a group of genes located on a single chromosome, the major histocompatibility complex (MHC) and, as their name implies, they provoke the strongest alloimmune responses. They are glycoproteins expressed on cell surfaces and, on the basis of structural and biological differences, are classified as Class I or Class II MHC molecules. There are a large number of minor histocompatibility antigens and these can also be important in transplantation. None of the gene products has yet been identified, but they are coded for by genes distributed throughout the genome and estimates of their number are in the hundreds.

In the context of organ transplantation it is important to realize that all the cellular constituents of a tissue are not equally immunogenic and that, at least partly, this is a consequence of differences in the amount, i.e. numbers, of MHC molecules on the constituent cell types. In the normal heart, which consists basically of myocardial cells, vascular endothelium and interstitial dendritic cells, myocardial cells express very few Class I MHC molecules and no Class II molecules. Vascular endothelium expresses Class I and, in some species only, e.g. human, Class II. Interstitial dendritic cells express both Class I and (relatively large amounts of) Class II. They have their counterpart in most other tissues[5], are bone marrow derived and have a comparatively short turnover time of days or weeks[6]. After transplantation, these cells are lost from the graft by replacement from the recipient bone marrow: loss of these 'passenger leukocytes' which are extremely potent stimulators of alloimmune responses from the graft leads therefore to a natural reduction in the immunogenicity of the graft.

In complete contrast to this reduction in MHC content which occurs as a result of normal cell turnover, the content of MHC antigen in tissues can be dramatically increased as a result of immune activation. *De novo* or increased expression of MHC antigens on cells *in vivo* was first described in rodents in the target organs of graft-versus-host disease[7,8] and more recently in rejecting cardiac[9] and skin[10] allografts. Numerous *in vitro* studies[11] then showed that the expression of MHC Class I and Class II antigens can be substantially altered on cells cultured from virtually every organ by exposure to immune interferon or to crude tissue culture supernatants obtained from activated lymphocytes. From all these studies has emerged the important concept that the amount of alloantigen contained within a particular tissue is not an unvarying quantity, and that the immunogenicity of a graft after transplantation may change as a consequence of the immune reaction to it. The extent of expression of MHC Class I or Class II antigens within an organ allograft at the time of transplant is of importance because each class of antigen tends to induce different types of immune response: in general, Class I MHC alloantigens induce cytotoxic T-cell responses and Class II antigens induce activation of the T-cells involved in delayed type hypersensitivity responses[12]. Subsequent increases in the expression of MHC molecules on the graft tissue following transplantation as a consequence of that immune activation will also have a profound effect on the susceptibility of the graft to immune-mediated damage. Effector mechanisms involving T cells directed at Class I and Class II differences are both involved in graft rejection[12,13] although the relative contribution of each may differ in different circumstances (see below).

Mechanisms of graft tissue injury

A great deal of work over the past decade has established the cellular basis for the immunological rejection of allografts. This has included detailed descriptions of the ways in which the immune system is stimulated by the presence of an organ or tissue allograft to produce a range of responses, and of the intragraft events which lead to its eventual destruction. Classical experiments in the 1950s and 1960s established that graft rejection cannot be passively transferred by immune serum but the transfer of lymphocytes from an animal which has rejected one allograft of a particular histocompatibility type to a naive recipient of a graft of the same histocompatibility type will result in an accelerated rejection of the graft. If a naive recipient of a graft is rendered incapable of rejecting the graft before transplantation, e.g. by irradiation, then transfer of T-lymphocytes alone from a previously sensitized animal will restore graft rejection. This type of experiment in a number of animal models including the rat cardiac allograft model[14] has established that graft rejection is primarily a cell-mediated reaction involving T-lymphocytes, although other cell types may be secondarily involved.

There are a number of ways in which the immune system can inflict damage on an allogeneic target organ. Specifically sensitized cytotoxic T-cells kill allogeneic target cells independently of alloantibody and complement: these cells are produced in response to cardiac allografts and can be recovered from the rejecting tissue itself[15]. A different cytotoxic cell, the killer or K-cell, destroys target cells only if they are coated with specific antibody, i.e. in a transplant situation if the graft cells are coated with alloantibody. This antibody dependent cell-mediated cytotoxicity (ADCC) has been demonstrated in cardiac allografts and, interestingly, it has been shown that different cells within cardiac tissue differ in their susceptibility to this kind of immune damage: vascular endothelial cells but not myocardial cells from rat heart were killed by cytotoxic T-cells, whereas the myocardial cells were more efficiently lysed by alloantibody dependent killing[16]. A third cytotoxic effector cell involved in cell-mediated cytotoxicity is the natural killer or NK-cell, and increased levels of NK-cell activity have been reported in rats rejecting cardiac allografts[17].

In addition to these direct mechanisms, graft tissue can be damaged indirectly by a number of inflammatory processes, probably mediated by various cytokines, and triggered coincidentally with and/or as a consequence of the specific immune response. For example, macrophages accumulate within rejecting cardiac tissue and exhibit some of the features of activation which suggest that they may be involved in graft destruction[18].

There has been much debate in recent years on the relative importance of each of these numerous effector systems to graft rejection[13,19]. It is most unlikely that any one mechanism of tissue destruction will always predominate, and highly likely that the importance of one or other will depend on the organ grafted, and the species involved. The relative importance of each mechanism may also change within the same organ with time after transplantation as a result of immune activation. The balance between the different effector mechanisms is also likely to be altered by different immunosuppressive strategies which may selectively inhibit one particular effector function and not another. More important, therefore, than trying to assign a rigid hierarchy of importance to the various mechanisms of rejection is to identify the detailed molecular and cellular events within each organ type in any particular species during uninterrupted graft rejection so that strategies for immune intervention can be designed.

RODENT MODELS OF CARDIAC GRAFTING

The availability of large numbers of different inbred strains of mice and rats has made these the species of choice for experimental transplantation. They are relatively inexpensive, easy to house, breed rapidly and efficiently. Grafts can be exchanged between individuals of different inbred strains which have well defined MHC disparities, and so the importance of genetic differences to the outcome of transplantation can be assessed. Much more is known about the genetics of the mouse MHC, the H-2 system, than the rat MHC and for this reason most of our knowledge has been obtained in the mouse.

However, although the study of the immune response in mice to allogeneic tissue, in the form of dissociated cell suspensions usually leukocytes, has furnished many of the basic facts of the immunobiology of transplantation, it is difficult to perform organ allografts in so small an animal. The rat is much more amenable to microsurgical techniques and this, together with the recent increase in the number of available inbred rat strains, has resulted in widespread use of rat cardiac graft models. The heart graft can be either adult heterotopic, i.e. placed surgically in an extra-thoracic site such as in the abdomen[20] or neck[21], or it can be neonatal. Fetal grafts can be placed, without microsurgery, in a highly vascularized tissue space such as the pinna of the ear, or the plantar space[22]. The amount of fetal tissue transplanted is very small, and gaseous exchange is achieved by simple diffusion.

The heterotopic adult abdominal model pioneered by Ono and Lindsey[20], and used in a modified form by many groups, involves the microsurgical end-to-side anastomosis of the aorta and pulmonary artery to the abdominal aorta and the inferior vena cava, respectively. It is this method which has been successfully adapted to the mouse[23] although there are only a handful of laboratories in which this extremely exacting technique is routinely carried out. One variation to the model in the rat uses end-to-end anastomoses, following unilateral nephrectomy, between the renal and left carotid arteries and between the pulmonary artery and the renal vein[9]. In a different heterotopic model, cuffing techniques are used to establish the vascular connections and the graft is placed in the neck[21]. The advantages are that difficult microsurgery is avoided, and the cervical site also makes the monitoring of gross graft function (visibly) easy. Both the abdominal and cervical sites have been used sequentially in the same animal to compare the immunological parameters of first and second set cardiac graft rejection[24].

As is the case with all experimental models, the questions asked of these cardiac allograft models must be carefully chosen. In many respects the immune response to allogeneic cardiac tissue is the same irrespective of the particular model used. For example, the rejection time is very similar for the same graft tissue placed in different anatomical sites if there are not substantial differences in blood flow. The antigenicity of adult compared to neonatal tissue is, at least where MHC differences are involved, essentially the same. Without exception, allogeneic cardiac tissue, whether adult or neonatal and irrespective of the transplant site, is infiltrated with leukocytes before rejection, and some or all of the immune effector functions described above have been identified in all the models described. However, in some respects the models differ from each other and the results obtained are not comparable.

Additionally, it should be remembered that in none of the experimental models described does the graft function as a normal heart, so although an assessment can be made of myocardial function at the cellular level, one cannot ask questions concerning organ function which are physiologically or clinically relevant. For the same reason results obtained from these experimental models can be of only limited usefulness in assessing for example which parameters of cardiac function might be most useful in the early diagnosis of clinical rejection: the criteria for defining useful cardiac function are very different for the orthotopic compared to the heterotopic auxiliary graft. Nevertheless, despite their limitations, these experimental models have furnished the basic facts of cardiac transplantation biology as described in detail in the following section.

INTRAGRAFT EVENTS DURING REJECTION

Uninterrupted rejection

One of the strategies used to identify which lymphocytes are involved in cardiac allograft rejection and to assign specific roles for the different populations of T-lymphocytes (viz. helper/inducer or suppressor/cytotoxic cells) has been to compare the capacity of the different subpopulations to restore graft rejection in grafted animals which are rendered unable to reject their grafts. The results obtained from a number of laboratories can be summarized as follows: purified populations of unsensitized T-cells, i.e. taken from naive animals, were found to be sufficient to restore acute first set cardiac graft rejection in lethally irradiated grafted recipients; B-lymphocytes were not effective[14]. In a similar system using T-cells sensitized to histocompatibility antigens of the same type as the graft, it was found that purified T-cells of either the helper/inducer T-cell subpopulation (also responsible for delayed-type hypersensitivity reactions[25]) or of the cytotoxic/suppressor subpopulation could, when transferred alone, restore first set cardiac rejection[26]. Subsequent studies, using monoclonal antibodies with specificity for the different T-cell subpopulations[27] to purify the T-cell subsets before transfer, confirmed that T-helper/inducer (CD4-positive) cells alone could bring about graft rejection[25] although, as had been described previously in mouse skin allografts[28], the grafts at rejection contained large numbers of the cytotoxic/suppressor (CD8-positive) cells[29], probably of host rather than donor origin. Using a different model it was shown that small numbers of sensitized T-cells injected together with IL2-containing lymphokine supernatants could adoptively restore heart graft rejection in T-cell-deprived rats[30]. More recently the same group reported that although CD4-positive T-cells alone restored rejection, they were less effective than unfractionated T-cell populations also containing CD8-positive cells[31]. Taken all together these studies suggest a necessary role for both the helper/inducer or DTH T-cell and the suppressor/cytotoxic T-cell subpopulations in rat cardiac rejection: it has been proposed that the relative importance of each may depend on the class of MHC disparity between donor and recipient[32,33]. This suggestion has recently been supported by direct evidence that CD4-positive T-cells respond to MHC Class II alloantigens whereas CD8-positive cells respond to Class I alloantigens[34] and by the elegant demonstration using monoclonal anti-CD4 and anti-CD8 antibodies *in vivo* as immunosuppressives that monoclonal anti-CD4 antibody is sufficient to prevent rejection of MHC Class II-disparate grafts and monoclonal anti-CD8 antibody is sufficient to prevent rejection of MHC Class I-disparate grafts[35].

Rat cardiac allograft rejection is invariably preceded by infiltration of the graft by leukocytes from the blood. The leukocyte infiltrate is composed mainly of lymphocytes although, particularly at later stages of rejection, other cell types, e.g. macrophages and platelets are also present. This lymphocyte infiltrate can be identified by routine histological techniques, but a more informative approach has been to use isotope-labelling of lymphocytes to obtain a dynamic picture of lymphocyte migration in recipients of cardiac allografts. Results from this laboratory[36] and elsewhere[37,38] using ^{111}In-labelled lymphocytes injected into recipients of cardiac allografts established that the rate of infiltration of the grafts was not uniform during the course of rejection, i.e. there were particular times during the rejection response at which the influx of cells was large and rapid and others at which few if any cells migrated into the graft. The extent to which the infiltrate consisted of lymphocytes with specificity for the antigens of the graft also varied at different stages of rejection[36]. The results of these and earlier migration studies which showed that sensitized lymphocytes accumulated to an only slightly preferential degree in grafts of the immunizing haplotype[39] established that the infiltrate in rejecting cardiac grafts comprises an immunologically specific population as well as a (sometimes substantial) population of cells recruited non-specifically to the site, probably as a result of the local release of inflammatory mediators.

More detailed analysis of the nature of the cellular infiltration into rejecting cardiac grafts became possible with the advent of monoclonal antibodies with specificity for different surface markers on different cell types and the development of techniques to visualize cells which express these markers in tissues. Phenotype analysis *in situ* of the lymphocyte infiltrate in cardiac allografts during the course of graft rejection confirmed to a large extent the results obtained in the adoptive transfer experiments: T-cells of both CD4 (helper/inducer) and CD8 (suppressor/cytotoxic) phenotype were present in the graft infiltrate[40], with a predominance of CD8-positive cells at the peak[41,42] or late stages[29] of rejection. This predominance of CD8 positive T-cells identified in situ at rejection correlated with earlier functional studies which had shown that the specific cytotoxic (CD8-positive) T-cell activity in leukocyte populations recovered from allogeneic cardiac grafts was maximal just before rejection[43]. More informative than simple phenotype analysis is the identification of activation markers as well as phenotype markers on the infiltrating cells[44]. Even more useful is the measurement of immunological function in graft-infiltrating cells but this has been feasible in only a few systems, e.g. in experimental kidney allografts[45] which can be readily disrupted by mechanical and enzyme treatment. Assessment of immunological function is particularly important to understanding the mechanism(s) of long-term graft survival obtainable in experimental models by a number of immunosuppressive strategies (see below).

Although it is not disputed that T-cells are responsible for initiating cardiac allograft rejection and can cause direct damage to the target organ, there is also no doubt that other cell types become secondarily involved in a cascade of inflammatory events triggered by the cell death and tissue injury in the grafted organ. The pathological changes which occur in the graft during uninterrupted rejection and which can be considered to be direct or indirect consequences of immune activation include a rise in graft tissue levels of prostacyclin and thromboxane[46], probably released from the macrophages or platelets which could result in vascular injury leading to ischaemic damage, deposition in the graft of fibrin[44], probably released by macrophages which would result in an elevated intragraft pressure and compromised contractile function, and an increase in the amount of MHC molecules expressed on the vascular endothelium and the myocardium[9], probably caused by local release of immune interferon. Increased expression of MHC antigens would make the cells of the graft substantially more susceptible to immune attack.

Interrupted rejection

Numerous strategies have been used in experimental models to prolong allograft survival, and some have been successfully used in experimental cardiac transplantation. Most involve manipulation of the immune system of the recipient in order to prevent either the induction of the immune response to the graft, or the proper development of the effector mechanisms responsible for graft destruction. This can be accomplished by treatment with immuno-suppressive drugs, or irradiation, or by active or passive immunization of the recipient at the time of grafting. Indefinite cardiac allograft survival in rats can be achieved by treatment of the recipient either before grafting with antidonor strain hyperimmune globulin (graft enhancement) or with donor antigen[47] given as whole blood (the transfusion effect) or purified cell preparations, or at the time of grafting with a short course of the immunosuppressive drug cyclosporine[48]. A more recent strategy has been to treat graft recipients with monoclonal anti-T-cell antibodies in order to inactivate, by depletion or simple blockade, the cells involved in graft rejection[49]. Using monoclonal antibodies which bind only to activated T-cells e.g. anti- interleukin 2 receptor (anti-IL2R) antibodies[50] makes the immunosuppression even more selective. The combination of donor antigen pretreatment[51] or anti-IL2R antibodies[52] with cyclosporine has the advantage that substantially lower doses of the drug can be used. In all these models the state of immunological unresponsiveness in the graft recipients can be maintained for long periods of time without further immunosuppression.

Treatment of graft recipients with immunosuppressive doses of cyclosporine alone from the time of grafting or with donor antigen before grafting are both effective means of preventing graft rejection. Analysis of the graft tissue in both these systems compared to rejecting cardiac tissue identified important differences between them: in the enhanced cardiac graft there were fewer T-cells, and the cell populations recoverable by enzyme digestion showed no specific cytotoxic T-cell activity[15]. During the prevention of acute graft rejection by continuous treatment of the recipient with cyclosporine there was no large influx of lymphocytes which occurred in rejecting grafts[36], although the grafts did contain infiltrating cells. There was no preponderance of CD8 positive cells in these grafts compared to rejecting grafts[41], and no fibrin deposition or prostaglandin release within the graft[44,46]. Neither was there induction of Class II MHC antigen on the constituent cells of the graft[6]. This is in contrast to long-standing enhanced kidney allografts in which donor type Class I and Class II MHC antigens were induced to the same extent as in rejecting grafts[53]. Interestingly, in the grafts of cyclosporine treated cardiac grafted rats during the early graft period there were substantial numbers of Class II MHC positive T-cells and macrophages[44], suggesting that some degree of immune activation did occur during the acute phase. Taken together, these findings suggest that cyclosporine acts in the early post-grafting period to prevent the release from activated cells of the soluble mediators responsible for tissue injury and necessary for the development of fully differentiated immune effector function. This hypothesis is supported by the finding that spleen cells taken during this acute phase from rats bearing CS-maintained allografts have a greatly impaired capacity for interleukin synthesis and release[54].

In contrast to the reasonably clear understanding of the mechanism of action of cyclosporine in the prevention of acute graft rejection, it is not clear why short term treatment with the drug results in indefinite survival of the graft[48,55]. Similarly, it is not fully understood why enhancement protocols or treatment with donor antigen at the time of grafting results in long term graft survival. When long standing grafts achieved by a short course of cyclosporine were retransplanted into normal syngeneic animals they were rejected acutely, showing that the grafts had not lost their immunogenicity[15], although a more recent study demonstrated that there is an eventual reduction in immunogenicity[56]. Adoptive transfer of very large numbers of normal lymphocytes to rats bearing these long-term grafts did not cause rejection, which suggested that the unresponsive state was being maintained by active suppression[57]. Cells from rats with long surviving grafts could not restore rejection of donor strain heart grafts in adoptive hosts and, significantly, inhibited the capacity of simultaneously transferred normal lymphocytes to do so[58]. More recent work from the same group has shown that the suppressor cells involved are CD4-positive[59] and that they develop in the recipient at the same time as CD4-positive cells capable of specific positive responses to the graft alloantigens in vitro disappear[60]. Another group has however obtained perhaps conflicting results using an adoptive transfer system to demonstrate functional donor-specific T-helper cells in these animals[61]. This was in support of their earlier observation that spleen cells from these rats had fully recovered their potential for lymphokine production[54]. On balance, it seems likely that rats bearing cyclosporine-induced long-term cardiac allografts have both functional suppressor and functional helper T-cells with specificity for the graft alloantigens and that the tolerant, i.e. unresponsive state is maintained by a dominance of the former over the latter.

A consensus has emerged that long-term cardiac allograft survival can be achieved in rodents by a number of different immunosuppressive strategies. The grafts function apparently indefinitely without the need for further manipulation of the host immune system, the state of unresponsiveness is stable and the recipient is immunocompetent in respect to all other antigens with which he is challenged. Some of these strategies could be directly applicable to clinical transplantation, e.g. the combination of donor-specific antigen pretreatment by blood transfusion or anti-interleukin monoclonal antibody treatment with low dose cyclosporine. Current experimental research is directed towards achieving a better understanding of these particular models, towards identifying new and more effective combinations of existing immune strategies and to trying completely novel approaches in the search for a clinically useful means of obtaining long term transplant survival. A significant problem in clinical heart transplantation which has become evident only in the past few years is late failure of the graft as a consequence of graft atherosclerosis and the experimental rodent cardiac allograft model is now being used to try to understand its immunopathology[62]. Experimental models have been instrumental in identifying the mechanisms of graft rejection and in devising the means to prevent it; they will almost certainly contribute to the solution of the future problems in clinical heart transplantation.

ACKNOWLEDGEMENTS

Some of the work described on the rat model has been carried out in my laboratory over the past few years in collaboration with colleagues at this and other institutions. Grateful thanks to Josephine Cox, Debbie Bevan, Tai Ping Pan and Sally Darracot-Cankowic. I acknowledge financial support from the British Heart Foundation and the Wellcome Trust.

References

1. Proceedings of the International Congress of the Transplantation Society, Helsinki, Finland, 1986. (1987) *Transplant. Proc.*, 19
2. Proceedings of the International Congress of the Transplantation Society, Sydney, Australia 1988. (1989) *Transplant. Proc.* 21
3. Moller, G. (ed.). (1984). Intragraft rejection mechanisms. *Immunol. Rev.*, 77 (Copenhagen: Munksgaard)
4. Morris, P.J. and Tilney, N.L. (Eds.) (1987). *Transplantation Reviews*, 1. (Grune and Stratton, New York.)
5. Hart, D.N.J. and Fabre, J.W. (1981). Demonstration and characterization of Ia-positive dendritic cells in the interstitial connective tissues of rat heart and other tissues, but not brain. *J. Exp. Med.*, **153**, 347–61
6. Milton, A.D., Spencer, S.C. and Fabre, J.W. (1986). The effects of cyclosporin A on the induction of donor class I and class II MHC antigens in heart and kidney allografts in the rat. *Transplantation*, **42**, 337–47
7. Lampert, I.A., Suitters, A.J. and Chisholm, P.M. (1981). Expression of Ia antigens on epidermal keratinocytes in graft-versus-host disease. *Nature*, **293**, 149–50
8. Mason, D.W., Dallman, M. and Barclay, A.N. (1981). Graft-versus-host disease induces expression of Ia antigen in rat epidermal cells and gut epithelium. *Nature*, **293**, 150–1
9. Milton, A.D. and Fabre, J.W. (1985). Massive induction of donor-type histocompatibility complex antigens in rejecting cardiac allografts in the rat. *J. Exp. Med.*, **161**, 98–112
10. de Waal, R.M.W., Bogman, M.J.J., Maass, C.N., Cornelisson, L.M.H., Tax, W.J.M. and Koene, R.A.P. (1983). Variable expression of Ia antigens on the vascular endothelium of mouse skin allografts. *Nature*, **303**, 426–7
11. Pober, J.S., Collins, T., Gimbrone Jr., M.A., Libby, P. and Reiss, C.S. (1986). Inducible expression of class II major histocompatibility complex antigens and the immunogenicity of vascular endothelium. *Transplantation*, **41**, 141–6
12. Mason, D.W., Dallman, M.J., Arthur, R.P. and Morris, P.J. (1984). Mechanisms of allograft rejection: the roles of cytotoxic T-cells and delayed-type hypersensitivity. *Immunol. Rev.*, 77, 167–84
13. Loveland, B.E. and McKenzie, I.F.C. (1982). Which T cells cause graft rejection? *Transplantation*, **33**, 217–21
14. Hall, B.M., Dorsch, S. and Roser, B. (1978). The cellular basis of allograft rejection in vivo. I. The cellular requirements for first-set rejection of heart grafts. *J. Exp. Med.*, **148**, 878–89
15. Tilney, N.L., Kupiec-Weglinski, J.W., Heidecke, C.D., Lear, P.A. and Strom, T.B. (1984). Mechanisms of rejection and prolongation of vascularized organ allografts. *Immunol. Rev.*, 77, 185–216
16. Parthenais, E., Soots, A. and Hayry, P. (1979). Sensitivity of rat heart endothelial and myocardial cells to alloimmune lymphocytes and to alloantibody-dependent cellular cyto-toxicity. *Cell. Immunol.*, **48**, 375–82
17. Soulillou, J.P., Vie, H., Moreau, J.F., Peyrat, M.A. and Blandin, F. (1983). Increased NK cell activity in rats rejecting heart allografts. *Transplantation*, **36**, 726–7
18. MacPherson, G.G. and Christmas, S.E. (1984). The role of the macrophage in cardiac allograft rejection in the rat. *Immunol. Rev.*, 77, 143–66
19. Dallman, M.J. and Mason, D.W. (1982). Role of thymus-derived and thymus-independent cells in murine skin allograft rejecton. *Transplantation*, **33**, 221–3
20. Ono, K. and Lindsey, E.S. (1969). Improved technique of heart transplantation in rats. *J. Thorac. Cardiovasc. Surg.*, **57**, 225–9
21. Heron, I. (1971). A technique for accessory cervical heart transplantation in rabbits and rats. *Acta Pathol. Microbiol. Scand.*, **79**, 366–72
22. Wotherspoon, J.S. and Dorsch, S.E. (1986). The mechanism of prolonged graft survival following removal of the regional lymph node. *Transplantation*, **42**, 532–7
23. Corry, R.J., Winn, H.J. and Russell, P.S. (1973). Primarily vascularized allografts of hearts in mice. The role of H-2D, H-2K, and non-H-2 antigens in rejection. *Transplantation*, **16**, 343–50
24. Stewart, R., Butcher, G., Herbert, J. and Roser, B. (1985). Graft rejection in a congenic panel of rats with defined immune response genes for MHC class I antigens. I. Rejection of and priming to the RTIA antigen. *Transplantation*, **40**, 427–31

11

25. Lowry, R.P., Gurley, K.E. and Forbes, R.D.C., (1983). Immune mechanisms in organ allograft rejection: I. Delayed type hypersensitivity and lymphocytotoxicity in heart graft rejection. *Transplantation*, 36, 391–401
26. Lowry, R.P., Gurley, K.E., Blackburn, J. and Forbes, R.D.C. (1983). Delayed-type hypersensitivity and lymphocytotoxicity in cardiac allograft rejection. *Transplant. Proc.*, 15, 343–6
27. Mason, D.W., Arthur, R.P., Dallman, M.J., Green, J.R., Spickett, G.P. and Thomas, M.L. (1983). Functions of rat T-lymphocyte subsets isolated by means of monoclonal antibodies. *Immunol. Rev.*, 74, 57–82
28. Dallman, M.J., Mason, D.W. and Webb, M. (1982). The roles of host and donor cells in the rejection of skin allografts by T cell-deprived rats injected with syngeneic T cells. *Eur. J. Immunol.*, 12, 511–18
29. Clarke Forbes, R.D., Lowry, R.P., Gomersall, M. and Blackburn, J. (1985). Comparative immunohistologic studies in an adoptive transfer model of acute rat cardiac allograft rejection. *Transplantation*, 40, 77–85
30. Lear, P.A., Heidecke, C.D., Kupiec-Weglinski, J.W., Araneda, D., Strom, T.B. and Tilney, N.L. (1983). Restoration of allograft responsiveness in B rats II. Requirements for lymphoid populations and lymphokine. *Transplantation*, 36, 412–17
31. Heidecke, C.D., Kupiec-Weglinski, J.W., Lear, P.A., Abbudfilho, M., Araujo, J.L., Araneda, D., Strom, T.B. and Tilney, N.L. (1984). Interactions between T lymphocyte subsets supported by interleukin 2-rich lymphokines produce acute rejection of vascularized cardiac allografts in T cell deprived rats. *J. Immunol.*, 133, 582–8
32. Lowry, R.P., Clarke Forbes, R.D., Blackburn, J.H. and Marghesco, D.M. (1985). Immune mechanisms in organ allograft rejection. V. Pivotal role of the cytotoxic suppressor T cell subset in the rejection of heart grafts bearing isolated class I disparities in the inbred rat. *Transplantation*, 40, 545–50
33. Lowry, R.P. and Gurley, K.E. (1983). Immune mechanisms in organ allograft rejection. III. Cellular and humoral immunity in rejection of organ allografts transplanted across MHC subregion disparity RT1.B (RT1.D). *Transplantation*, 36, 405–11
34. Sprent, J., Schaeffer, M., Lo, D. and Korngold, R. (1986). Properties of purified T cell subsets. II In vivo responses to Class I vs. Class II H-2 differences. *J. Exp. Med.*, 163, 998–1011
35. Wheelahan, J. and McKenzie, I.F.C. (submitted for publication).
36. Cox, J.H., Forsyth, A.T., De Villiers, J.S., Yacoub, M.H. and Chisholm, P.M. (1984). The kinetics and specificity of lymphocyte infiltration of cardiac allografts in unmodified and cyclosporine-treated rats. *Transplantation*, 38, 17–22
37. Oluwole, S., Wang, T., Fawwaz, R., Satake, K., Nowygrod, R., Reemtsma, K. and Hardy, M.A. (1981). Use of indium-111-labeled cells in measurement of cellular dynamics of experimental cardiac allograft rejection. *Transplantation*, 31, 51–5
38. Kupiec-Weglinski, J.W. de Sousa, M. and Tilney, N.L. (1985). The importance of lymphocyte migration patterns in experimental organ transplantation. *Transplantation*, 40, 1–6
39. Tilney, N.L., Notis-McConarty, J. and Strom, T.B. (1978). Specificity of cellular migration into cardiac allografts in rats. *Transplantation*, 26, 181–6
40. Clarke Forbes, R.D., Guttmann, R.D., Gomersall, M. and Hibberd, J. (1983). Leukocyte subsets in first-set rat cardiac allograft rejection. A serial immunohistologic study using monoclonal antibodies. *Transplantation*, 36, 681–6
41. Chisholm, P.M., Cox, J.H. and Yacoub, M.H. (1985). The effect of cyclosporine on the nature and extent of lymphocyte infiltration in rat cardiac allografts. *Transplant. Proc.*, 17, 1357–61
42. Araujo, J.L., Kupiec-Weglinski, J.W., Araneda, D., Towpik, E., Heidecke, C. D., Williams, J.M. and Tilney, N.L. (1985). Phenotype, activation status, and suppressor activity of host lymphocytes during acute rejection and after cyclosporine-induced unresponsiveness of rat cardiac allografts. *Transplantation*, 40, 278–84
43. Tilney, N.L., Strom, T.B., Macpherson, S.G. and Carpenter, C.B. (1975). Surface properties and functional characteristics of infiltrating cells harvested from acutely rejecting cardiac allografts in inbred rats. *Transplantation*, 20, 323–30
44. Cox, J.H. and Chisholm, P.M. (1987). Mechanism of action of cyclosporine in preventing cardiac allograft rejection. I. Rate of entry of lymphocytes from the blood, fibrin deposition and expression of Ia antigens on infiltrating cells. *Transplantation*, 43, 340–42

45. Dallman, M.J., Wood, K.J. and Morris, P.J. (1988) Cytotoxicity and IL2 Reactivity of cells from rejected and nonrejected allografts. *Transplant. Proc.*, **20**(2), 226–28
46. Fan, T.P.D., Cox, J.H. and Chisholm, P.M. (1987). The mechanism of action of cyclosporine in preventing cardiac allograft rejection. II. Graft tissue levels of prostacyclin and thromboxane. *Transplantation*, **43**, 343–45.
47. Tilney, N.L., Bancewicz, J., Rowinski, W., Notis-McConarty, J., Finnegan, A. and Booth, D. (1978). Enhancement of cardiac allografts in rats. Comparison of host responses to different treatment protocols. *Transplantation*, **25**, 1–6
48. Nagao, T., White, D.J.G. and Calne, R.Y. (1982). Kinetics of unresponsiveness induced by a short course of cyclosporin A. *Transplantation*, **33**, 31–5
49. Madsen, J.C., Peugh, W.N. and Morris, P.J. (1987). The effect of anti-L3T4 monoclonal antibody treatment on first set rejection of murine cardiac allografts. *Transplantation*, **42**, 849–52
50. Kupiec-Weglinski, J.W., Diamanstein, T., Tilney, N.L. and Strom, T.B. (1986). Therapy with monoclonal antibody to interleukin 2 receptor spares suppressor T cells and prevents or reverses acute allograft rejection in rats. *Proc. Natl. Acad. Sci. USA*, **83**, 2624
51. Oluwole, S.F., Wasfie, T., Fawwaz, R., Reemstma, K. and Hardy, M. (1989). Functional and phenotype characteristics of suppressor T cells in unresponsive rats pretreated with UV-B irradiated donor lymphocytes combined with peritransplant cyclosporine. *Transplant. Proc.*, **21**(1), 484
52. Tellides, G., Dallman, M. J. and Morris, P.J. (1988). Synergistic interaction of cyclosporine with interleukin 2 receptor monoclonal antibody therapy. *Transplant. Proc.*, **22**, 202
53. Wood, K.J., Hopley, A., Dallman, M.J. and Morris, P.J. (1988). Lack of correlation between induction of donor Class I and Class II major histocompatibility antigens and graft rejection. *Transplantation*, **45**(4), 759–67
54. Abbud-Filho, M., Kupiec-Weglinski, J.W., Araujo, J.L., Heidecke, C.D., Tilney, N.L. and Strom, T.B. (1984). Cyclosporine therapy of rat heart allograft recipients and release of interleukins (IL 1, IL 2, IL 3): A role for IL 3 in graft tolerance? *J. Immunol.*, **133**, 2582–6
55. Hall, B.M., Roser, B.J. and Dorsch, S.E. (1979). A model for study of the cellular mechanisms that maintain long-term enhancement of cardiac graft survival. *Transplant. Proc.*, **11**, 958–61
56. Klempnauer, J. and Steiniger, B. (1990). Depletion of donor Class II MHC positive passenger cells and reduction in immunogenicity in longstanding rat heart allografts. (in press)
57. Kupiec-Weglinski, J.W., Lear, P.A., Bordes-Aznar, J., Tilney, N.L. and Strom, T.B. (1983). Acute rejection in cyclosporin A-treated graft recipients occurs following abrogation of suppressor cells. *Transplant. Proc.*, **15**, 531–4
58. Hall, B.M., Jelbart, M.E. and Dorsch, S.E. (1984). Suppressor T cells in rats with prolonged cardiac allograft survival after treatment with cyclosporine. *Transplantation*, **37**, 595–600
59. Hall, B.M., Jelbart, M.E., Gurley, K.E. and Dorsch, S.E. (1985). Specific unresponsiveness in rats with prolonged cardiac allograft survival after treatment with cyclosporine. *J. Exp. Med.*, **162**, 1683–94
60. Hall, B.M., Gurley, K.E., Pearce, N. and Dorsch, S.E. (1989). Specific unresponsiveness in rats with prolonged cardiac allograft survival after treatment with cyclosporine. II Sequential changes in alloreactivity of T cell subsets. *Transplantation*, **47**(6), 1030–3
61. Kupiec-Weglinski, J.W., Heidecke, C.D., Araujo, J.L., Abbud-Filho, M., Towpik, E., Araneda, D., Strom, T.B. and Tilney, N.L. (1985). Behavior of helper T lymphocytes in cyclosporine-mediated long-term graft acceptance in the rat. *Cell. Immunol.*, **93**, 168–77
62. Cramer, D.V., Qian, S., Harnaha, J., Chapman, F.A., Estes, L.W., Starzl, T.E. and Makowka, L. (1989). Cardiac transplantaion in the rat. I The effect of histocompatibility differences on graft arteriosclerosis. *Transplantation*, **47**(3), 414

2
Cardiopulmonary resuscitation

D.A. ZIDEMAN

There are three irregularities of the heart beat which result in no cardiac output and thus require immediate treatment if permanent damage to the brain is to be prevented. The three irregularities of rhythm are:
(1) Ventricular fibrillation,
(2) Asystole,
(3) Electromechanical dissociation.

Their management is described under the global term of cardiopulmonary resuscitation.

Unlike the treatment of many other abnormal cardiac rhythms, the treatment or correction of these rhythms may not be immediately possible. Thus the priority becomes the maintenance of life by providing an artificially driven circulation by external chest compression and, if required, the maintenance of the oxygenation of blood by artificial respiration (expired air resuscitation). This is known as basic life support. Even the shortest of delays in the initiation of basic life support cannot be tolerated especially when this may be as a result of waiting for specific equipment and drugs to treat the particular arrhythmia. The use of equipment and drugs in resuscitation is known as advanced life support. Should such adjuncts be immediately available it may be more appropriate not to delay the implementation of advanced life support whilst establishing basic life support. The linking of basic and advanced life support is therefore of outstanding importance and it requires training, practice and experience to achieve the best results.

BASIC LIFE SUPPORT

Basic life support is classically described as an Airway, Breathing, Circulation sequence. It is used to maintain a flow of oxygenated blood to the various vital organs of the body until a more definitive therapy, advanced life support, is available. In hospital this period may be short, if at all. In the out-of-hospital situation basic life support techniques may be carried out for prolonged periods

15

of time. Cummins and Eisenberg[1] examined the determinants of survival in nine studies of pre-hospital resuscitation. They found that the chance of survival was improved in witnessed arrests, where the emergency medical system (the ambulance/paramedic system) had been activated, and in the early arrival (within 4 minutes) and implementation of advanced life support procedures. Tweed and Wilson[2] in another analysis of survival similarly found that the time to the initiation of basic life support was a highly significant factor. Furthermore, they found that the time to arrival of the emergency medical team and the time to the first defibrillation of ventricular fibrillation was even more highly significant to eventual survival. Thus basic life support 'buys time' until the arrival of definitive therapy. Some authors believe that this time may be as short as 4–6 minutes, and that prolonged basic resuscitation produces similar results to no resuscitation[3].

Airway

In the unconscious victim of a cardiac arrest the muscles of the tongue, neck and pharynx relax resulting in the tongue and/or epiglottis obstructing the upper airway[4]. Furthermore, if respiratory efforts continue in the victim with a fully or a partially obstructed airway, then the negative inspiratory pressures created may suck the tongue or epiglottis into a position where they occlude the upper airway[5]. Guildner[6] showed that the best ways of opening and monitoring the airway were the dual manoeuvres of tilting the head back, thus extending the head on the neck, plus lifting the jaw forward to displace the tongue away from the posterior pharyngeal wall. The upper airway should then be briefly inspected for any obvious obstruction and vomit or foreign material carefully removed by finger sweeps.

Breathing

Having opened the airway, as described above, it is a simple matter to check whether the victim is still breathing. Breathing is checked in three ways: by looking for chest wall movement, by listening for breathing and by feeling over the mouth to see if these movements are effective in moving air. If there is no effective respiration then expired air resuscitation must be commenced. Mouth to mouth, mouth to nose or mouth to stoma are all methods of expired air resuscitation. Initially, two normal individual breaths should be given by the rescuer to the victim. With each breath the rescuer should observe the chest rise and fall thus confirming successful ventilation. High inspiratory pressures and gas flow rates, excessive inspiratory volumes or not allowing for full expiration between breaths should be avoided as they will result in gastric inflation, distension and vomiting[7].

Circulation

In basic life support the circulation is assessed by palpating a major pulse, preferably the carotid pulse. If there is no palpable pulse then the circulation is temporarily maintained by external chest compressions. Compressions are performed on the lower third of the victim's sternum, two fingers breadth above the xiphisternum, with the heel of one hand superimposed on the other hand and stabilized by interlocking the fingers. Compressions should be 4 to 5 cm in depth and carried out at a rate of 80 compressions per minute. After 15 compressions, the rescuer should give two expired air ventilations as described above. If two rescuers are present then one should perform chest compression at a rate of 60 per minute whilst the second rescuer performs a single expired air ventilation after every fifth compression. The second rescuer should also check that the chest compressions are achieving a palpable pulse.

Chest compressions were originally described by Kouwenhoven and his colleagues in 1960[8], and have become part of conventional or standard cardiopulmonary resuscitation (CPR). They postulated that during compressions the heart was compressed between the sternum and the vertebral bodies of the spine. This has been described as the heart pump theory[9]. More recently, Maier and his colleagues[10] have used moderate force, brief duration chest compressions, performed at high rates and demonstrated higher stroke volumes and improved coronary blood flow. In 1976, Criley et al.[11] found that vigorous coughing by a cardiac arrest victim was able to sustain consciousness for 92 seconds before successful defibrillation. He proposed that the rise in intrathoracic pressure that resulted from coughing provided a significant cerebral blood flow. Other authors[12,13] have taken this 'thoracic pump' theory further. In this theory it has been proposed that external chest compressions will raise the intrathoracic pressure thus increasing the pressure in all intrathoracic structures. This increased pressure is transmitted from the intrathoracic great vessels to the extrathoracic arteries as these arterial vessels have relatively thick and rigid walls. The returning veins, on the other hand, which are relatively thin walled, collapse. This creates an extrathoracic arterial to venous pressure gradient and results in the forward flow of blood. The passive role of the heart as a conduit during CPR[14] was further supported by pressure-synchronized cineangiography in dogs[15] and 2D-echo-cardiography in man[16,17]. These techniques have demonstrated little change in cardiac chamber volume during external chest compressions; that the aortic and mitral valves open simultaneously during compressions; and that the pulmonary valve prevents retrograde blood flow by closing during compression and opening during relaxation. More recently, a preliminary report has challenged these findings by demonstrating motion of the heart valves and chamber compression during the initial four minutes of external chest compression[18].

Chandra and her colleagues converted the thoracic pump theory into a practical treatment schedule and applied it initially to dogs[19] and then to man[20].

They synchronized prolonged slow chest compressions, a 60% downstroke at a rate of 40/minute, with ventilations performed at a high airway pressure of 40–100 mmHg. They alternated this synchronized compression ventilation CPR ('New CPR') with conventional CPR every 30 seconds. Provided the high airway pressure was maintained they achieved an improvement in systolic pressure of 13 mmHg and a 250% increase in carotid blood flow using this 'New CPR'. Interposed abdominal compression CPR[21] has also been tested as a method of augmenting intrathoracic pressure during cardiopulmonary resuscitation. A clinical trial in Milwaukee did not demonstrate any significant improvement in results over conventional methods[22]. Furthermore, Martin et al.[23] have recently confirmed the fear of others[24,25] that there is a deterioration in myocardial perfusion pressure in patients undergoing synchronized compression and ventilation resuscitation. In Martin et al.'s study, no patient receiving 'New CPR' was successfully resuscitated. The newer methodologies need much more research in humans, including further evaluation of survival, before they can be recommended.

ADVANCED LIFE SUPPORT

The use of equipment and drugs during resuscitation is called advanced life support. It is essential to initiate and continue basic life support until these adjuncts arrive and their use is established.

Airway management and ventilation

A detailed examination of this topic in this chapter is probably inappropriate. Tracheal intubation is the definitive method of airway management. Not only does it guarantee an established airway, but it will also protect the airway from the aspiration of vomit. Hess and Baran[26] have shown that the alternative methods of mouth to mask and bag–valve–mask provide inadequate tidal volumes even in experienced hands.

The increase in awareness of infectious diseases in the community has led to unfounded fears of the passage of infection from the victim to the rescuer during mouth to mouth resuscitation. There has followed a demand for airway adjuncts to separate the victim from the rescuer. At the time of writing there has been no reported case in the world literature of any serious infectious disease being transmitted by mouth to mouth resuscitation. The Centres for Disease Control report of 1988[27] emphasized the fact that blood was the infective medium in the two infectious diseases of most concern, hepatitis and human immuno-deficiency virus (HIV). Thus with regard to mouth to mouth resuscit- ation only saliva contaminated with visible blood should be considered a risk. If the prevalence of these infectious diseases is high in the community being served or there is a high incidence of trauma resuscitation, there probably is a justifiable case for providing protective airway adjuncts. It is essential that effective devices, both in terms of infection protection and in the ability to ventilate the victim, should be selected. Furthermore formal training and testing of rescuers in the use of the selected adjunct is vitally important so that resuscitation is not compromised by lack of experience.

Drug therapy

The administration of drugs during resuscitation requires the resuscitator to establish a reliable and safe intravenous route at an early stage. Cannulation of a central vein is the most ideal and access can be achieved via the internal or external jugular veins, subclavian or femoral vein. A recent study has shown that there is a significant delay in drugs reaching the heart, and a lower peak drug level when drugs are administered via a peripheral rather than central route, even with effective chest compressions[28].

An alternative is to administer drugs via the tracheal tube[29-31]. This route is often considered preferable, especially when there is a delay in establishing intravenous access. Lignocaine, atropine and adrenaline can all be given by the tracheal route, instillation being followed by 5 to 10 rapid ventilations. The intracardiac route must be considered a poor third, and is probably only indicated if the intravenous and endotracheal routes are not available. Sabin and his colleagues[32] showed that, when using the left sternal edge approach, only 11% of intracardiac injections entered the left ventricle and in 25% the needle had lacerated the left anterior descending coronary artery. The intraosseous infusion of fluids[33] and drugs[34,35] is a route used in children[36], yet to be properly evaluated in adults.

Specific arrhythmia therapies

Effective treatment of the arrhythmias of cardiac arrest requires the initiation of basic life support to be co-ordinated with specific arrhythmia therapies. Specific preplanned regimens have been recommended in the United Kingdom and the North American literature (see 'Further Reading') for the treatment of ventricular fibrillation, asystole and electromechanical dissociation. Training and practice in these protocols is essential in order to co-ordinate the resuscitation team and to allow the rapid establishment of an effective treatment policy with minimal delay.

Ventricular fibrillation (and pulseless ventricular tachycardia)

Ventricular fibrillation represents the total breakdown of ordered electrical conduction within the myocardium. The result is a heart with no cardiac output and a pulseless patient. It is the commonest of the pulseless rhythms in patients with ischaemic heart disease and although it may be heralded by the signs and symptoms of a myocardial infarction, heart failure or cardiogenic shock, it sometimes occurs without any warning causing sudden cardiac death.

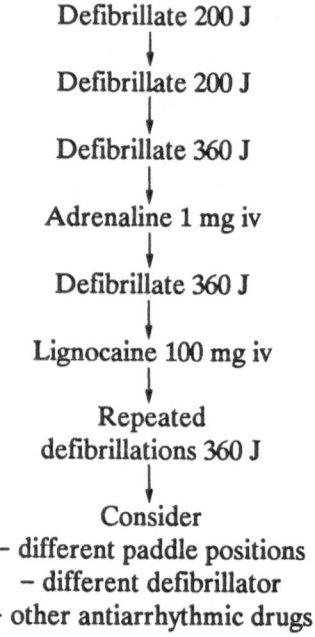

The treatment of ventricular fibrillation is to convert the fibrillation, as rapidly as possible, to a more ordered rhythm with a cardiac output. The definitive treatment is electrical defibrillation. Caldwell and his colleagues[37] have defended mechanical cardioversion of monitored or 'in-hospital' patients. Five out 248 had ventricular fibrillation terminated and 17 out of 68 had ventricular tachycardia converted by a simple cough or chest thump. Fifteen of these 22 patients survived to discharge. In another study[38], looking at the 'out-of-hospital' patient, the chest thump was found a less useful technique. Of the 23 patients that were thumped for ventricular fibrillation, none were converted, but 10 were later converted by electrical defibrillation. In the same study 15 of the 27 thumped for ventricular tachycardia changed rhythm, but only three changed to an improved rhythm, of which two were successfully resuscitated.

The importance of the use of electrical defibrillation in the termination of ventricular fibrillation is reflected in its repeated occurrence in the recommended treatment schedule (see scheme above). Defibrillation should be attempted as rapidly as possible with 200 J of electrical energy. This initial defibrillation level was set following out-of-hospital[39] and in-hospital studies[40] showing that eventual survival and subsequent discharge was the same for those patients receiving either 175 J or 320 J of energy. The lower level of energy was recommended as it seemed safer because the higher level may cause myocardial cell damage. Following defibrillation external chest compressions must be continued until the 'recovery' of the electrocardiographic trace. Should fibrillation continue then a second 200 J defibrillation followed by a 360 J defibrillation is recommended. It was originally believed that repeated electrical energy discharge across the thoracic cavity decreased transthoracic resistance[41]; thus defibrillating with the same energy would deliver more current to the heart. Kerber and his colleagues[42] found that transthoracic resistance varied considerably in humans, but that it was best related to chest size. Furthermore, they found that repeated shocks of the same energy level had minimal and unpredictable effects on the transthoracic resistance.

If the heart does not respond to this initial therapy then it becomes necessary to improve the cardiac output and blood pressure which are being maintained by external chest compressions. Adrenaline, 10 ml of 1 in 10,000 (1.0 mg), is administered via the intravenous or the endotracheal route. By stimulating the α-adrenergic receptors, adrenaline will increase the peripheral vascular tone, raise the end diastolic pressure, increase the myocardial perfusion pressure and the central nervous system blood flow[43]. It will also stimulate β-adrenergic receptors, thus increasing inotropy and coarsening the ventricular fibrillation[44]. Two minutes of basic life support should follow the administration of adrenaline. A further attempt at defibrillation (360 J) should then be made.

If ventricular fibrillation persists then the administration of lignocaine, either intravenously or via the endotracheal tube, may improve the response to the next defibrillation attempt. Lignocaine raises the ventricular fibrillation threshold, suppresses automaticity, decreases action potential amplitude and shortens the action potential duration and the effective refractory period in the Purkinje fibres[45]. When given as a bolus or as a constant infusion, lignocaine has been found to raise the electrical energy threshold to defibrillate the heart[46].

Bretylium tosylate has been reported as producing chemical defibrillation[47]. Bretylium releases noradrenaline from adrenergic nerve endings and blocks the reuptake mechanism. In electrophysiological terms it increases the action potential duration, prolongs the effective refractory period in the Purkinje cells and raises the ventricular fibrillation threshold[48]. Other antifibrillatory agents that may be considered useful are procainamide, verapamil, flecainide and β-adrenergic blocking drugs, such as propranolol. Administration of any of these drugs must be accompanied by careful monitoring of the blood pressure as they may cause a precipitous fall in blood pressure.

Should resuscitation continue for a prolonged period, then repeat doses of adrenaline, 1 mg, should be administered every five minutes. It may also be necessary to administer sodium bicarbonate, 1 mmol/kg intravenously in prolonged resuscitation, or if there is inadequate ventilation or a period of prolonged hypoxia. Large doses of sodium bicarbonate are detrimental as they can cause hypercarbia (by the metabolic conversion of bicarbonate to carbon dioxide), paradoxical cerebrospinal spinal fluid acidosis, hyperosmolarity and may inactivate simultaneously administered catecholamines[49]. Sodium bicarbonate should not be considered routine but should only be given if indicated. Sodium bicarbonate should only be given following the measurement of blood gases and pH, and when effective ventilation of the lungs has been established.

The above recommendations for the treatment of ventricular fibrillation are the same for the treatment of pulseless ventricular tachycardia.

Asystole

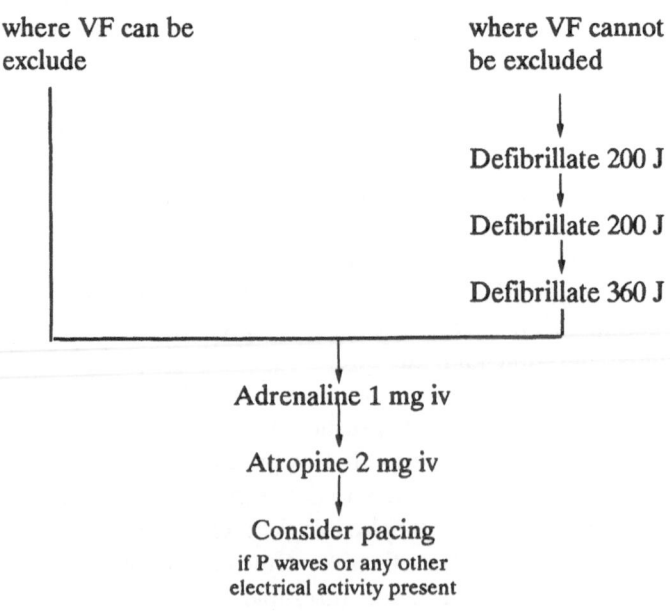

Apparent asystole
isoelectric ECG

where VF can be exclude

where VF cannot be excluded

Defibrillate 200 J
Defibrillate 200 J
Defibrillate 360 J

Adrenaline 1 mg iv

Atropine 2 mg iv

Consider pacing
if P waves or any other
electrical activity present

Asystole is the cessation of electrical and mechanical ventricular activity. It is estimated that 10% of out-of-hospital cardiac arrests and 25% of in-hospital cardiac arrests are asystolic. As asystole has a worse prognosis than ventricular fibrillation and the distinction between them, and thus the appropriate treatment, is made by monitoring the ECG, it is essential when a flat ECG trace is obtained that the switches, connections and gain of the monitoring system are carefully checked. If there is any doubt as to the electrocardiographic rhythm or if ventricular fibrillation cannot be excluded, then the patient must be defibrillated immediately as described in the algorithm in the previous section.

As in ventricular fibrillation the first drug to be administered is adrenaline, 1mg. Atropine, a parasympathetic blocking drug, in a dose of 2 mg, via the intravenous or endotracheal route is recommended as being effective in asystole[50]. Parasympathetic overactivity, especially in the presence of depressed sympathetic tone (e.g. ischaemia, infarction or β-blockade) may cause asystole by depression of the sinus and atrioventricular nodes. Ventricular fibrillation and tachycardia have been reported following the administration of atropine[51].

The further treatment of asystole depends on the maintenance of the circulation by external chest compressions together with the aid of the adrenergic stimulation of adrenaline. Sodium bicarbonate may be given to correct any measured acidosis that has occurred, but with the same provisos as in the previous section. The advent of transthoracic pacing, using large high-impedance electrodes applied to the thoracic wall, has been reported as being effective in those patients in asystole but with 'P-wave activity', especially when used early in the treatment[52]. Others have found that pacing in the out-of-hospital situation was disappointing and have not recommended its routine use[53].

Electromechanical dissociation

Electromechanical dissociation is the failure of the heart to pump blood despite organized electrical activity. It is usually seen as an in-hospital phenomenon; less than 3% of cardiac arrests occurring outside hospital are due to electromechanical dissociation. The prognosis for survival is very poor.

Adrenaline, 1 mg, is the first drug of choice. It is then necessary to exclude the pharmacological and physiological causes of electromechanical dissociation: drugs, hypovolaemia, severe acidosis, cardiac tamponade, pulmonary embolism, tension pneumothorax, intracardiac tumour or thrombus, myocardial rupture or exsanguination. It may also be seen as the final event in a prolonged ventricular fibrillation. The mechanism is not fully understood, but it is believed to be, in part, due to inadequate myocardial blood flow, intracellular acidosis and autonomic causes.

Electromechanical dissociation

QRS without palpable pulse

↓

Adrenaline 1 mg iv

↓

Consider specific therapy
for – hypovolaemia
  – pneumothorax
  – cardiac tamponade
  – pulmonary embolism

↓

Consider calcium
chloride (10 ml of 10%)
for – hyperkalaemia
  – hypocalcaemia
  – calcium antagonists

Calcium chloride, 10 ml of a 10% solution, may be used to improve myocardial contraction. Dembo found that calcium may increase coronary artery spasm and increase myocardial ischaemia[54]. Hyperkalaemia, hypocalcaemia, and the prior use of calcium antagonists are specific indications for the use of calcium chloride.

CONCLUSION

The foregoing text has described the management of the arrhythmias associated with cardiac arrest and resuscitation. It is of great concern that recent studies have shown that doctors[55–57] and nurses[58] perform poorly when tested in their theoretical and practical knowledge of resuscitation. Only regular formal training[59] in these resuscitation procedures will improve the management of this life and death medical emergency.

REFERENCES

1. Cummins, R. O. and Eisenberg, M. S. (1983). Prehospital cardiopulmonary resuscitation. Is it effective? *J. Am. Med. Assoc.*, **253**, 2408-12
2. Tweed, W. A. and Wilson, E. (1984). Is CPR on the right track? (Editorial). *Can. Med. Assoc. J.*, **131**, 429-33
3. Krause, G. S., Kumar, K., White, B. C., Aust, S. D. and Wiegenstein, J. G. (1986). Ischemia, resuscitation and reperfusion. Mechanisms of tissue injury and prospects for protection. *Am. Heart J.*, **111**, 768-80
4. Boidin, M. P. (1985). Airway patency in the unconscious patient. *Br. J. Anaesth.*, **57**, 306-10

5. Ruben, H., Elam, J. O. and Ruben, A. M. (1961). Investigation of upper airway problems in resuscitation. *Anaesthesiology*, **22**, 271-9
6. Guildner, C. W. (1976). Resuscitation – opening the airway. A comparative study of techniques for opening an airway obstructed by the tongue. *JACEP*, **5**, 588-90
7. Melker, R. (1985). Recommendations for ventilation during cardiopulmonary resuscitation. Time for change? *Crit. Care Med.*, **13**, 882-3
8. Kouwenhoven, W. B., Jude, J. R. and Knickerbocker, G. G, (1960). Closed-chest cardiac massage. *J. Am. Med. Assoc.*, **173**, 1064-7
9. Babbs, C. F. (1980). New versus old theories of blood flow during CPR. *Crit. Care Med.*, **8**, 191-5
10. Maier, G. W., Tyson, G. S. and Olsen, C. O. (1984). The physiology of external cardiac massage: High impulse cardiopulmonary resuscitation. *Circulation*, **70**, 86-101
11. Criley, J. M., Blaufass, A. H. and Kissel, G. L. (1976). Cough-induced cardiac compression. Self-administered form of cardiopulmonary resuscitation. *J. Am. Med. Assoc.*, **236**, 1246-50
12. Niemann, J. T., Rosborough, J., Garner, D. and Criley, J. M. (1979). The mechanism of blood flow in closed chest cardiopulmonary resuscitation. *Circulation*, **60**, (Suppl 2), 74
13. Rudikoff, M. T., Maughan, W. L., Effron M., Freund, P. and Weisfeldt. M.L. (1980). Mechanisms of blood flow during cardiopulmonary resuscitation. *Circulation*, **61**, 345-52
14. Criley, J. M., Niemann, J. T., Rosborough, J. P., Ung, S. and Suzuki, J. (1984). The heart is a conduit in CPR. *Crit. Care Med.*, **9**, 373-4
15. Niemann, J. T., Rosborough, J. T., Hausknecht, M., Gardner, D. and Criley, J. M. (1981). Pressure-synchronised cineangiography during experimental cardio-pulmonary resuscitation. *Circulation*, **64**, 985-91
16. Werner, J. A., Green H., Janko, C. L. and Cobb, L. A. (1981). Visualization of cardiac valve motion during external chest compression using two dimensional echocardiography. Implications regarding the mechanisms of blood flow. *Circulation*, **63**, 1414-21
17. Rich, S., Wix, H. L. and Shapiro, E. P. (1981). Clinical assessment of heart chamber size and valve motion during cardiopulmonary resuscitation by two dimensional echocardiography. *Am. Heart J.*, **102**, 368-73
18. Deshmukh, H., Weil, M. H. and Swindall, A. (1985). Echocardiographic observations during cardiopulmonary resuscitation: A preliminary report. *Crit. Care Med.*, **13**, 904-6
19. Chandra, N., Rudikoff, M. T., Tsitlick, J. and Weisfeldt, M. L. (1979). Augmentation of carotid flow during cardiopulmonary resuscitation in the dog by simultaneous compression and ventilation with high airway pressure. *Am. J. Cardiol.*, **43**, 422
20. Chandra, M., Radikoff, M. T. and Weisfeldt, M. L. (1980). Simultaneous chest compression and ventilation at high airway pressure during cardiopulmonary resuscitation. *Lancet*, **1**, 175-8
21. Ralston, S. H., Babbs, C. F. and Niebauer, M. J. (1982). Cardiopulmonary resuscitation with interposed abdominal compression in dogs. *Anesth. Analg.*, **61**, 645-51
22. Mateer, J. R., Stueven, H. A., Thompson, B. M., Aprahamian, C. and Davin, J. (1985). Prehospital IAC-CPR versus standard CPR. Paramedic resuscitation of cardiac arrests. *Am. J. Emerg. Med.*, **3**, 143
23. Martin, G. B., Carden, D. L., Nowak, R. M., Johnston, W. and Tomlanovich, M. C. (1985). Aortic and right atrial pressures during standard and simultaneous ventilation and compression CPR in human beings. *Ann. Emerg. Med.*, **14**, 497
24. Sanders, A. B., Ewy, G. A. and Taft, T. (1983). The importance of aortic diastolic blood pressure during cardiopulmonary resuscitation. *J. Am. Coll. Cardiol.*, **1**, 609
25. Niemann, J. T., Criley, J. M. and Rosborough, J. P. (1985). Predictive indices of successful cardiac resuscitation after prolonged arrest and experimental cardiopulmonary resuscitation. *Ann. Emerg. Med.*, **14**, 521
26. Hess, D. and Baran, C. (1985). Ventilatory volumes using mouth-to-mouth, mouth-to-mask and bag-valve-mask techniques. *Am. J. Emerg. Med.*, **3**, 292
27. Centres for Disease Control (1988). Update: Universal precautions for prevention of transmission of human immunodeficiency virus, hepatitis B virus and other blood born pathogens in health care settings. *Morbid. Mortal. Weekly Rep.*, **37**, 377-88
28. Kahn, G. J., White, B. C. and Swetnam, R. E. (1981). Peripheral vs central circulation times during CPR: A pilot study. *Ann. Emerg. Med.*, **10**, 417-19
29. Greenberg, M. I. (1984). The use of endotracheal medication in cardiac emergencies. *Resuscitation*, **12**, 155-65

30. Quinton, D. N., O'Byrne, G. and Aitkenhead, A. R. (1987). Comparison of endotracheal and peripheral intrvanous adrenaline in cardiac arrest. Is the endotracheal route reliable? *Lancet*, **1**, 828

31. Hoernchen, U., Schuettler, J. and Stoekel, H. (1987). Endobronchial instillation of epinephrine during cardiopulmonary resuscitation. *Crit. Care Med.*, **15**, 1037

32. Sabin, H. I., Coghill, S. B., Khunti, K. and McNeil, G. O. (1983). Accuracy on intracardiac injections determined by a post-mortem study. *Lancet*, **2**, 1054-5

33. Iserson, K. V. and Criss, E. (1986). Intraosseous infusions, a usable technique. *Am. J. Emerg. Med.*, **4**, 540

34. Prete, M. R., Hannan, C. J. and Burkle, F. M. (1987). Plasma atropine concentrations via intravenous, endotracheal and intraosseous administration. *Am. J. Emerg. Med.*, **5**, 101

35. Spivey, W. H., Lathers, C. M. and Malone, D. R. (1985). Comparison of the intraosseous, central and peripheral routes of sodium bicarbonate administration during CPR in pigs. *Ann. Emerg. Med.*, **14**, 1135

36. Glaeser, P. W. and Losek, J. D. (1986). Emergency intraosseous infusion in children. *Am. J. Emerg. Med.*, **4**, 34

37. Caldwell, G., Millar, G., Quinn, E., Vincent, R. and Chamberlain, D. A. (1985). Simple mechanical methods for cardioversion: defence of the precordial thump and cough version. *Br. Med. J.*, **291**, 627-30

38. Miller, J., Tresch, D., Horwitz, L., Thompson, B. M., Aprahamian, C. and Davin, J. C. (1984). The precordial thump. *Ann. Emerg. Med.*, **13**, 791-4

39. Weaver, W. D., Cobb, L. A., Copass, M. K. and Hallstrom, A. P. (1982). Ventricular defibrillation – a comparative trial using 175J and 320J shocks. *N. Engl. J. Med.*, **307**, 1101-6

40. Kerber, R. E., Jensen, S. R. and Gascho, J. A. (1983). Determinants of defibrillation: Prospective analysis of 183 patients. *Am. J. Cardiol.*, **52**, 739-45

41. Dahl, C. F., Ewy, G. A. and Ewy, M. D. (1976). Transthoracic impedance to direct current discharge: Effect of repeated countershocks. *Med. Instrum.*, **10**, 151-5

42. Kerber, R. E., Grayzel, J., Hoyt, R., Marcus, M. and Kennedy, J. (1981). Transthoracic resistance in human defibrillation. *Circulation*, **63**, 676–82

43. Redding, J. S. and Pearson, J. W. (1963). Evaluation of drugs for cardiac resuscitation. *Anesthesiology*, **24**, 203-7

44. Livesay, J. J., Follette, D. M. and Fey, K. H. (1978). Optimizing myocardial supply/demand balance with adrenergic drugs during cardiopulmonary resuscitation. *J. Thorac. Cardiovasc. Surg.*, **76**, 244-51

45. Rosen, M. R., Hoffman, B. F. and Wit, A. L. (1975). Electrophysiology and pharmacology of cardiac arrhythmias versus cardiac antiarrhythmic effects of lidocaine. *Am. Heart J.*, **89**, 526-36

46. Babbs, C. F., Yim, G. K. W. and Whistler, S. J. (1979). Evaluation of ventricular defibrillation threshold in dogs by antiarrhythmic drugs. *Am. Heart J.*, **98**, 345-50

47. Sanna, G. and Arcidiacono, R. (1973). Chemical ventricular defibrillation of human heart with bretylium tosylate. *Am. J. Cardiol.*, **32**, 982-7

48. Bacaner, M. (1968). Quantitative comparison of bretylium with other antifibrillatory drugs. *Am. J. Cardiol.*, **21**, 504-21

49. Jaffe, A. S. (1986) Cardiovascular pharmacology 1 – Bicarbonate. *Circulation*, **74**, Suppl. IV, 70-1

50. Myerburg, R. J., Estes, D. and Laman, L. (1984). Outcome of resuscitation from bradyarrhythmic or asystolic prehospital cardiac arrest. *J. Am. Coll. Cardiol.*, **4**, 1118

51. Cooper, M. J. and Abinader, E. G. (1979). Atropine induced ventricular fibrillation: Case report and review of the literature. *Am. Heart J.*, **97**, 225-8

52. Zoll, P. M., Zoll, R. H. and Falk, R. H. (1985). External non-invasive temporary cardiac pacing: Clinical trials. *Circulation*, **71**, 937-44

53. Falk, R. H., Jacobs, L. and Sinclair, A. (1983). External non-invasive cardiac pacing in out-of-hospital cardiac arrest. *Crit. Care Med.*, **11**, 779-82

54. Dembo, D. H. (1981). Calcium in advanced life support. *Crit. Care Med.*, **9**, 358

55. Lowenstein, S. R., Hansbrough, J. F., Libby, L. S., Hill, D. M., Mountain, R. D. and Scoggin, C. H. (1981). Cardiopulmonary resuscitation by medical and surgical house officers. *Lancet*, **2**, 679-81

56. Casey, W. F. (1984). Cardiopulmonary resuscitation: a survey of standards among junior hospital doctors. *J. R. Soc. Med.*, **77**, 921-4

57. Skinner, D. V., Camm, A. J. and Miles, S. (1985). Cardiopulmonary resuscitation skills of pre-registration house officers. *Br. Med. J.*, **290**, 1549
58. Wynne, G., Marteau, T. M., Johnston, M. and Evans, T. R. (1987). Inability of trained nurses to perform basic life support. *Br. Med. J.*, **294**, 1198
59. Kaye, W., Mancini, M. E., Rallis, S. F. and Mandel, L. P. (1989). Resuscitation training and evaluation. *Clin. in Crit. Care Med.*, **16**, 177-222

Further reading

(A) *National Guidelines*

Evans, T. R. (ed.) (1990). *ABC of Resuscitation*. (London: British Medical Journal)

Standards and Guidelines for Cardiopulmonary Resuscitation and Emergency Cardiac Care (1986). *J. Am. Med. Assoc.*, **255**, 2841-3044.

(B) *Other*

Safar, P. and Bircher, N. G. (eds.) (1988). *Cardiopulmonary Cerebral Resuscitation*, 3rd Edn. (W.B. Saunders Company Ltd and Laerdal Medical)

Baskett, P. (ed.) (1989). Cardiopulmonary resuscitation. In *Monographs in Anaesthesiology*, **17**. (Elsevier Science Publishers BV)

Kaye, W. and Bircher, N. G. (eds.) (1989). Cardiopulmonary resuscitation. In *Clinics in Critical Care Medicine*, **16**. (Churchill Livingstone Inc, New York)

3
Practical cardiac pacing

J. PERRINS

Modern cardiac pacing is a highly specialized and technical area of cardiology. Cardiac pacemakers and their associated programming devices are becoming ever more complex and sophisticated, in addition the rapid evolution of sensor driven rate responsive pacemakers has added a new dimension to the problem of fine tuning a device to a patient's individual physiological needs. The combination of multiple sensors and dual chamber cardiac pacemakers will represent a further technological escalation. In this chapter I hope to give a broad outline to the subject covering device technology as well as clinical issues but only bradycardias and their allied conditions will be considered.

Pacemaker implantation rates vary widely between countries and although there is a tendency for the most affluent societies to have the highest rates there are glaring exceptions, for example the United Kingdom. Approximately 10,000 pacemaker implants are performed in the UK each year which represents only 160 implants per million population. This contrasts with considerably higher rates in USA, Canada and West Germany of up to 500 per million[1]. This almost certainly represents underdiagnosis and referral in this country, particularly of patients suffering from sick sinus syndrome and carotid sinus syndrome. A recent survey carried out in the UK by the British Society of Pacing and Electrophysiology suggested that there was a surprisingly poor level of general knowledge concerning pacing in GPs, general physicians and even 'specialized' cardiologists, and although funding problems are often blamed as the main reason for low implant rates this clearly is not the only factor. A sustained programme of postgraduate education will be required to bring pacemaker implantation and practice up to an acceptable level.

INDICATIONS

Pacemakers are generally implanted either for symptomatic bradycardia, for prophylaxis against sudden death or for both. There are three major causes of bradycardia: (1) atrioventricular block (AVB), (2) sick sinus syndrome (SSS) and (3) carotid sinus syndrome (CSS). Their respective incidence is shown in Figure

3.1. It is important to note that there is some overlap in diagnosis between SSS and AVB but much less between CSS and the other two.

There are a few miscellaneous indications for pacing of which the most important are dual chamber pacing for prevention of atrial dysrhythmias (particularly atrial fibrillation), treatment of the malignant vaso-vagal syndrome, and treatment of hypertrophic cardiomyopathy.

BRADYCARDIAC SYMPTOMS

The symptomatology is similar regardless of aetiology. A significant number of patients with bradycardias are asymptomatic, many of these will still require pacing.

Syncope

This is the most important symptom and classically is termed Adams–Stokes attacks[2,3]. Typically the patient looses consciousness without warning, usually falling to the ground and sustaining self-injury. The patient is at first very pale then cyanosed. Consciousness is regained rapidly, often accompanied by facial flushing due to reactive hyperaemia. The patient is rarely confused for longer than a few minutes and then recovery is complete. The attacks coincide with either asystole, extreme bradycardia or occasionally ventricular fibrillation. Although typically many patients have variations of this pattern some undoubtedly do get a warning and clonic-tonic convulsions may ensue if cerebral anoxia is prolonged and occasionally sphincter incompetence can occur but this is rare. Similarly confusion may be prominent but it is unusual to get sustained neurological deficit after an attack. Attacks of prolonged unresponsiveness have been described in sick sinus syndrome and are thought to be due to persistent extreme sinus bradycardia[4]. They have been called hibernation attacks and have been reported to last for up to one and a half hours but they are unusual and such symptoms would normally suggest an epileptic syndrome or hysteria. It must be remembered that in sick sinus syndrome there is probably an increased incidence of systemic embolism so that occasionally true cerebral ischaemic symptoms may occur in addition to bradycardia.

Dizziness

Transient dizziness is common between major attacks described above but a significant number of patients only experience dizziness and this is more a feature of sick sinus syndrome. There are usually no features of vertigo but as with syncope neurological syndromes may co-exist with the attack leading to erroneous diagnoses of cerebral ischaemia. Dizziness is usually associated with extreme bradycardia although it may also be caused by reflex hypotension either in patients with carotid sinus syndrome or in patients with pacemaker syndrome (see below).

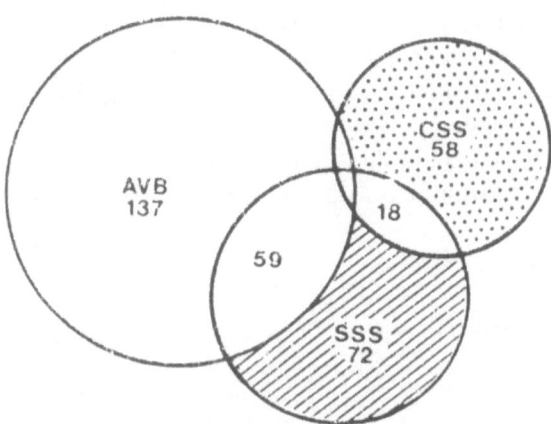

CSS only n = 58   30(2-74)months

SSS only n = 72   30(2-62)months

Figure 3.1 Venn diagram showing relative frequency of electrophysiological diagnoses in 352 patients presenting for pacing (1977-83). Note the overlap between sick sinus syndrome (SSS) and atrioventricular block (AVB) both overlap much less with carotid sinus syndrome (CSS)

Minor symptoms

Patients often complain of palpitations (which are usually tachycardias in patients with SSS). Chest discomfort is common though rarely is it typically anginal. There is a very rare condition of true bradycardiac angina where the ischaemia only occurs during severe and sustained bradycardia. Neck pulsation is an important symptom often overlooked or attributed to hysteria (often in women) but due to venous cannon waves during atrioventricular dissociation. This symptom may also occur during ventricular pacing.

Heart failure

Sustained bradycardia in the context of normal ventricular function never causes heart failure; however a significant number of patients with bradycardias have myocardial disease and in them the symptoms of heart failure may be exacerbated. Tiredness is a common complaint in patients unable to increase their cardiac output during exercise and is occasionally the only symptom of bradycardia present.

Unexplained or 'difficult' syncope

Even after routine clinical and electrophysiological examination there remains a small core of patients with unexplained syncope[5,6]. Detailed examination with intracardiac electrophysiology, prolonged Holter monitoring and specialist neurological examination will occasionally produce a diagnosis but often not. Prolonged head-up tilt (see below) may yield results. In those patients with totally negative results a history of injury (even relatively minor) is a strong pointer to an arrhythmia as the cause and pacemaker implantation can be justified particularly if symptoms are frequent. In patients whose diagnosis is unclear it is vital to implant a dual chamber device to minimize the possibility of subsequent pacemaker syndrome which could appear to duplicate the original symptoms. Approximately 50% of patients paced for unexplained syncope will become completely free of attacks.

CLASSIFICATION OF BRADYCARDIAS

Atrioventricular block

This is the commonest indication for pacemaker implant in the UK but worldwide the incidence of sick sinus syndrome is slightly greater.

Complete heart block

All patients with wide complex CHB require pacing for prognostic reasons irrespective of whether they have symptoms. This also applies to wide complex CHB (QRS > 0.12 ms) which is intermittent. The only possible exceptions are asymptomatic patients with narrow complex complete heart block proven to be congenital through prolonged observation and not associated with structural heart disease. Many cardiologists would still insist on thorough assessment of these patients with stress testing and Holter monitoring before finally withholding a pacemaker. It must be stressed that patients with asymptomatic CHB must be paced unless there are overwhelming reasons not to. Saventrine therapy is now discredited and must not be used, patients receiving this drug for bradycardia should be considered for pacing.

Mobitz type II AVB

All symptomatic patients and those asymptomatic patients with persisting block should be paced unless there has been a very recent myocardial infarction. It may be reasonable to withhold pacing in asymptomatic patients with intermittent

Mobitz type II block although if additional cardiac disease is present a pacemaker is probably indicated. Second degree block which either increases in severity or stays constant during exercise testing generally indicates severe conduction disease and such patients should be considered for a pacemaker irrespective of symptoms.

Mobitz type I AVB

Wenkebach block has been thought to be a benign arrhythmia but recent evidence would suggest this is not the case[7]. All symptomatic patients should be paced.

Sick sinus syndrome

This condition is characterized by periods of sinus arrest or SA block causing either intermittent or sustained severe bradycardia. The bradycardia may exist alone or in combination with paroxysmal atrial flutter/fibrillation, sinus tachycardia or atrial tachycardia. There is an increased incidence of systemic embolism in this condition. All symptomatic patients benefit from pacing and this often reduces the subsequent incidence of tachycardias although some patients require additional drug therapy[8,9]. There is as yet no clear evidence that asymptomatic patients with SSS derive prognostic benefit from pacing and this should probably be withheld unless the associated tachycardias are troublesome, drug therapy on its own for these patients will often precipitate severe bradycardia. It is widely believed, largely from retrospective data, that atrial fibrillation is reduced in frequency by atrial pacing either alone or in a dual chamber mode. A large prospective controlled trial is urgently needed to substantiate these observations.

Carotid sinus syndrome

This condition is now being increasingly recognized as a cause of symptomatic bradycardia. Its true incidence is difficult to assess but may be as high as 30 new patients per million per year. It is caused by overactivity·of the carotid sinus baroreflex arc. The exact site of the abnormality is not known although the available evidence suggests a central disorder[10]. The reflex arc causes sinus arrest and often atrioventricular block due to intense vagal activity (cardioinhibitory). In addition peripheral vasodilatation leading to hypotension may occur (vasodepressor). Some patients may have a mixed cardioinhibitory and vasodepressor response. The condition is often overlooked as in between attacks the heart rhythm is almost invariably normal. Carotid sinus massage for 6 seconds with the patient resting and recumbent will often reveal the diagnosis, a pause of greater than 3.5 seconds being significant. In patients with a high level of sympathetic activity the reflex may be masked. The test should be repeated when the patient is relaxed if there is a high index of suspicion. The reflex can be further revealed by autonomic blockade with atropine and propranolol without loss of specificity and some authors advocate performing the carotid massage cautiously with the patient upright although severe syncope may ensue. It must be emphasized that the reflex can be activated spontaneously in many ways, the patient's symptoms do not normally relate to neck movement or pressure and in fact are frequently indistinguishable from Adams Stokes syncope.

Patients with CSS are particularly susceptible to pacemaker syndrome (see below) and atrioventricular pacing is the mode of choice.

Malignant vasovagal syndrome

This syndrome has recently been recognized as an occasional but important cause of syncope. It tends to be commoner in the younger patient and is generally revealed by prolonged 70 degree head-up tilt using a tilt-table[11]. The patient usually has a short prodrome followed by syncope. Careful observation of heart rate and blood pressure during the attack is essential. In those patients who demonstrate marked bradycardia during the attack a dual chamber pacemaker (programmed to DDI mode) will often abort or modify the symptoms.

Hypertrophic cardiomyopathy

There have been a number of anecdotal and short reports of the benefits of dual chamber pacing in patients with HOCM even in the absence of documented bradycardia. A short A–V delay seems to improve LV performance perhaps by lowering LVEDP. In patients with severe symptoms unresponsive to other treatments pacing is worth considering[19]. My own experience has been very favourable.

PACEMAKER TECHNOLOGY

A pacemaker is an implantable electronic device consisting of a battery and an electronic circuit usually totally encapsulated in a metallic can and connected to the heart by one or more leads (Figure 3.2). The connections to the myocardium may be made entirely within the lead (BIPOLAR) or alternatively the pacemaker can may form one part of the circuit (UNIPOLAR).

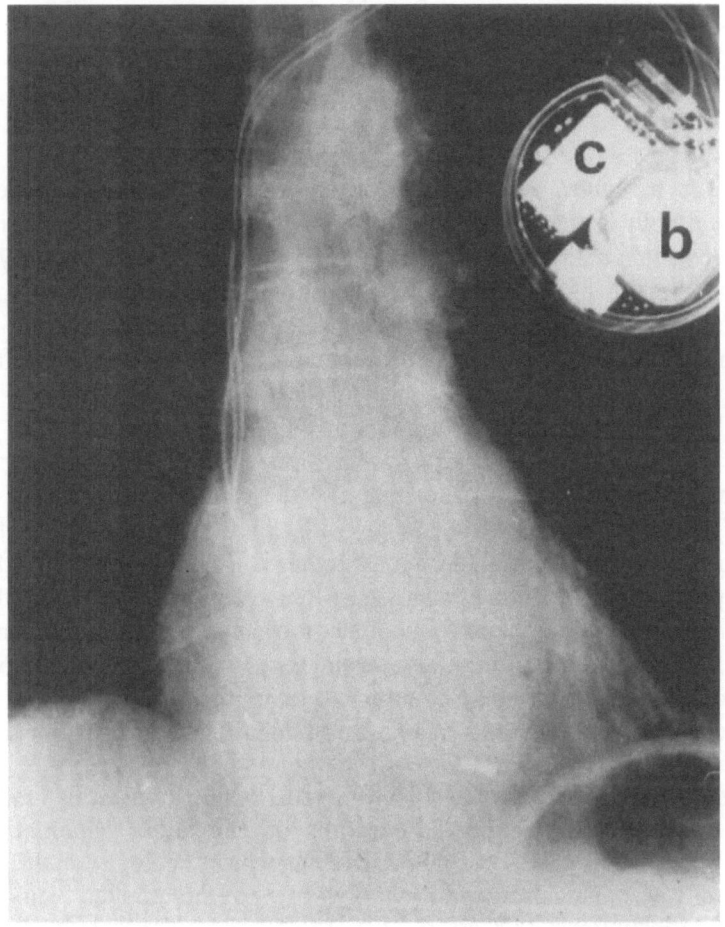

Figure 3.2 This X-ray of an implanted pacemaker clearly shows the battery (b) and the micro-circuit (c). In this older design there is a lot of empty space in the can, in newer designs specially shaped batteries and circuits allow very efficient packing of the components within the can contributing to the size reduction

Pacemaker batteries are usually of lithium iodine type and have a very high power to weight ratio. They also have extremely predictable discharge characteristics with a gradual rise in internal impedance which allows accurate and safe end-of-life calculation often with as much as one year safety margin. In addition the cells do not self discharge so that if the current drawn by a pacemaker circuit is reduced this will be reflected in a longer unit life.

The pacemaker circuit is functionally divided into a central timing or control block, sensing amplifiers and output circuits which produce the pacemaker impulse. The heart of any pacemaker is the timing and control circuitry which triggers the output circuits at the appropriate time and responds to the information from the sensing circuits.

Output circuits

These form a square wave signal of accurately defined pulse-width and amplitude usually in the region of 5 volts. The output is electronically regulated to ensure constant energy delivery in the face of gradually falling battery voltage during the lifetime of the pacemaker. The output is generally by a capacitive discharge mechanism. This has two advantages: first, by allowing gradual recharging of the capacitor between output pulses the current drain from the battery is kept constant which allows optimal discharge conditions for the battery. Secondly the capacitor minimizes DC leakage currents from flowing through the lead which can cause corrosion of the electrode surface by electrolysis. The output capacitance and also the capacitance of the lead/tissue interface may however allow 'ringing', a gradually decaying oscillation, to occur after stimulation and careful design is required to minimize this effect. In addition polarization potentials may persist long after the applied stimulus. The polarization potential is caused by ionic movements across the small gap between the lead surface and the myocardial tissues. These after-potentials may persist long enough and be of sufficient amplitude to be sensed by the pacemaker and there is the possibility of self-inhibition leading to dangerous loss of output.

The situation is worse in two lead systems where 'cross talk' may occur leading to false triggering or inhibition of the other channel. Many manufacturers incorporate 'recharge' circuits which apply a small potential (similar to the polarization voltage) opposite to the applied voltage after stimulation to minimize this effect. Atrial and ventricular output circuits are essentially the same. Although the timing and control blocks incorporate circuitry to limit the upper rate of the pacemaker the output circuit will generally incorporate a further rate limiting circuit to operate in the event of catastrophic failure of the control block. Finally in multiprogrammable devices both the pulse-width and output voltage or current may be selectable.

Sensing amplifiers

Sensing circuits are high sensitivity amplifiers which have to detect endocardial P-waves and QRS complexes reliably whilst rejecting other extraneous signals such as radio frequency or electromagnetic interference, muscle potentials (EMG), after-potentials, T-waves and in dual chamber modes interference from the other channel. As the amplitude of P-waves is in the region of 0.5–5 mV and the QRS complex 2.5–15 mV considerable problems with interference exist and the design of the sensing circuits is correspondingly complex. Two principal mechanisms are employed to optimize sensing: signal filtering and periods during which normal sensing is disabled (refractory periods). The incoming signal first passes through a RF filter to remove radiofrequency interference (low-pass filter), then a tuned filter to detect particular characteristics of the P-wave or QRS complex (bandpass filter) and finally through a noise detection circuit which if activated by high frequency noise (usually greater than 8 impulses per second) will disable sensing (see below). However despite complex filters the high sensitivity of the amplifiers makes the removal of after-potentials and T-waves very difficult. Accordingly a refractory period is required to disable the sensing amplifier for a short period after a paced or sensed event (150–350 ms).

Refractory periods

The operation of refractory periods is crucial to understanding complex pacemaker function and electrocardiograms. During the refractory period any signal which appears at the input must not be interpreted as either a P-wave or QRS complex by the device. The simplest (and earliest) approach was to disconnect totally sensing during the refractory period; however this had the disadvantage that if for example a QRS complex occurred just at the end of the refractory period (in a ventricular channel) then the amplifier would be switched back on in time to detect the following T-wave, similarly if noise occurred during the refractory period and continued when sensing was re-started it might then be detected as a QRS complex and cause inappropriate inhibition. Some modern sensing circuits therefore continue to sense during the terminal part of the refractory period. If a sensed event occurs during this 'noise sampling period' then the refractory period is re-set but no signal is passed to the pacemaker timing circuits. If interference continues then the refractory period is continuously reset so that no sensing occurs and the pacemaker automatically reverts to fixed rate asynchronous stimulation. This mechanism prevents continuous inhibition of the pacemaker by high levels of continuous noise. In some designs this noise sampling period is only activated by a signal from the noise detection circuitry which in addition may trigger a refractory period if noise is detected outside of the refractory period. Noise inhibition was a significant problem with early designs when pacemaker dependent patients encountered high levels of interference such as microwave ovens and airport security devices. Atrial sensing requires different filtering to ventricular sensing and requires a separate atrial amplifier.

Timing circuits

These circuits define the basic escape intervals for pacemaker operation. In the earliest devices they were simple transistor oscillators. Modern designs use a highly stable crystal controlled master oscillator. The timing circuits operate by counting a pre-determined number of master clock pulses. When the count is finished (times-out) the counter signals the control circuitry. In multi-programmable units where many individual timing intervals are adjustable this system allows easy alteration of the timing period by changing the number of pulses to be counted.

Control circuitry

In simple non-programmable VVI, VOO, AAI and AOO devices no separate control circuits were required as the operation of the device was defined by a single parameter: the escape interval of the R–R timer. In any unit incorporating programmability and in all dual chamber or rate responsive units control circuits are required. These circuits are extremely complex and in multiprogrammable DDD pacemakers are of equivalent complexity to a microprocessor chip. The large development costs of these chips are causing a trend towards full microprocessor control of the pacemaker controlled by both read only and externally programmable random access memory. New pacemaker modes and operating parameters may then be developed by changing the operating program (software) which is cheaper than building a new chip. The advent of software controlled pacemakers is bringing new problems of long term reliability not previously encountered by so called 'hard-wired' devices (i.e. the operation of the device is totally defined by the physical configuration of the circuit). The long term reliability of software and of memory devices within the chip is difficult to define. Most microprocessor based pacemakers therefore incorporate a separate failsafe ventricular pacemaker which will maintain ventricular pacing in the event of a microprocessor malfunction. It must be emphasized however that the large scale integrated circuits are inherently more reliable than designs using discrete components and that the increased complexity of the DDD device does not render it more susceptible to random failure than a VVI pacemaker.

Communications

In programmable devices a communications link is required between programmer and pacemaker. Early designs used various forms of electro-magnetic induction or even the simple opening and closing of a reed switch by a pulsed magnetic field to produce programming pulses[12]. Radio- frequency digital communication is the most frequently used system now. Most systems require the transmission to the pacemaker of a long binary word which may be from 10 to 30 bits long. The transmitted word will contain check digits to ensure security. In other designs the programming word is transmitted twice and only accepted by the pacemaker if both signals match. In addition the receiver circuitry is generally only switched on by the presence of a high magnetic field (provided by the programming 'head') which activates an internal reed switch. These features allow a very high degree of programme security and resistance to 'phantom programming'. Further refinements have included the provision of bi-directional telemetry. This allows the internal settings of the pacemaker to be read by the programming device which in turn allows proper confirmation of programming and is essential if a malfunction is suspected. A number of units also allow the real-time telemetry of endocardial signals. Some systems use simple amplitude modulated radiofrequency signals whilst others have opted for analogue to digital conversion within the pacemaker and subsequent digital transmission. Real-time endocardial recordings may be helpful in the diagnosis of arrhythmias. In addition some models provide timing markers which indicate when the pacemaker is sensing and pacing in atrium and ventricle. This latter feature may be helpful in ECG interpretation and may ultimately be developed into fully automatic ECG analysis by the programmer.

Programmers

As the complexity of pacemakers has increased their size has decreased. This cannot be said of programmers which have in many cases become very large and unwieldy microcomputers (Figure 3.3). The development of really simple to operate but effective programmers is still lagging far behind the pacemaker designs. As the different manufacturers' pacemakers become more and more similar due to the adoption of microprocessor controlled circuits it will ultimately be the programming and telemetry systems which really distinguish the different devices. At present mis-programming is far more likely to occur due to incorrect operation of the programmer than to any other cause and very detailed records of programming operations must be kept. The ability to interrogate the pacemaker as to its programmed settings is of great assistance in this respect.

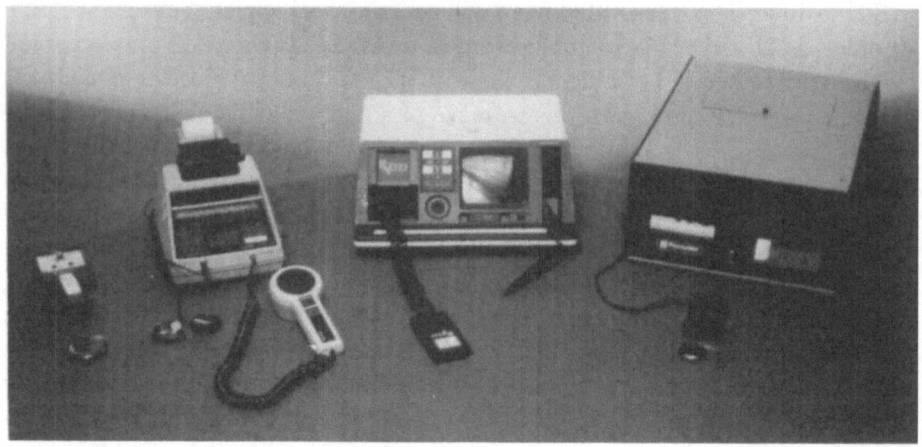

Figure 3.3 Pacemakers with their programmers. As pacemakers became smaller and more' sophisticated their programmers became large and complex (left to right)

TYPES OF PACEMAKER

Pacemaker modes are described by a three letter code with optional fourth and fifth positions. The first letter is the chamber paced (V-ventricle, A-atrium, D-both, O-none), the second letter is the chamber sensed (A,V,D,O) and the third letter is the mode of sensing (I-inhibit, T-trigger, D-trigger and inhibit, O-none). An optional fourth letter describes whether the unit has rate response (R). The fifth letter relates to tachycardia functions. A simple ventricular inhibited pacemaker is therefore VVI, a dual chamber pacemaker DDD, and a ventricular rate responsive unit VVIR.

Pacemakers conveniently divide into single chamber fixed rate devices (VVI, [ventricular inhibited], AAI [atrial inhibited]) dual chamber devices (DVI [A–V sequential pacing], DDD dual chamber physiological with atrial rate response) and sensor driven single chamber rate responsive units which are basically VVI pacemakers whose basic rate is altered according to some sensed parameter, e.g. Q–T interval, temperature, respiration and body activity. Other sensors are under active development such as mixed venous oxygen saturation. Dual chamber rate responsive units combine the functionality of a DDD pacemaker with an additional sensor. Currently available units employ activity but other sensors for DDR such as temperature and minute volume are under active development.

A block diagram of a dual chamber pacemaker (DDD) is shown in Figure 3.4. The unit functions as an A–V sequential pacemaker when the atrial spontaneous rate is below the programmed lower rate. When the atrial rate is between the low rate and the upper rate then each P-wave is followed by a QRS (either paced or sensed). If the P-wave rate is above the upper rate then the pacemaker introduces some form of A–V block (often similar to Wenkebach block) to limit the upper rate (Figure 3.5).

A block diagram of a rate responsive pacemaker is shown in Figure 3.6. The principle is the same regardless of the sensor system employed but the complexity of the algorithm relating the sensed parameter to the predicted heart rate is very dependent on the sensor used. Q–T for example is very complex whereas respiration is relatively simple. The pacemaker has programmable upper and lower rates and usually has at least a slope or sensitivity adjustment which changes the rate of change of rate with exercise.

Dual chamber sensor driven units combine the features of both DDD and rate responsive pacemakers. The sensor indicator can be programmed to function in either single or dual chamber modes. These pacemakers find their principal indication in patients with severe chronotropic incompetence (inability to increase heart rate with exercise), particularly if there is co-existing atrioventricular block. DDDR pacemakers have only been available since 1989 and as yet published experience is preliminary.

It is beyond the scope of this article to go into detailed functional descriptions of each of the pacing modes.

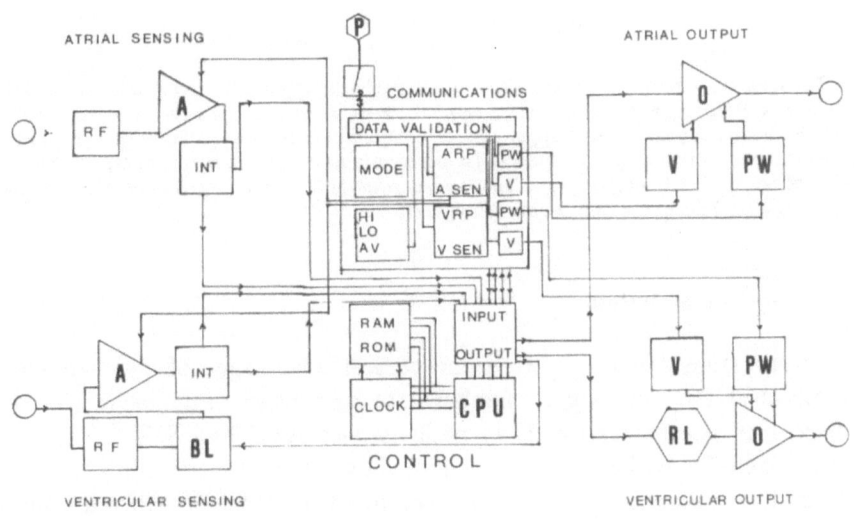

Figure 3.4 Block diagram of a multi-programmable DDD pacemaker. This is seen to be a highly sophisticated device. A, sensing amplifier; BL, blanking circuit; CPU, computer processing chip; O, output stage; V, voltage output control; PW, pulse-width output control; RL, hardware rate limiting circuit on the ventricular channel to protect against 'runaway'

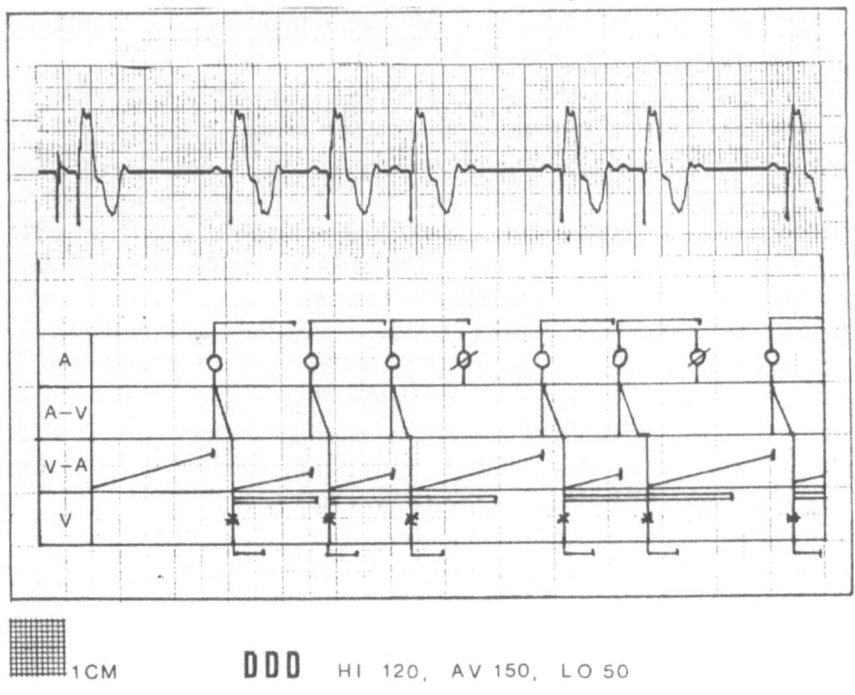

1 CM   **DDD**   HI 120, AV 150, LO 50

Figure 3.5 ECG and timing diagram showing Wenkebach upper rate behaviour of a DDD pacemaker. In QRS complexes 3 and 4 and 5 and 6 the P–R interval can be seen to lengthen, as the atrial rate is above the programmed upper rate of 120 bpm until the succeeding P wave is blocked by the lengthening atrial refractory period (upper line above the timing diagram). For a full discussion of pacemaker timing diagrams see Perrins *et al.* (1985) Interpretation of dual chamber electrocardiograms. *Pacing Clin. Electrophysiol.*, **8**, 6–16

Pacing mode/unit selection

Many recent studies have shown clear clinical advantages of dual chamber physiological (DDD) or single chamber rate responsive pacemakers (VVIR) over fixed rate pacemakers(VVI) in patients with AVB and SSS[13-16]. These units are selected in patients whom it is thought will benefit particularly from the increased effort tolerance. This is influenced by financial factors (they are more expensive) and the fact that the implant procedure for DDD is more complex. Younger patients are obvious candidates. In order to function correctly DDD pacemakers require normal sinus node function and particularly absence of atrial fibrillation. In these patients sensor driven rate responsive pacemakers will be required. In the UK at present about 20% of implants are with dual chamber or rate responsive units. Many cardiologists believe however that the majority of patients should in fact receive these complex devices so long as money is available to pay for them.

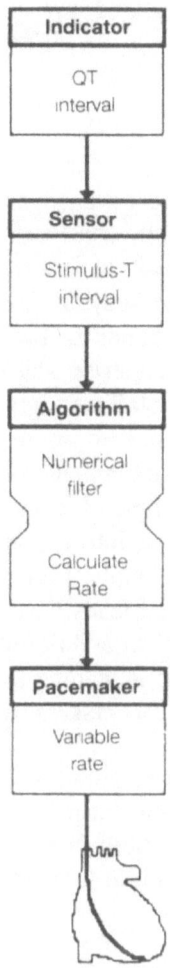

Figure 3.6 Block diagram of a rate responsive pacemaker

There has been much written discussion as to whether single chamber rate response (particularly VVIR) should be preferred to DDD. The arguments tend to be heavily biased towards the individual author's prejudice and experience. It is probably the case that in the majority of patients there is little to choose between systems, although in my own practice concern over avoiding atrial fibrillation and pacemaker syndrome cause me to favour the dual chamber approach[17,18]. Fortunately the advent of the dual chamber rate responsive pacemaker (DDDR) makes most of these arguments redundant.

There are still situations where the physical characteristics (e.g. size) are the most important. This is most evident in the very young and the very thin patient, and there is certainly no situation today where pacing is impossible due to technical factors.

Pacemaker leads

There have been very significant advances in pacemaker lead design over the past ten years. The lead is usually constructed from a plastic tube (silicone or polyurethane) in which is a coiled conductor (often multi-stranded). The tip of the lead is about 10 mm^2 and may be coated with carbon or some other compound or alternatively roughened or even porous. These 'tip technologies' result in lower threshold and superior sensing characteristics and are much superior to the older polished metallic designs. The most important advance has been 'active fixation' where at the lead tip an arrangement exists to temporarily lodge the lead until its fibrotic attachment is complete. This may be in the form of little projections (tines or fins, Figure 3.7) which entangle in the RV trabeculae or devices which screw into the myocardium itself. Fixation devices have dramatically reduced the complication rate so that less than 1% of leads displace after implantation. Atrial leads have been developed to the same state of reliability as ventricular leads. In addition it is now possible to construct thin diameter bipolar leads, and this is leading to increased use of bipolar systems particularly in dual chamber pacemakers where the sensing and cross-talk characteristics are improved.

Some sensors require the incorporation of a transducer into the lead (e.g. temperature, pressure, oxygen saturation); these approaches inevitably compromise lead characteristics both in terms of size and reliability but there are insufficient data to quantify this at present.

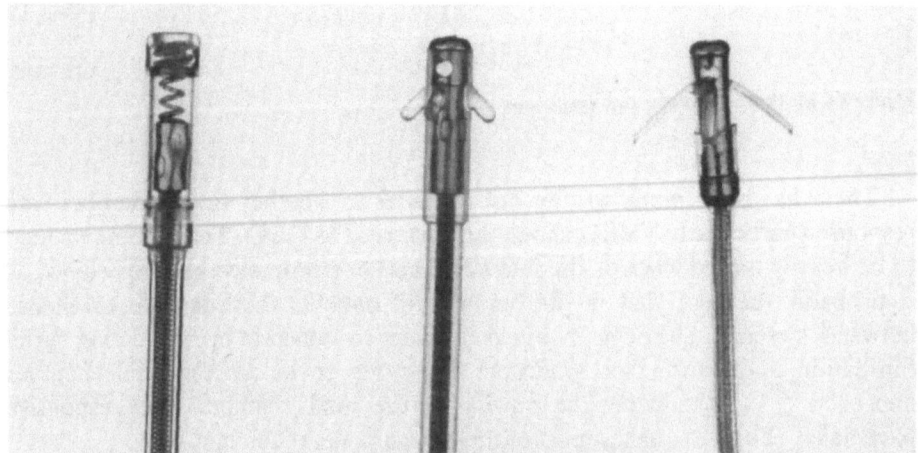

Figure 3.7 Three ventricular pacing leads showing screw and tine fixation

SURGICAL IMPLANTATION

Pacemakers are generally implanted under local anaesthetic and the vast majority are endocardial with venous access either to the cephalic vein by cut-down or to the subclavian vein by direct puncture. The leads are threaded through the vein into the heart under fluoroscopic control and positioned at the apex of the right ventricle and in the right atrial appendage (if an atrial lead is being used). The pulse generator itself is placed in a pocket fashioned between the surface of pectoralis major and the subcutaneous tissue. The implant procedure is extremely simple and rarely takes longer than 45 minutes. Epicardial systems are still implanted, usually in the presence of major congenital or valvular heart disease affecting the right side of the heart. Epicardial pacing generally requires a general anaesthetic and an approach to the heart which is xiphisternal. The procedure carries increased morbidity (and possibly mortality) compared to the endocardial approach. There is also unequivocal evidence that epicardial leads are less durable than endocardial ones, presumably related in part to greater mechanical stresses.

FOLLOW-UP

Once the unit is implanted and stitches have been removed the pacemaker has to be checked at 4–6 weeks initially. At follow-up clinics (which require specialized equipment and appropriately trained technicians) the pacemaker is tested and programmed. In simple terms this involves checking adequate capture and sensing in one or both chambers and in testing the battery. Battery tests may in-part be performed by the pacemaker programmer combination but in addition the state of the battery is often linked to the pulse width or basic pacing rate of the unit. In more complex devices considerable fine tuning may be required in order to maximize the haemodynamic advantages to the patient. After initial visits the pacemaker needs to be checked at 6–12 monthly intervals. The patient is advised that the pacemaker places no restrictions on him/her at all. Patients may drive once the first 4–6 week follow-up appointment has been satisfactory.

Modern pacemakers can be expected to last on average 7 years although many could last up to 15 years.

COMPLICATIONS

Complications during the implant are very rare and are generally related to venous access, a particularly with direct puncture of the subclavian vein which can result in pneomothorax or haemothorax or even laceration of the subclavian artery. For this reason many operators prefer the cephalic approach where it is possible although in reality a good operator must be competent at both techniques. It is possible for the pacing lead to perforate the heart acutely, often only resulting in a poor threshold, and this may go unrecognized. Acute tamponade can occur but is extremely rare. Primary infections are unusual but skin erosion at the sight of the implant (which may or may not be infective) can occur in up to 2% of implants. Prompt management of a suspicious wound may save the patient from having to have a complete explantation and such patients should be referred back immediately to their pacemaker clinic. Lead displacement occurs in less than 1% but the lead may become unsatisfactory for sensing (entrance block) or pacing (exit block) acutely without displacement. This is temporary in about half of cases and programmability to adjust output or sensitivity will cure the problem. Very occasionally patients consistently produce exit block and in them a new lead which slowly elutes a steroid from the tip is showing excellent results. Occasionally pectoral or diaphragmatic stimulation are caused (nearly always in unipolar pacemakers) this again can be generally remedied by programming. Random failure of either the pacemaker or lead is excessively rare (99.9% of pacemakers survive 5 years without technical faults).

An occasional long term complication is subclavian vein thrombosis on the side of the pacing lead. This does appear to be more common when the direct subclavian puncture technique is used. It usually responds to simple anticoagulation.

Pacemaker syndrome

This is an important condition which primarily affects patients with ventricular pacemakers[20,21]. It generally occurs in patients in whom retrograde atrioventricular conduction is intact. It is therefore common in patients with intact anterograde conduction (sick sinus syndrome and carotid sinus syndrome) although retrograde conduction can sometimes occur even in the presence of complete anterograde block. The retrograde p-waves during ventricular pacing cause cannon waves in the atria. In the right atria they may be felt in the neck by the patient whilst the left atrial cannon waves raise the pulmonary capillary pressure causing dyspnoea. In addition profound hypotension may occur at the onset of pacing, causing severe dizziness or syncope. The mechanism is thought to be due to the activation of atrial stretch receptors by the cannon waves causing reflex vasodilation.

Pacemaker syndrome generally occurs at rest when there is the greatest likelihood of pacing activity. Upgrading the patient to a dual chamber DDD[22] system will eliminate the problem and rate hysteresis programming may also help.

Rate responsive single chamber pacemakers also may cause pacemaker syndrome either by the above mechanisms or if the rate response is quite inappropriate to the physiological circumstances. These problems often reflect particular idiosyncrasies of the sensor system employed and are beyond the scope of this article.

CONCLUSIONS

Modern cardiac pacing is a highly effective and safe treatment modality. The mortality is negligible from the procedure and morbidity is low. Pacemakers may now be prescribed safely even in areas of clinical doubt. The complexity of operation and follow-up of these systems is challenging both to the clinician and to his/her supporting technicians. In the United Kingdom there is still considerable underdiagnosis and under-utilization of this treatment which although apparently expensive in fact represents excellent value for money and is one of the most clinically rewarding activities in cardiology today.

References

1. Feruglio, G.A. and Steinbach, K. (1983). World survey on Cardiac pacing. In Steinbach *et al.*(eds). *Cardiac Pacing.* pp. 953–68. (Darmstadt: Steinkopff).
2. Adams, R. (1827). Irregularity of breathing and remarkable slowness of pulse. Dublin hospital report, 4, 396
3. Stokes, W.(1846). Observations on some cases of permanently slow pulse. *Dublin Q. J. Med. Soc.*, 2, 73
4. Sutton, R. and Perrins, E.J. (1979). Neurological manifestations of the sick sinus syndrome. In Busse, E. (ed). *Cerebral Manifestations of Episodic Cardiac Dysrhythmias.* pp. 174–82. (Amsterdam: Excerpta Medica).
5. Kapoor, W.N., Hammill, S.C. and Gersh, B.J. (1989). Diagnosis and natural history of syncope and the role of invasive electrophysiologic testing. *Am. J. Cardiol.*, 63(11), 730–4
6. Scheinman, M. (1988). Evaluation of the patient with syncope [editorial]. *Clev. Clin. J. Med.*, 55(6), 503–4
7. Shaw, D.B., Kekwick, C.A., Veale, D., Gowers, J. and Whistance, T. (1985). Survival in second degree atrioventricular block. *Br. Heart J.*, 53(6), 587–93
8. Sasaki, Y., Shimotori, M., Akahane, K., Yonekura, H., Hirano, K., Endoh, R., Koike, S., Kawa, S., Furuta, S. and Homma, T. (1988). Long-term follow-up of patients with sick sinus syndrome: a comparison of clinical aspects among unpaced, ventricular inhibited paced, and physiologically paced groups. *Pace*, 11(11), 1575–83
9. Rosenqvist, M., Brandt, J. and Schuller, H. (1988). Long-term pacing in sinus node disease: effects of stimulation mode on cardiovascular morbidity and mortality. *Am. Heart J.*, 116(1), 16–22
10. Baig, M.W., Kaye, G.C. and Perrins, E.J. (1989). Can central neuropeptides be implicated in the syndrome of carotid sinus reflex hypersensitivity? *Medical Hypotheses*, 28(4), 255–65
11. Kenny, R.A., Ingram, A., Bayliss, J. and Sutton, R. (1986). Head-up tilt: a useful test for investigating unexplained syncope. *Lancet*, 1, 1352–5
12. Tarjan, P. (1973). Engineering aspects of implantable cardiac pacemakers.. In Samet, P. (ed.), *Cardiac Pacing*, p. 47. (New York: Grune and Stratton)
13. Kruse, I. *et al.* (1988). A comparison of the long term effects of ventricular inhibited and atrial synchronous ventricular inhibited pacing. *Circulation*, 65, 846–55
14. Perrins, E.J., Morley, C.A., Chan, S.L. and Sutton, R. (1982). A randomised controlled trial of physiological and ventricular pacing. *Br. Heart J.*, 50, 112–17
15. Byrd, C.L., Schwartz, S.J., Gonzales, M., Byrd, C.B., Ciraldo, R.J., Sivina, M., Yahr, W.Z. and Greenberg, J.J. (1988). DDD pacemakers maximize hemodynamic benefits and minimize complications for most patients. *Pace*, 11(11), 1911–6

16. Ebagosti, A., Gueunoun, M., Saadjia, A., Dolla, E., Gabriel, M., Levy, S. and Torresani, J. (1988). Long-term follow-up of patients treated with VVI pacing and sequential pacing with special reference to VA retrograde conduction. *Pace*, 11(11), 1929–34
17. Langenfeld, H., Grimm, W., Maisch, B. and Kochsiek, K. (1988). Atrial fibrillation and embolic complications in paced patients. *Pace*, 11(11), 1667–72
18. Mitsuoka, T., Kenny, R.A., Yeung, T.A., Chan, S.L., Perrins, J.E. and Sutton, R. (1988), Benefits of dual chamber pacing in sick sinus syndrome. *Br. Heart J.*, 60(4), 338–47
19. McDonald, K., McWilliams, E., O'Keeffe, B. and Maurer, B. (1988). Functional assessment of patients treated with permanent dual chamber pacing as a primary treatment for hypertrophic cardiomyopathy. *Eur. Heart J.*, 9(8), 893–8
20. Ausubel, K. and Furman, S. (1985). The pacemaker syndrome. *Ann. Intern. Med.* 103, 420–9
21. Alicandri, C., Fouad, F.M., Tarazi, R.C., Castle, L. and Mourant, V. (1978). Three cases of hypotension and syncope with ventricular pacing. Possible role of atrial reflexes.
22. Morely, C.A., Perrins, E.J., Grant, P., Chan, S.L., McBrien, D. and Sutton, R. (1982). Carotid sinus syncope treated by pacing. Analysis of persistent symptoms and the role of atrio-ventricular sequential pacing. *Br. Heart J.*, 47, 411–18

4

The pathology of immunological injury to the heart

E.G.J. OLSEN

INTRODUCTION

Immunological mechanisms have been demonstrated or presumed to be involved in almost all diseases that affect the cardiovascular system. The varieties of immunological pathways detailed elsewhere in this volume find morphological expression in many instances. Frequently the changes are non-specific and 'chronic inflammation' is all that can be observed. Special staining techniques have been applied to distinguish the subsets of lymphocytes and other cellular components. Monoclonal and polyclonal techniques, and immunohistology have all widened the horizon of examination of tissue. The application of molecular probes linking morphological changes with the presence of virus has also recently been applied.

An immense amount of work has been undertaken since the first publication of this chapter in 1987, especially in the field of dilated cardiomyopathy and myocarditis.

The pathology may be sufficiently characteristic to permit diagnosis by morphological examination alone. In this chapter the pathology of immunological injury will briefly be described together with an indication as to the possible immunological pathways involved. The disease entities are grouped according to the morphological features: those with diagnostic or characteristic changes, and those in which the features are non-specific.

DISEASES OF THE HEART AND VESSELS WITH DIAGNOSTIC OR CHARACTERISTIC MORPHOLOGICAL CHANGES

Rheumatic heart disease

In the acute phase, morphological characteristics readily provide easy diagnosis. The valve leaflets of the mitral valve – the most frequently involved valve – are covered by fibrin excrescences along the line of closure which can best be seen with the naked eye by placing the heart in water.

Histologically, beneath the fibrin cap the reactive cellular infiltrate found in the oedematous valve tissue consists of Anitschkow cells, and Aschoff cells as well as lymphocytes and other mononuclear cells, Aschoff nodules do not usually form in valvar tissue.

In the myocardium Aschoff bodies, a granulomatous myocarditis, are evident, and form the pathognomonic features of acute rheumatic heart disease. The formation and resolution of Aschoff bodies proceeds sequentially. The early, formative, stage is characterized by swelling and degeneration and increased eosinophilia of collagen tissue, together with a sparse cellular infiltrate consisting predominantly of lymphocytes and plasma cells. Increased basophilia and metachromasia of the ground substance of the connective tissue are also observed.

Approximately one month after infection by β-haemolytic streptococcus Lancefield Group A, the Aschoff nodules begin to form with the appearance of Anitschkow cells which have characteristic chromatin bars within their nuclei. Two to three of these cells condense to form multinucleate Aschoff cells. These cells, together with chronic inflammatory cells, constitute the Aschoff nodule which assumes different patterns and measures approximately 80 x 800 μm. This size is sufficient to enable one to see Aschoff bodies on macroscopic inspection.

The cellular components disappear in reverse order of their appearance, so that by 3–6 months after infection, non-specific changes consisting of fibrous tissue, often in onion-skin formation, and some chronic inflammatory cells are all that can be seen[1,2].

Recurrent rheumatic heart disease shows valvar thickening, commissural fusion and thickening and shortening of the chordae tendineae which ultimately result in the chronic phase of the disease. Not all the characteristic features may be observed and predominantly valvar or commissural or chordal changes are well recognized[3].

With the advance of cardiac surgery part of the atrial appendages are often excised. These have shown endocardial Aschoff nodules in between 37–75% of cases, even though no clinical manifestation of active disease is recognized. This indicates that when the heart has been affected, the disease process is a continuing one, finding occasional, or perhaps even no, clinically recognizable expression[4(a)].

The nature of the Aschoff nodule has been controversial. Among various suggestions that have been advanced[5] the connective tissue theory and the myogenic theory[6] have received most attention. Electron microscopy has provided proof that the connective tissue theory is likely.

In addition to the pathognomonic changes, non-specific myocarditis is also evident. Furthermore, the pericardium is frequently involved in rheumatic heart disease, resulting in fibrinous pericarditis, which eventually heals giving rise to either a milky spot or fibrous adhesions.

The mechanisms that result in the morphological changes are far from solved. The relationship between rheumatic fever and an upper respiratory infection by β-haemolytic streptococci Lancefield Group A is established. What has, so far, not been established is the exact mechanism of interaction between the organism and the host. Among the numerous hypotheses that have been proposed the 'toxic-immunological hypothesis' seems to be the most likely mechanism[7]. Antigenic constituents of the bacterial wall such as the M protein, and constituents of the cell membrane, cross-react with the host tissue such as the myocardium (subsarcolemma or sarcolemma) and also with glycoproteins of the valves[8]. Conversely, antisera against human heart muscle may cross-react with the same antigen of the wall of the bacterium[9]. These immunological responses occur at the onset of rheumatic fever but may also occur during the attack. Fragments of streptococci may directly be responsible for myocarditis without mediation of hypersensitivity[10].

The complicated immunological pathways that may exist resulting in the morphologically recognizable Aschoff bodies and other manifestations, are far from solved.

Chagas' disease

The heart is affected in African trypanosomiasis and in Chagas' disease which forms a major public health and social problem on the South American continent[11]. Infection is transmitted by arthropod vectors: some 90 species of *Triatoma* have been recorded. Three major phases are recognized. The acute phase is characterized by myocarditis which macroscopically results in a slightly enlarged and overweight heart, and in the early phases the inflammatory cells in the myocardium consist of neutrophils, which are soon replaced by chronic inflammatory cells. A careful search will be rewarded by the finding of pseudo-Leishmanic cysts. These are usually located within the myocardial fibres, and contain innumerable *Trypanosoma cruzi* – the infective organism. Accompanying degenerative changes and eventual fibrosis complete the myocardial changes observed in this phase, and neuronal cell loss also begins at this stage. Most patients survive the acute involvement of the heart

Little is known of the latent phase. In the chronic phase, hypertrophy and dilatation, with apical aneurysm formation and lymphatic hyperplasia are the macroscopic hallmarks. Histology shows extensive fibrosis of the myocardium and a non-specific mononuclear cellular infiltrate of varying intensity is discernible. Pseudo-Leishmanic cysts are usually not found.

An immense literature exists on the possible pathogenetic mechanisms, based on clinico-pathological studies and experimental investigations. A constant finding in the chronic phase[12] is the depopulation of neurons in the ganglia, which are usually easily located in right atrial strips between the venae cavae. The data suggest that in chronic infection the continuous liberation of auto-antigens from injured neurons and myocardial tissue may constitute a stimulus for the perpetuation of an auto-immune response[13]. Immunoglobulins and EVl antibodies on the plasma membrane of the myocardial cells have been demonstrated on tissue obtained by biopsy[14]. Electron microscopic evidence of invasion of the plasma membrane by lymphocytes suggests that a cell-mediated immune response may be implicated in Chagas' disease. In addition to the presence of anti-tissue auto-antibodies or self-reactive T-lymphocytes, a genetic predisposition is also likely to exist[15].

Endomyocardial fibrosis

This is a type of cardiomyopathy the pathology of which was first described by Davies in 1948, and was considered initially to be confined to the African continent. Subsequently, reports suggested that the disease existed in other tropical regions. In Switzerland, Löffler in 1936 described a disease entity called Löffler's endocarditis parietalis fibroplastica which was associated with an eosinophila and believed to be confined to the temperate zones[16]. A retrospective study showed that irrespective of the geographical origin, endomyocardial fibrosis and Löffler's disease belong to the same disease spectrum, originating in an inflammatory process in the myocardium rich in eosinophils[17]. This unitarian approach has been widely accepted.

From a morphological standpoint three major phases could be identified:

(1)   The *necrotic phase* is characterized by an often intense myocarditis rich in eosinophils, and this was found when the average length of history was 5 weeks.

(2)   If the history had extended to an average period of 10 months the *thrombotic phase* was observed. In this phase the inflammatory cell infiltrate was greatly reduced, and some endocardial thickening was present, but thrombus superimposition on the endocardium dominated the morphological picture.

(3)   Finally, after an average length of history of 2.5 years the *fibrotic phase* was reached. This consisted of extremely thick endocardium, frequently exceeding 5000 μm in thickness (normal for the left ventricular outflow tract = 20 μm). Usually the inflow tract, apex and outflow tracts were involved in left ventricular disease. When the region of the anterior mitral valve leaflet was reached the thick endocardium often ceased abruptly in a thick rolled edge. The papillary muscles and posterior mitral valve leaflets were also frequently involved by the disease process. The region beneath the anterior mitral valve leaflet was usually spared.

In right ventricular involvement, an area beneath the tricuspid valve (posterior leaflet) and the apex is involved, and as the disease progresses the apex becomes progressively drawn towards the atrioventricular valve ring resulting in the characteristic W shape of the cardiac silhouette[16]. Right (11%), left (38%) or both (51%) ventricles are involved, but in the cases recently studied in the United Kingdom all patients showed bilateral involvement. The distribution of endocardial thickness varies in the ventricles and five patterns have been described[18]. The atria may also be involved in endomyocardial fibrosis.

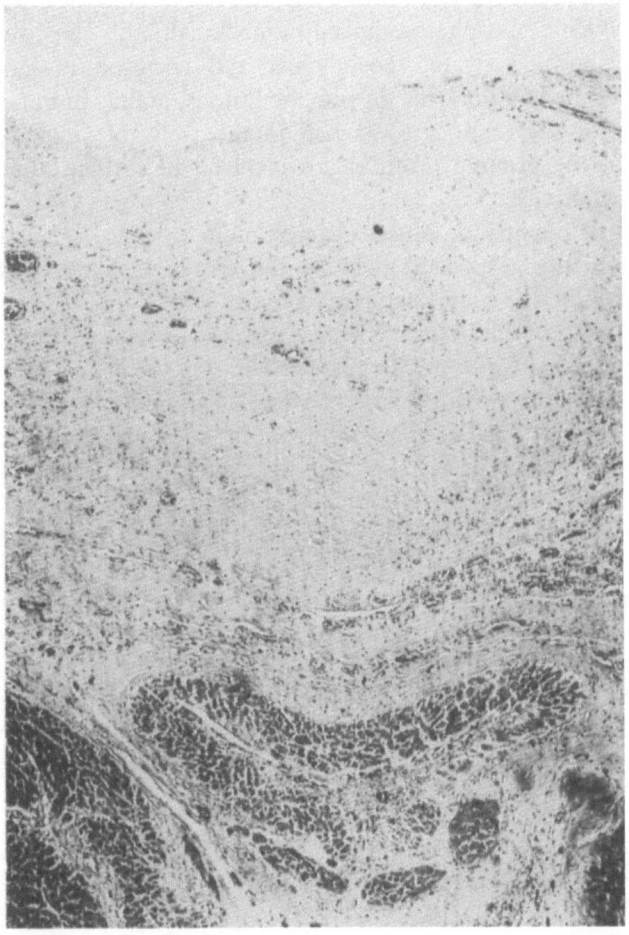

Figure 4.1 Endomyocardial disease. The extremely thickened endocardium is arranged in layers. Beneath the organizing thrombus (top right) a layer of dense fibrous tissue is followed by the granulation tissue layer in which blood vessels and some chronic inflammatory cells are seen. This layer abuts on to the myocardium. Haematoxylin and eosin × 40

Histologically, the thick endocardium is arranged in layers (Figure 4.1). Superficial fibrin or thrombus covers a layer of often dense connective tissue. The deepest layer, the so-called, 'granulation tissue layer' is composed of loosely arranged connective tissue, in which vascular channels abound and chronic inflammatory cells can be identified[19]. Not infrequently, even at this late stage of the disease, eosinophils can also be found[16]. In studies between the Hammersmith Hospital, the Mayo Clinic and the National Heart Hospital[20], tissue obtained from postmortem or by biopsy were stained for eosinophil major basic protein by indirect immunofluorescence. For eosinophil cationic protein and eosinophil protein X (now known to be a neurotoxin) and for activated eosinophils, alkaline phosphatase-linked monoclonal antibodies were used. The results have shown activated eosinophils and secreted eosinophil granule proteins in necrotic and the later thrombotic lesions, mainly in the areas of acute tissue damage in the endocardium and in the walls of small blood vessels, suggesting that the granule proteins are involved in cardiac injury leading to endomyocardial disease.

Since the first publication of this chapter, much work has been undertaken by Spry and co-workers, especially defining the nature of cationic proteins. The reader is referred to the monograph on the eosinophil[21].

The causes of eosinophilia could not be ascertained in about half of the patients. In 25% of patients eosinophilia was ascribed to eosinophilic leukaemia[17], though some doubt existed whether all patients were leukaemic. In the remaining 25% eosinophilia occurred in conjunction with polyarteritis nodosa, anti-tubercular treatment, asthma, Hodgkin's disease and tumours. More recently this has been extended to include myeloproliferative diseases, other vascular diseases, acute T-lymphocytic leukaemia, and carcinoma of the lung[16].

The eosinophils in patients with heart disease have shown abnormal morphology taking the form of degranulation and vacuolation[16] (Figure 4.2).

An immunological pathogenesis is likely. Serum cryoglobulins containing both IgG and IgM and auto-antibodies to the heart[22] and deposition of γ-globulin[23] have been demonstrated. Studies have also shown that blood eosinophils have an increased binding capacity for IgG and their phagocytic capacity was also increased. This was due to unmasking of Fc receptors. This suggests that with increased Fc receptors eosinophils may bind IgG-coated particles more effectively and this leads to a secretion of the eosinophilic constituents inducing a cytotoxic response[16].

Vascular diseases

Many diseases of the arteries (and veins) may affect the heart, though the brunt of the lesion may fall on other organs. In arterial diseases such as Buerger's disease or syphilis, morphological changes are typical so that recognition is easy.

In many instances the aetiology and pathogenesis are unknown and not infrequently an immunological basis has been suggested. Vascular diseases in which a possible immunological mechanism has been proposed are briefly described in the following sections.

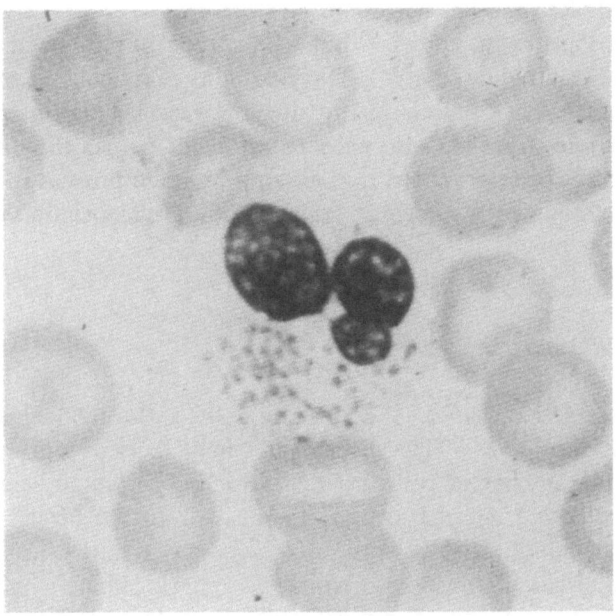

Figure 4.2 A degranulated eosinophil in the blood film from a patient with biopsy-proven endomyocardial disease. May Grunwald and Giemsa × 800

Takayasu's disease (pulseless disease, primary aortiis)

This disease affects mostly the aorta and large systemic and pulmonary arteries. Coronary arteries may, however, also be involved leading to myocardial infarction[24]. Macroscopically, the entire aorta or segments of that vessel may be involved, showing localized fusiform dilatation with white intimal thickening which may show wrinkling not unlike that seen in syphilis. Medial destruction may be discerned with the naked eye, and classically the adventitia is enormously thickened, anchoring the vessel to surrounding tissue so that sharp dissection may be necessary for its removal. As far as the coronary arteries or similar sized vessels are concerned, their appearance is that of extremely thick-walled white, rigid tubes. Irrespective of the size of vessel involved, histologically severe intimal thickening – which may exceed medial thickness – is composed of loosely arranged connective tissue devoid of elastic fibres, distinguishing this form of arteritis from all other forms of vascular disease in which the intima is involved. Destruction of the media by inflammation results in fibrous replacement and in some cases there is extreme fragmentation or disappearance of the elastic component. The inflammatory cell infiltrate is often mixed, and giant cells may be observed at the interface between medial destruction and relatively normal media. The thick adventitia is composed of dense connective tissue, and is ill-defined and often reaches neighbouring structures.

The aetiology is unknown, but the process has been linked with rheumatic–rheumatoid disease[25,26]. The possibility of it being a connective tissue disease expressed as an immunopathy affecting vascular elastin and aggravated by haemodynamic stress has also been entertained[26,27]. As the disease is often widespread it has been proposed that an auto-immune process is responsible[28]. Anti-aortic antibodies have been demonstrated[29]. An association with HLA A9 and B5 has been noted[30].

Thromboangiitis obliterans

A similar association has also been found with thromboangiitis obliterans (Buerger's disease)[30,31]. This disease is characterized morphologically by occlusion of the arteries or veins by non-retracting thrombus, and in the early phase giant cells and microabscesses are present. In the healed phase typical features are capillary sized vessels surrounded by a thick muscular coat. In contrast to other vascular diseases, the internal elastic lamina is thick and intact. A panarteritis or panphlebitis is present, and adjacent nerves are usually involved due to this vasculitic process resulting in the typical triad. Medium sized vessels of the lower and upper limbs are the most commonly affected. Isolated cases with coronary arterial disease have been documented[32].

Syphilis

Macroscopically, aortic involvement by syphilis may mimic Takayasu's disease, but histological differentiation is possible usually affording a correct diagnosis. Endocardial thickening, which may be severe, consists of fibro-elastic tissue. Patchy destruction of the medial elastic tissue by vascular fibrous tissue and perivascular cuffing of the vasa vasorum in the adventitia by lymphocytes and plasma cells constitute points of differentiation. Furthermore, the aortic valve leaflets are frequently involved in syphilis resulting in separation at the commissures and valvar deformities. Immunological studies show a varied antibody response, and the infective agent may act as a polyclonal B cell activator, as in infective endocarditis, initiating the proliferation of self-reacting antigen-binding and antibody-forming cells. Although humoral immunity may only play a minor role in the tissue damage, and cell mediated immunity may be important, circulating immune complexes have been found in the secondary stage of the infection.

Ankylosing spondylitis

The cardiovascular system is involved in this chronic disease of the sacro-iliac and synovial joints. Heart block, non-specific myocarditis (*vide infra*) and pericarditis have all been noted[33]. Aortic insufficiency is seen in 12% of patients particularly when it has been present for as long as 30 years, but occasionally aortic valve symptoms may precede spondylitis[34].

The aortic valve leaflets are thick and often have a rolled edge. Commissural fusion does not occur, mimicking syphilis macroscopically. Histologically, the normal architecture is distorted by an increase in collagen tissue which is particularly marked in the distal half of the valve leaflets. Increased vascularity may be observed, and in typical cases, chronic inflammatory cells are present. In the aorta, involvement is often limited to its ascending part. Cicatrization of the aortic media is a typical feature with destruction of the elastic component. Intimal thickening may be severe, but is non-specific consisting of fibro-elastic tissue. The vasa vasorum in the adventitia show severe intimal thickening, and chronic inflammatory cells are seen in the aorta and adventitia. An association with HLA B27 has been found consistently in this disease, and in Reiter's syndrome and other related disorders[35]. IgG[36] and circulating immune complexes and complement inactivation products have been found[37,38]. Reduction of inhibition of the cellular products of leukocytes has also been demonstrated[39].

Vasculitides

Polyarteritis nodosa, Wegener's granulomatosis (which may cause myocardial infarction[40]), vasculitides accompanying the hypereosinophilic syndrome, including granulomatous vasculitis (Churg–Strauss) and giant cell arteritis, are vascular diseases which may involve the coronary arteries. They all have certain morphological characteristics in common. These consist of the presence of giant cells, fragmentation of the internal elastic lamina and varying numbers of eosinophils forming part of the inflammatory process associated with the vascular disease as well as fibrinoid necrosis of the wall. The diseases attack different types of vessels. For example, polyarteritis nodosa affects medium sized and small vessels, whilst giant cell arteritis affects the temporal, cranial and large vessels, including the aorta. In Wegener's granulomatosis vessels of the lungs and kidneys are usually involved.

The size of the vessel involved and the site provides, therefore, some diagnostic hints. Morphological overlap is, however, encountered. For example, in polyarteritis nodosa giant cells are usually absent but have occasionally been described[41], whilst in giant cell arteritis fibrinoid necrosis – usually not a feature of this disease – has also been noted[42]. There are additional diagnostic features in giant cell arteritis. The intimal thickening, which is a constant feature, is arranged in two layers: an inner layer consisting of loosely arranged collagen tissue, whilst the outer layer is composed of dense fibrous tissue (Figure 4.3). Even in the healed phase this characteristic finding is evident[4(b)].

Vasculitis is also a morphological expression of allergic and hyper-sensitivity states, including those induced by drugs. No specific changes are present and the interpretation of vascular changes necessitates a detailed clinical history.

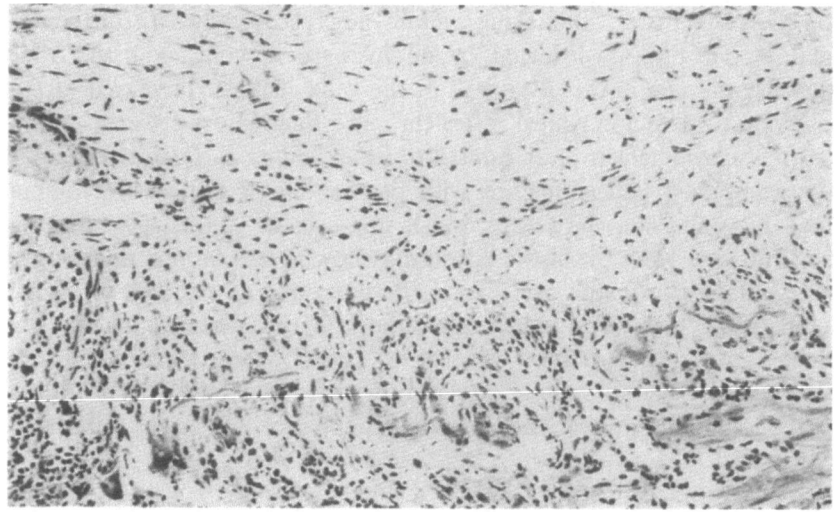

Figure 4.3 Giant cell arteritis. The thick intima is arranged in two layers, the inner one of which consists of dense collagen tissue in which inflammatory cells abound. The outer layer, occupying the upper half of the illustration, consists of loosely arranged connective tissue. Fragments of the internal elastic lamina can be seen. Haematoxylin and eosin × 227

It is not always clear whether a hypersensitivity reaction involves the heart by direct injury or whether it is secondary to vascular damage. Interstitial myocarditis is found which may be granulomatous, and eosinophils may dominate the inflammatory cell infiltrate. Anaphylaxis triggered by IgE, immune complexes and cell mediated immune reactions may all be implicated. The reason as to why various sizes of vessels are affected is not known.

Immunological investigations are also often not helpful in distinguishing between the various types of vascular diseases. Necrotizing angiitis occurs, for example in metamphetamine abusers[43] and in rheumatoid arthritis and can be indistinguishable from polyarteritis nodosa[44]. It is likely that damage due to immune complexes might be the common denominator for all the angiitides based on the observation that the presence of rheumatoid factors, hypergamma-globulinaemia and hypocomplementaemia are seen in a variety of arteritic lesions[45]. The part played by the physical properties of proteins or by cryoglobulins which cause hyperviscosity[46] is not fully resolved.

Granulomatous vasculitis (Churg–Strauss)[46]

Though morphological criteria alone may make this condition indistinguishable from polyarteritis nodosa, certain characteristics can make distinction possible. These include giant cell granulomata, not confined to the vessel wall but also involving the connective tissue of the body, and the presence of severe asthma, fever, hypereosinophilia and raised serum levels of IgE.

Rheumatoid arthritis

Although rheumatoid arthritis predominantly affects the synovial tissue of peripheral joints, the heart can be involved, especially the pericardium and the rings of the aortic and mitral valves. Typical rheumatoid nodules consist of a central area of necrosis which is surrounded by a layer of mononuclear cells, often showing palisading. An overlap between rheumatic fever and rheumatoid arthritis is recognized[47]. Apart from these typical nodules, vasculitis is widespread including involvement of the vasa vasorum of the aorta. Initial changes include fibrinoid necrosis, and a predominantly neutrophilic cellular infiltrate followed by a lymphocytic cellular infiltrate – a non-specific appearance.

Humoral reactions have received most attention. Immunoglobulin containing complexes in the synovial tissue from affected joints may be the key to the pathogenetic mechanism, but whether these complexes consist exclusively of autologous protein or in part of exogenous antigen including microbial agents – is not solved. Cellular immunity, including cytotoxicity may also play a role in the pathogenetic mechanism of rheumatoid arthritis[48].

Sjögren's syndrome

Kerato-conjunctivitis sicca, xerostomia and rheumatoid arthritis constitute the triad of Sjögren's syndrome. Fibrinous pericarditis is most frequently found when the cardiovascular system is affected. The association with rheumatoid arthritis suggests a similar immunological pathogenesis, but the reasons why only some patients with rheumatoid arthritis are affected is not solved. HLA B8 is commonly present in patients with this syndrome, and this may be the explanation for the association[49].

Polymyositis and dermatomyositis

Cardiovascular involvement may occur in these inflammatory disorders of skeletal muscle. Children are more frequently involved than adults[50]. A non-specific vasculitis is typical with lymphocytes and plasma cells dominating the morphological picture. Cell mediated cytotoxicity is likely to explain the morphological changes[51]. Deposits of IgG, IgM and C3 have been identified in vessels of skeletal muscles[52] and abnormal T-cells have also been demonstrated[53].

Thrombotic thrombocytopaenic purpura

This condition is characterized by vascular damage and thrombocytopaenia, and it is similar to the haemolytic–uraemic syndrome, sparing the nervous system. Small vessels in the kidney and the heart are involved. The vessels are occluded by a hyalin material which is most likely to be fibrin. Fibrinoid necrosis of the vascular walls is present, but it lacks the cellular infiltrate commonly encountered when fibrinoid necrosis is present in other diseases.

An immunological pathogenesis has been postulated but not proven. It can occur in conjunction with autoimmune disorders such as systemic lupus erythematosus. Immunoglobulins and complement have been found, but not immune complexes.

A plasma factor may be absent which normally stimulates a prostacyclin-like activity, and inhibits excessive platelet aggregation[54].

Amyloid

The time-honoured sub-division of amyloid into primary, secondary, familial and senile types is a useful classification, which has been retained by the World Health Organization/International Society and Federation of Cardiology Task Force recommendation on the definition and classification of cardiomyopathies and specific heart muscle diseases[55].

Classical primary amyloid affects the heart in approximately 90% of cases, although it is rarely confined to this site. The heart is also often affected in secondary amyloid which is associated with a number of other diseases. A classification based on organ distribution is, therefore, not reliable. Sub-division of amyloid into peri-reticular and peri-collagenous types[56], is also unsatisfactory, because when deposition is severe, this difference may be impossible to recognize, even though it is likely that peri-reticular and peri-collagenous forms originate from different cell types.

Although most forms of amyloid give similar staining reactions, they do not consist of a uniform material. A classification based on the different components in amyloid has also been proposed[57]. Its resistance to digestion, histological appearance and ability to persist in the tissue are all due to the physical chemical structure, namely that of a β-pleated sheet fibrils[58].

Macroscopically the walls of the heart are rigid and have a glassy appearance. With the naked eye greyish-yellow streaks may be discerned and soaking the tissue in iodine gives a mahogany brown discoloration. Deposition is not confined to the myocardium: the valves and epicardium as well as atria, coronary arteries and conduction tissue do not escape. In senile amyloidosis nodules in atrial endocardium can often be discerned macroscopically.

Histologically deposition occurs in the connective tissue surrounding myocardial fibres, and in the wall of the vessels. Recognition is effected by staining with Congo Red giving an apple green fluorescence on viewing under crossed polaroids. Staining with thioflavine T results in a yellow-green discoloration under ultraviolet light, and sulphated Alcian Blue stain results in bright green discoloration[4(c)].

Electron microscopy

The most reliable way to confirm amyloid is at the ultrastructural level. The fibrillary structure is diagnostic. Each fibril is 5–30 nm in width, and consists of up to eight laterally aggregated filaments showing a periodicity of 10 nm. Deposition occurs in relation to the basement membrane of muscle cells, blood vessels and connective tissue[4(c)].

As indicated above, the chemical composition of amyloid can vary. In primary amyloid and in amyloid associated with multiple myeloma, the fibres consist predominantly of immunoglobulin-light chains[59] and are closely related to the existing collagen tissue[60]. On the other hand the secondary form consists mainly of AA protein, unrelated to immunoglobulin[61]. Amyloid in familial Mediterranean fever is rich in fibrinogen but contains little γ-globulin[62]. Conversely, in patients with hypergammaglobulinaemia little fibrinogen is evident. Another protein (AP), showing no cross-reaction with immunoglobulin, is a consistent component in all forms of amyloid[63].

Plasma cells are responsible for the formation of amyloid. When this cell is under persistent antigenic stimulation the immunoglobulin function is disturbed and pyronin positivity is lost. Lysosomes increase and destroy cellular structure releasing cell fractions from which amyloid is derived[64].

Sarcoid

Sarcoidosis is a systemic granulomatous disease, the aetiology of which is not yet solved. The heart is involved in about 20% of patients, usually secondary to disease elsewhere[65]. Before a morphological diagnosis can be substantiated diseases giving rise to granulomata in the heart, such as tuberculosis, leprosy, fungal infection, cat-scratch disease and exposure to beryllium, must be excluded[4(d)].

With the naked eye fibrous areas may be discernible which can be massive. The interventricular septum is often severely involved[66] but lesions may be found anywhere in the heart; the atria are usually spared. Histologically, sarcoid resembles tuberculosis but caseation is absent. Lymphocyte reaction is less severe and giant cells tend to be larger. Furthermore, nodules tend to be separate rather than confluent. The lesion consists of a central zone in which epithelioid cells and macrophages are in close contact with lymphocytes. In the periphery, active exchange takes place, new macrophages enter and altered epithelioid cells leave that area.

An immunological pathogenesis seems likely and a depression of a delayed-type hypersensitivity suggesting impaired cell mediated immunity and raised or abnormal immunoglobulins have been noted[4(d)]. A significant reduction in the number of circulating lymphocytes has also been described[67] which may be due to coating of T-cell membranes with antilymphocyte antibody preventing recognition or leading to destruction of the cells[68]. A possible triggering mechanism by virus is not yet fully substantiated[69]. The role of immune complexes is also not yet defined. Total serum complement is frequently raised. Platelet aggregates, and complement conversion from C3 to C3b has been demonstrated[70].

Systemic lupus erythematosus

The heart is involved in about 50% of patients with systemic lupus erythematosus, which can give rise to myocarditis, endocarditis, and pericarditis[71]. Small intramyocardial arteries may be involved. Classical Libman–Sacks endocarditis is found in approximately 60% of patients[72]. The mitral valve is most frequently involved; the aortic valve rarely.

The vegetations have a dry appearance and show a greyish-pink or yellow discoloration. They are often arranged along the line of closure, rarely gaining large proportions. Characteristically, the under surface of the posterior mitral valve leaflet is involved, and the inflammatory process may extend on to the mural endocardium[73]. The core of the verrucae consists of vascularized fibrous tissue and an inner zone of neovascularization (Figure 4.4). Fibrinoid necrosis and inflammatory cells are usually present in these areas. Fibrin deposition on the surface containing nuclear debris, haematoxyphil bodies and inflammatory cells complete the typical changes of the endocarditic process[74]. Occasionally aortic insufficiency may manifest itself together with perforation of the leaflets[75].

Pericarditis is a frequent accompaniment of systemic lupus erythematosus and may be fibrinous or fibrous, rarely purulent. Myocarditis is non-specific, and may not be the sole cause of heart failure[76]. In about half of the patients small intramyocardial vessels may show narrowing of the lumina by cellular intimal thickening which is rarely associated with areas of fibrosis[77].

Deposits of IgG, IgM, IgA and C3 have been demonstrated in the wall of the vessels in the neovascular zone[74], and Clq deposits have also been found in the pericardium, myocardium and valves[78] suggesting that deposition of immune complexes plays an important role in the pathogenesis of systemic lupus erythematosus. Morphologically this is represented by fibrinoid necrosis. As a triggering mechanism for the immunological idiosyncracy, virus or drugs have been suggested[79]. Auto-antibodies against intracellular antigens, cell surface antigens and DNA in inverse relationship with suppressor activity of T-cells have been demonstrated[79,80].

Myocardial infarction in a patient with a variant form of systemic lupus erythematosis showing increased DNA binding, thrombocytopenia, positive antinuclear antibodies and immunoglobulin A deficiency has recently been documented[81]. Myocardial infarction was attributed to antiphospholipid antibodies.

Infective endocarditis

Despite modern therapeutic approaches and diagnostic tools, infective endocarditis has remained a world-wide problem[82]. Any bacterium, fungus or rickettsia may affect normal or previously damaged valves and may complicate congenital heart disease. Specific antibacterial antibodies have been demonstrated as well as high titres of rheumatoid factors[83]. Concurrent immune complexes may be released[84]. Rheumatoid factors may show autospecificity for autologous complexes[85]. Other examples of autoantibody products have been demonstrated[86], and may reflect polyclonal B-cell stimulation by bacterial antigens.

Focal glomerulonephritis has been ascribed to injury by immune complexes[87]. Skin manifestations in infective endocarditis may be related to localization of immune complexes, but microemboli and abscesses with pathogenetic organisms have been identified[88].

Morphologically it is often impossible to be certain of the type of infective organism that has given rise to vegetations. These may attain large proportions, are usually ragged and friable and have a variegated appearance. The process begins along the line of closure (the rough zone) of the valve leaflets. Histologically, vegetations consist predominantly of fibrin, and the infective organism may be identified often requiring special staining techniques. The response in the underlying valve tissue is variable. For example, in rickettsial endocarditis (Q-fever) the reaction may be sparse, or absent, whereas in bacterial endocarditis due to *Staphylococcus aureus* it may be intense. Palisading of the reacting cells in the valve leaflets may be observed.

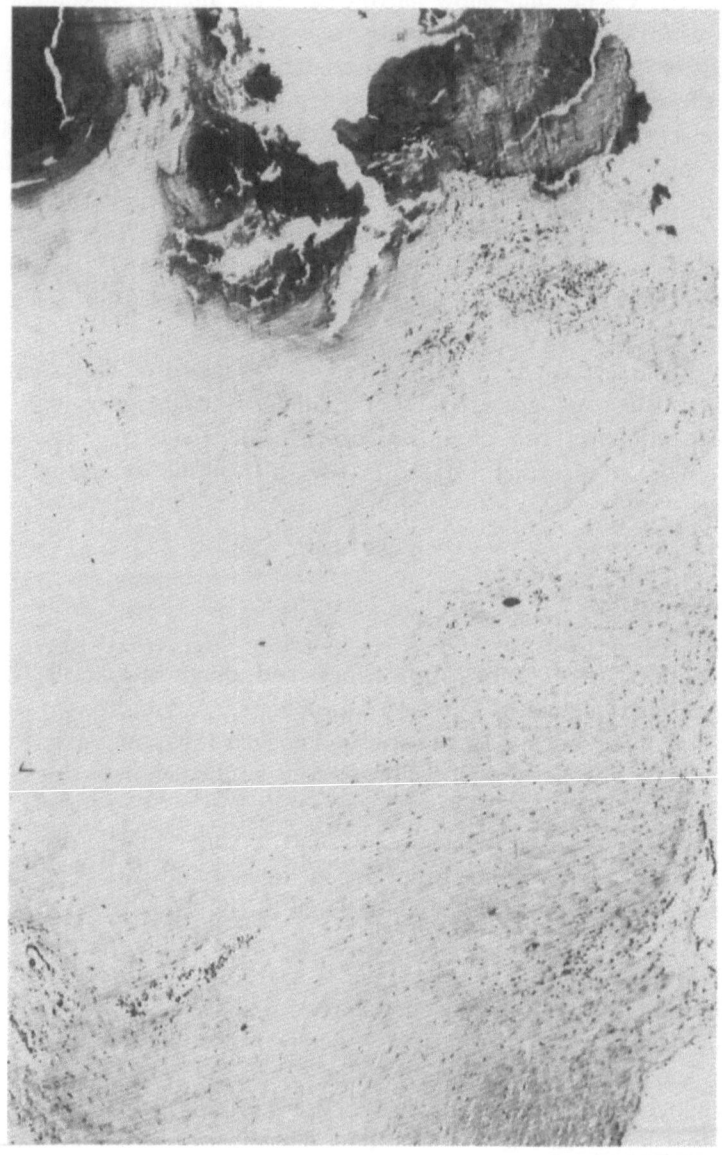

Figure 4.4 Vegetation of the mitral valve from a patient with systemic lupus erythematosus. The fibrous core shows vascularization. Superimposition of fibrin is striking. Martius Scarlet Blue × 45

DISEASES OF THE HEART AND PERICARDIUM WITH NON-SPECIFIC MORPHOLOGICAL CHANGES

Dilated cardiomyopathy

This is the most commonly encountered form of heart muscle disease of unknown cause. Little is known about the natural history of the disease, and patients usually only come under medical care when serious symptoms have appeared. About 10 in 100,000 people are affected[89,90].

There are no specific morphological features, and the diagnosis can only be made after excluding conditions that can result in a hypertrophied, dilated heart. All chambers are affected, often being dilated to a severe degree, and the cardiac muscle may be pale and flabby on macroscopic examination. Endocardial thickening may be widespread, and thrombus may be superimposed. Histologically, when patients die, usually after several years of symptoms, no clues can be identified as to the possible aetiology. Myocardial fibres are in normal alignment, show evidence of hypertrophy and attenuation and varying degrees of increase of interstitial fibrous tissue or fibrous replacement in which a few chronic inflammatory cells can sometimes be found. Small vessels are often normal, and when intimal thickening is found it is unlikely to be responsible for the global involvement of the myocardium. Endocardial thickening is also non-specific, and an increase in the smooth muscle component indicates long-standing dilatation[91].

Histochemical analysis of substances such as glycogen or succinic dehydrogenase which may be increased, normal, or decreased, depending on the duration and severity of heart failure, have contributed little towards establishing a pathogenetic mechanism.

Electron microscopy shows evidence of hypertrophy and varying degrees of degeneration of actin and myosin and alteration in mitochondria, but examination at this level has not provided useful aetiological clues[92].

With the increasing use of the bioptome which permits the recovery of fresh endomyocardial tissue[93,94], myocarditis has been found with varying frequency (2–63%)[95] in patients clinically suspected of having dilated cardiomyopathy. Based on persuasive evidence that a virus, especially Coxsackie B1–6 is implicated in the pathogenesis of this type of cardiomyopathy, treatment by immuno- suppressive agents and corticosteroids has led to sequential biopsy examination in patients thus treated. This has permitted classification of myocarditis into active, healing and healed forms[96].

Active myocarditis is characterized by an interstitial chronic inflammatory infiltrate, necrosis of myofibres adjacent to the infiltrate but usually little or no increase in interstitial connective tissue. Healing myocarditis is recognized by a diminution of the inflammatory cell infiltrate and a mild to moderately severe increase in interstitial fibrous tissue (Figure 4.5). A very occasional focus of necrosis of adjacent myocardial fibres may be found. In the healed phase an often severe increase in interstitial fibrous tissue is present, as well as areas of fibrous replacement of myocardial fibres. In these areas some chronic inflammatory cells may be present. Should this be the patient's first biopsy a myocarditic process can only be surmised.

More recently the basic classification has been extended and amended. Healing myocarditis is denoted by 'resolving (healing)' and the healed phase by 'resolved (healed)' myocarditis[97].

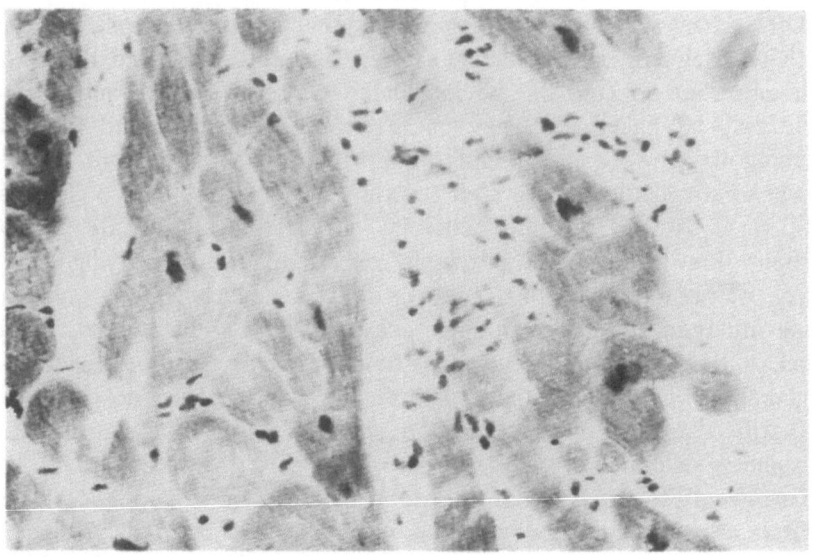

Figure 4.5 Endomyocardial biopsy showing healing myocarditis in a patient clinically suspected of having dilated cardiomyopathy. Haematoxylin and eosin × 250

During the last few years intensive investigations have been undertaken combining morphological examination with virological and immunological studies. It has been postulated that an infectious–immune mechanism is likely to be operative in a substantial number of patients with dilated cardiomyopathy. In a study of 74 patients clinically thought to suffer from dilated cardiomyopathy, neutralizing antibody titres to Coxsackie B virus has shown rising or significant levels in 10 of 22 patients with acute myocarditis, in 3 out of 16 patients with healing or healed myocarditis and in 7 of 36 patients showing non-specific changes consisting of a hypertrophied, dilated myocardium only[96]. In another study investigating neutralizing antibody to Coxsackie B virus in 50 patients with dilated cardiomyopathy, titres of 1 in 1024 were found in 15 of the 50 cardiomyopathic patients compared with only 1 patient of 50 age and sex matched controls[98].

Virus-specific cDNA hybridization probes have detected Coxsackie B virus RNA sequences in over 50% of patients, not only in those showing evidence of myocarditis, but also in patients where biopsy examination showed non-specific changes of a hypertrophied dilated myocardium (dilated cardiomyopathy)[99].

Heart reactive antibodies, evidence of cell mediated immunity, cytotoxity and defective T-suppressor cell function have all been demonstrated with varying degrees of significance. It has been postulated that there is an immunological process in up to 40% of patients with dilated cardiomyopathy, which may have been triggered by an initial viral infection[96].

Evidence in experimental animals of an autoimmune process in myocarditis has been provided by several authors. These have been detailed in a publication entitled *New Concepts in Viral Heart Disease*[100] based on a symposium held in Tergernsee, Germany in 1988. The interested reader is referred to this publication.

Other highlights of the work in animals and man include the following.

Fragments of tissue from endomyocardial biopsies were cultured in the presence of interleukin (IL-2) to ascertain the functional characteristics and the specificity of infiltrating T lymphocytes in myocarditis in man. Phenotyping was undertaken and in view of the absence of an identifiable antigen or appropriate target cell T cell receptor gene, re-arrangements were elected to detect selective T lymphocyte cells in myocarditis.

The results indicated that in patients with myocarditis a small number of T lymphocyte clones dominated. The authors concluded that it may be possible to utilise IL-2 cultured lymphocytes to identify specific antigens involved in the pathogenesis of myocarditis. The value of therapeutic approaches was emphasized[101].

Experimental work in mice has been reported by Schultheiss and colleagues, demonstrating antibodies primarily directed against ADP/ATP carriers reacting with the surface of cardiac myocytes. This has resulted in impairment of contractility and a cytotoxic effect dependent on extracellular calcium, which was prevented by calcium channel blocks[102].

Diagnosis of myocarditis by endomyocardial biopsies is now well established, though conflicting reports as to the incidence continues to be reported. Immune markers and identification of the expression of classes I and II and major histocompatible complexes have been shown to be helpful in categorization of cellular and humoral immune markers and therefore, aiding in defining acute or resolved immunological processes even in the absence of infiltrating lymphocytes. These findings suggest that functional abnormalities are not only attributable to inflammation, but also to non-cell mediated immune processes[103].

These various mechanisms which may play a role in the pathogenesis of dilated cardiomyopathy have been shown to find another form of morphological expression. A significant decrease in neuronal cells in the ganglia of right atrial strips (between the venae cavae) has been observed, but the reduction is not as severe as in chagasic heart disease[104].

Viral myocarditis

The description that has been given of myocarditis was based on findings in Coxsackie virus infections but any virus may affect the myocardium. By the time morphological examination is possible either post-mortem, or on biopsy, the changes that are evident are usually totally non-specific.

Macroscopically, haemorrhagic depressions, which are often serpiginous in shape, can be discerned. In long-standing cases, areas of fibrosis are all that can be seen. In the active phase, a mononuclear cell infiltrate of varying intensity is present which may have resulted in individual cardiocyte necrosis or affecting groups of myocardial fibres resulting in myocytolysis. As the pericardium is often involved (unlike in patients with suspected dilated cardiomyopathy even though they show inflammation in the myocardium) the term peri-myocarditis has been applied.

Peripartal heart disease

Unexplained cardiac dilatation or heart failure occurring during late pregnancy or within 3 months of childbirth[105] is, from a morphological point of view, identical to the changes described in dilated cardiomyopathy including the presence of myocarditis in some of the patients.

Though heart failure may occur in pregnancy or follow childbirth in toxaemia of pregnancy, or be related to nutritional deficiency, or as a result of local customs, this form of peripartal heart disease appears to be unassociated with any of these factors, and like dilated cardiomyopathy is of unknown aetiology.

In a recent study from Africa, 5 of 11 patients who had undergone investigation by bioptome had shown evidence of myocarditis. Lymphocytes dominated the morphological picture. In 9 of 11 patients T-lymphocyte cell subsets were measured using monoclonal antibodies to identify the total number of T-cells (OKT3), the percentage of helper T-cells (OKT4) and suppressor–inducer T-cells (OKT8). The helper–suppressor ratios (OKT4/OKT8) were found to be high in three of these patients[106].

Evidence of virus in the myocardium

Despite many attempts, there has been a lack of success in isolating a virus from patients with dilated cardiomyopathy (and in patients with peripartal heart disease). This was attributed to the delay that occurs after the appearance of the symptoms, so that by the time a biopsy had been undertaken, the virus has disappeared. It has been assumed that replication takes place during the early phase of infection[107]. Recently, a molecular probe technique has been applied. A 1.6 kb Coxsackie B virus-specific cDNA clone derived from the conserved 3' region of the virus genome was used as a hybridization probe to test for the presence of virus nucleic acid sequences in myocardial biopsies. Positive hybridization signals, quantitated by densitometry, were obtained in 9 of 17 patients, some of whom showed only the non-specific changes of dilated cardiomyopathy[108]. These findings indicate that virus may persist long after the initial infection and implies that perhaps therapy should be directed to antiviral medication.

Endocardial fibroelastosis

Two forms of this disease of unknown aetiology are recognized. One occurs in the neonatal period, the other in the adolescent age group. In the former the affected ventricles (usually the left, but the right may also be involved) are small and covered with thick, white endocardium. Histologically, the severely thickened endocardium shows an immense increase in elastic fibres which are often in regular alignment.

In the adolescent form, dilatation of the affected ventricles may be severe. The endocardial thickening may extend from the atria, involve valve cusps and the entire ventricular cavity surrounding each individual trabeculum so that they clearly stand out on macroscopic examination. Histologically, identical changes to those described under the neonatal form are present.

An intrauterine infection with mumps virus has been postulated as a cause of this disease[109], and interstitial myocarditis has been found in 41 of 64 children[110]. Virus-like particles have been identified in one case[111]. The suggestion that a delayed type of hypersensitivity reaction to mumps could be responsible in the absence of circulating antibodies (split immunological recognition) runs counter to established concepts; however, persuasive experimental evidence of its occurrence has been demonstrated[112]. Occlusive vascular disease following a viral infection has also been advanced as a possible pathogenic mechanism[111].

Post-cardiac injury syndrome

The post-pericardiotomy syndrome, and the post-myocardial infarction syndrome (Dressler's syndrome) are included under this term. It is characterized by pericarditis, pleuritis and a pericardial and pleural effusion[113].

Irrespective whether damage occurs following a surgical operation, or in association with myocardial infarction, the morphological features are similar. The pericardium can only react in a limited way to injury, and in this syndrome the morphological features are non-specific. Macroscopically, the pericardium has a shaggy appearance and may be haemorrhagic. It resembles other forms of serous or fibrinous pericarditis. The effusions may be clear, containing chronic inflammatory cells, or may be haemorrhagic.

Histological examination shows oedema of the epicardial and pericardial surfaces, and a chronic cellular infiltrate, consisting predominantly of lymphocytes and plasma cells but also other mononuclear cells. Fibrin deposition may be extensive. Vascularity is increased (Figure 4.6). Subsequently the collagen content of the pericardium increases, the inflammatory cells decrease and fibrin becomes organized and may result in fibrous adhesions. These adhesions may be numerous and obliterate the entire pericardial cavity.

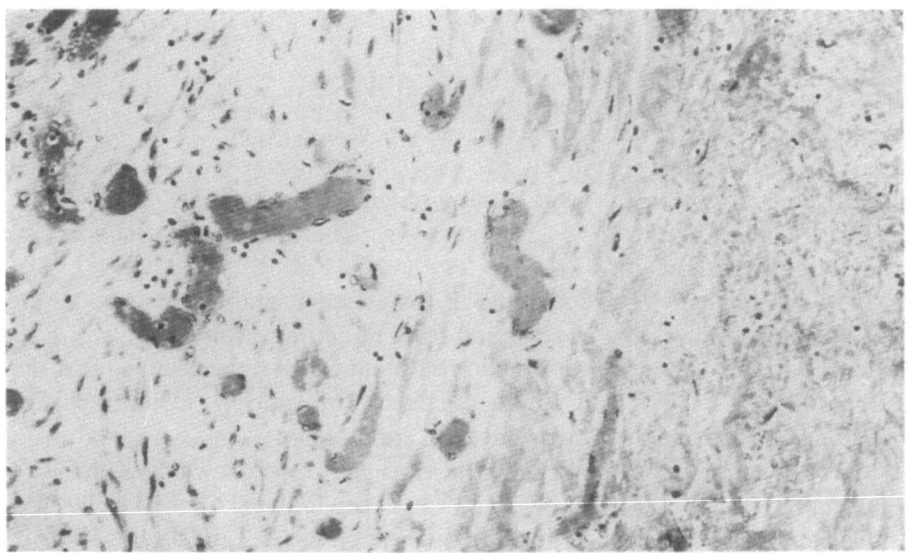

Figure 4.6 Post-pericardiotomy syndrome showing loose connective tissue, numerous dilated vascular channels, inflammatory cells and fibrin (right side of the illustration). Haematoxylin and eosin × 210

The immunological background to this syndrome is likely to be auto-immune[114]. Heart reactive antibodies have also been demonstrated indicative of a cellular type of immunity specific for heart and skeletal muscle. They have been found in serum and in the pericardial fluid[115]. It is likely that the syndrome results from an exaggerated immunological response to cardiac damage[116], but the presence of antiheart antibodies cannot account for the cardiac damage. It was suggested that they lack specificity or occur secondarily to damaged heart muscle.

Reactivation of a latent virus infection when the heart is traumatized has been implicated in the pathogenesis, but the basic mechanisms of this syndrome are still not solved.

CONCLUSIONS

In this chapter, the morphology of many different diseases of the heart and vessels has been described, in which an immunological pathogenesis has been proven or persuasively demonstrated. The various entities documented here do not by any means constitute a complete list, as, for almost every disease of the heart and vessels, such a pathogenesis has been suggested at one time or another.

In those diseases not included in this chapter, such as atherosclerosis, evidence of the role that immunological factors play in their pathogenesis is incomplete or circumstantial and they have therefore not been included in this review.

References

1. Gross, L. and Ehrlich, J. C. (1934). Studies on the myocardial Aschoff body. I. Descriptive classification of lesions. *Am. J. Pathol.*, **10**, 467–87
2. Gross, L. and Ehrlich, J. C. (1934). Studies on the myocardial Aschoff body. II. Life cycle, sites of predilection and relation to clinical course of rheumatic fever. *Am. J. Pathol.*, **10**, 489–504
3. Rusted, I. E., Scheifley, C. H. and Edwards, J. E. (1956). Studies of the mitral valve. II. Certain anatomic features of the mitral valve and associated structures in mitral valve stenosis. *Circulation*, **14**, 398–406
4. Olsen, E. G. J. (ed.). (1980). *The Pathology of the Heart*, 2nd edn. (a) p. 141, (b) p. 105, (c) pp. 65–8, (d) pp. 181–2. (London and Basingstoke: Macmillan Press)
5. Ferrans, V. J. and Roberts, W. C. (1980). Pathology of rheumatic heart disease. In Gotsman, M. and Borman, J. B. (eds.). *Rheumatic Valvular Disease in Children*. pp. 25–58. (Berlin, Heidelberg, New York: Springer)
6. Murphy, G. E. and Becker, C. G. (1966). Occurrence of caterpillar nuclei within normal immature and normal appearing and altered heart muscle cells and the evolution of Anitschkow cells from the latter. *Am. J. Pathol.*, **48**, 931–57
7. El Kholy, A., Rotta, J., Wannamaker, L. M., Strasser, T., Bytchenko, Ferreira, W., Houang, L. and Liisberg, E. (1978). Recent advances in rheumatic fever control and future prospects: a WHO Memorandum. *Bull. World Health Org.*, **56**, 887–912
8. Kaplan, M. H. (1963). Immunologic relation of streptococcal and tissue antigens. I. Properties of antigen in certain strains of group A streptococci exhibiting an immunological cross-reaction with human heart tissue. *J. Immunol.*, **90**, 595–606
9. Kaplan, M. H. and Suchy, M. L. (1964). Immunologic relation of streptococcal and tissue antigens. II. Cross-reaction of antisera to mammalian heart tissue with a cell wall constituent of certain strains of Group A streptococci. *J. Exp. Med.*, **119**, 643–50
10. Hadler, N. M. and Granovetter, D. A. (1978). Phlogistic properties of bacterial debris. *Sem. Arthritis Rheum.*, **8**, 1–16
11. Amorim, D. S. (1978). Special problems in COCM: South America. *Postgrad. Med. J.*, **54**, 462–7
12. Koberle, F. (1974). *Pathogenesis of Chagas' disease*. Ciba Foundation Symposium 20 [n.s.], 137–52
13. Amorim, D. S. (1979). Chagas' Disease. In Yu, P.N. and Goodwin, J. F. (eds.). *Progress in Cardiology*. Vol 8, pp. 235–79. (London: Henry Kimpton)
14. Cossio, P. M., Laguens, R. P., Kreutzer, E., Diez, C., Segal, A. and Arana, R. M. (1977). Chagasic cardiopathy. Immunopathologic and morphologic studies in myocardial biopsies. *Am. J. Pathol.*, **68**, 533–44
15. Fudenberg, A. H. (1978). Molecular theology, immunophilosophy and autoimmune disease. *Scand. J. Immunol.*, **7**, 351–5

16. Olsen, E. G. J. and Spry, C. J. F. (1979). The pathogenesis of Löffler's endomyocardial disease, and its relationship to endomyocardial fibrosis. In Yu, P. N. and Goodwin, J. F. (eds.). *Progress in Cardiology*, Vol 8, pp. 281–303. (London: Henry Kimpton)
17. Brockington, I. F. and Olsen, E. G. J. (1973). Löffler's endocarditis and Davies' endomyocardial fibrosis. *Am. Heart J.*, **85**, 308–22
18. Shaper, A. G., Hutt, M. S. R. and Coles, R. M. (1968). Necropsy studies of endomyocardial fibrosis and rheumatic heart disease in Uganda. *Br. Heart J.*, **30**, 391–401
19. Olsen, E. G. J. and Spry, C. J. F. (1985). The relation between eosinophilia and endomyocardial disease. *Prog. Cardiovasc. Dis.*, **27**, 241–54
20. Tai, po-Chun, Ackerman, S. J., Spry, C. J. F., Dunnette, Sandra, Olsen, E. G. J. and Gleich, G. J. (1987). Deposits of eosinophil granule proteins in cardiac tissues of patients with eosinophilic endomyocardial disease. *Lancet*, **1**, 643–7
21. Spry, C.J.F. (1988). *The Eosinophil. A Comprehensive Review, and Guide to the Scientific and Medical Literature*, pp. 502. (Oxford: Oxford University Press)
22. Shaper, A. G., Kaplan, M. H., Foster, W. D., MacIntosh, D. M. and Wilks, N. E. (1967). Immunological studies in endomyocardial fibrosis and other forms of heart disease in the tropics. *Lancet*, **1**, 598–600
23. Van der Geld, H., Peetom, F., Somers, K. and Kanyerczi, B. R. (1966). Immunohistological and serological studies in endomyocardial fibrosis. *Lancet*, **2**, 1210
24. Clinico-Pathological Conference (Royal Postgraduate Medical School) (1969). A case of aortitis with nephrotic syndrome. *Br. Med. J.*, **2**, 359–65
25. Falicov, R. E. and Cooney, D. R. (1964). Takayasu's arteritis and rheumatoid arthritis. *Arch. Int. Med.*, **114**, 594–600
26. Munoz, N. and Correa, P. (1970). Arteritis of the aorta and its major branches. *Am. Heart J.*, **80**, 319–28
27. Judge, R. D., Currier, R. D., Gracie, W. A. and Figley, M. M. (1962). Takayasu's arteritis and the aortic arch syndrome. *Am. J. Med.*, **32**, 379–92
28. Riehl, J-L. and Brown, W. J. (1965). Takayasu's arteritis: An auto immune disease. *Arch. Neurol.*, **12**, 92–7
29. Ueda, H., Saito, Y., Ito, I., Yamaguchi, H., Takeda, T. and Morooka, S. (1971). Further immunological studies of aortitis syndrome. *Jpn. Heart J.*, **12**, 1–21
30. Naito, S., Arakawa, K., Kanaya, H., Doi, H., Sasaki, Y., Skai, T., Akaiwa, H., Takeshita, A., Saito, S. and Toyoda, K. (1978). HLA and cardiovascular disease. *Jpn. Circ. J.* [Engl. edn.], **42**, 1196–9
31. McLoughlin, G. A., Helsby, C. R., Evans, C. C. and Chapman, D. M. (1976). Association of HLA-A9 and B5 with Buergers disease. *Br. Med. J.*, **2**, 1165–6
32. Fischer, C. M. (1957). Cerebral thromboangiitis obliterans (including a critical review of the literature). *Medicine*, **36**, 169–209
33. Takkunen, J., Vuopala, U. and Isomaki, H. (1970). Cardiomyopathy in ankylosing spondylitis. *Ann. Clin. Res.*, **2**, 106–12
34. Graham, D. C. and Smythe, H. A. (1958). The carditis and aortitis of ankylosing spondylitis. *Bull. Rheum. Dis.*, **9**, 171–4
35. Ehlers, N., Kissmeyer-Nielsen, F., Kjerbye, K. E. and Lamm, L. U. (1974). HL-A27 in acute and chronic uveitis. *Lancet*, **1**, 99
36. Arana, R. M., de la Vega, M. T., Porrini, A. and Morteo, O. G. (1975). Antiglobulins in ankylosing spondylitis. *J. Rheum.*, **2**, 303–7
37. Corrigall, V., Panayi, G. S., Unger, A., Poston, R. N. and Williams, B. D. (1978). Detection of immune complexes in serum of patients with ankylosing spondylitis. *Ann. Rheum. Dis.*, **37**, 159–63
38. Sturrock, R. D., Barrett, A. J., Versey, J. and Reynolds, P. (1974). Raised levels of complement inactivation products in ankylosing spondylitis. *J. Rheum.*, **1**, 428–31
39. Buisseret, P. D., Pembrey, M. E. and Lessof, M. H. (1977). a-1-Antitrypsin phenotype variations in rheumatoid arthritis and ankylosing spondylitis. *Lancet*, **2**, 1358–9
40. Gatenby, P. A., Lytton, D. G., Bulteau, V. G., O'Reilly, B. and Basten, A. (1976). Myocardial infarction in Wegener's granulomatosis. *Aust. N.Z. J. Med.*, **6**, 336–40
41. Holland, L. K. (1976). polyarteritis nodosa with peripheral gangrene and myocardial infarction. *Proc. R. Soc. Med.*, **69**, 580–1

42. Heptinstall, R. H., Porter, K. A. and Barkley, H. (1954). Giant cell (temporal) arteritis. *J. Pathol. Bacteriol.*, **67**, 507–19

43. Citron, B. P., Halpern, M., McCarron, M., Lundberg, G. D., McCormic, R., Pincus, J., Tatter, D. and Haverback, B. J. (1970). Necrotizing angiitis in drug addicts. *N. Engl. J. Med.*, **283**, 1003–11

44. Theofilopoulos, A. N., Burtonboy, G., LoSpalluto, J. J. and Ziff, M. (1974). IgG rheumatoid factor and low molecular weight IgM: An association with vasculitis. *Arthritis Rheum.*, **17**, 272–84

45. Lessof, M. H. and Olsen, E. G. J. (1981). The cardiovascular system in connective tissue disease. In Lessof, M. H. (ed.). *Immunology of Cardiovascular Disease, Basic and Clinical Cardiology.* Vol 1, pp. 189–250. (New York: Marcel Dekker)

46. Churg, J. and Strauss, L. (1951). Allergic granulomatosis, allergic angiitis, and periarteritis nodosa. *Am. J. Pathol.*, **27**, 277–301

47. Bywaters, E. G. L. (1950). The relation between heart and joint disease including 'rheumatoid heart disease' and chronic post-rheumatic arthritis (type Jaccoud). *Br. Heart J.*, **12**, 101–31

48. MacLennan, I. C. M. and Loewi, G. (1970). The cytotoxic activity of mononuclear cells from joint fluid. *Clin. Exp. Immunol.*, **6**, 713–20

49. Fye, K. H., Terasaki, P. I., Montsopoulos, H., Daniels, T. E., Michalski, J. P. and Talal, N. (1976). Association of Sjogren's syndrome with HLA–B8. *Arthritis Rheum.*, **19**, 883–6

50. Banker, B. Q. and Victor, M. (1966). Dermatomyositis (systemic angiopathy) of childhood. *Medicine (Baltimore)*, **45**, 261–89

51. Dawkins, R. L. and Mastaglia, F. L. (1973). Cell-mediated cytotoxicity to muscle in polymyositis: Effect of immunosuppression. *N. Engl. J. Med.*, **288**, 434–8

52. Whitaker, J. N. and Engel, W. K. (1972). Vascular deposits of immunoglobulin and complement in idiopathic inflammatory myopathy. *N. Engl. J. Med.*, **286**, 333–8

53. Currie, S., Saunders, M., Knowles, M. and Brown, A. E. (1971). Immunological aspects of polymyositis. *Q. J. Med.*, **157**, 63–84

54. Editorial. (1979). Plasma exchange in thrombotic thrombocytopenic purpura. *Lancet*, **1**, 1065–6

55. WHO/ISFC. Report of the Task Force on the definition and classification of cardiomyopathies. *Br. Heart J.*, **44**, 672–3

56. Missmahl, H. P. (1976). Amyloidosis. In Miescher, P. A. and Muller-Eberhard (eds.), *Textbook of Immunopathology*, 2nd edn, pp. 607–18. (New York: Grune and Stratton)

57. Stirling, G. A. (1975). Amyloidosis. In Harrison, C. V. and Weinbren, K. (eds.). *Recent Advances in Pathology*, Vol 9, pp. 249–272. (Edinburgh: Churchill Livingstone)

58. Glenner, G. G. and Page, D. L. (1976). Amyloid, amyloidosis, and amyloidogenesis. *Int. Rev. Exp. Pathol.*, **15**, 1–92

59. Glenner, G. G., Terry, W., Harada, M. and Isersky, C. (1971). Amyloid proteins: Proof of homology with immunoglobulin light chains by sequence analyses. *Science*, **172**, 1150–1

60. Aly, F. W., Braun, H. J. and Missmahl, H. P. (1968). Dys- und Paraproteinamien bei Amyloidbefall. *Klin. Wochenschr.*, **46**, 762–8

61. Husby, G. and Natvig, J. B. (1974). A serum component related to non-immunoglobulin amyloid protein AS, a possible precursor of the fibrils. *J. Clin. Invest.*, **53**, 1054–61

62. Horowitz, R. E., Stuyvesant, V. W., Wigmore, W. and Tatter, D. (1965). Fibrinogen as a component of amyloid. *Arch. Pathol.*, **79**, 238–44

63. Cathcart, E. S., Mullarky, M. and Cohen, A. S. (1970). Amyloidosis: An expression of immunological tolerance? *Lancet*, **2**, 639–40

64. Teilum, G. (1964). Pathogenesis of amyloidosis. The two-phase cellular theory of local secretion. *Arch. Pathol. Microbiol. Scand.*, **61**, 21–45

65. Longcope, W. T. and Freiman, D. G. (1952). A study of sarcoidosis based on a combined investigation of 160 cases including 30 autopsies from the Johns Hopkins Hospital and Massachussetts General Hospital. *Medicine (Baltimore)*, **31**, 1–132

66. Fleming, H. A. (1974). Sarcoid heart disease. *Br. Heart J.*, **36**, 54–68

67. Daniele, R. P. and Rowlands, D. T. (1976). Lymphocyte subpopulations in sarcoidosis: Correlation with disease activity and duration. *Ann. Intern. Med.*, **85**, 593–600

68. Daniele, R. P. and Rowlands, D. T. (1976). Antibodies to T cells in sarcoidosis. *Ann. NY Sci.*, **278**, 88–100

69. Byrne, E. B., Evans, A. S., Fouts, D. W. and Israel, H. L. (1973). A seroepidemiological study of the Epstein–Barr virus and other viral antigens in sarcoidosis. *Am. J. Epidemiol.*, **97**, 355–63

70. Turner-Warwick, M. (1978). *Immunology of the Lung.* p. 155. (London: Arnold)
71. Estes, D. and Christian, C. L. (1971). The natural history of systemic lupus erythematosus by prospective analysis. *Medicine,* **50**, 85–95
72. Györkey, F. (1969). Systemic lupus erythematosus and myxovirus. *N. Engl. J. Med.,* **280**, 333
73. Libman, E. and Sacks, B. (1924). A hitherto undescribed form of valvular and mural endocarditis. *Arch. Intern. Med.,* **33**, 701–37
74. Shapiro, R. F., Gamble, C. N., Weisner, K. B., Castles, J. J., Wolf, A. W., Hurley, E. J. and Salel, A. F. (1977) Immunopathogenesis of Libman–Sacks endocarditis. *Ann. Rheum. Dis.,* **36**, 508–16
75. Bernhard, G. C., Lange, R. L. and Hensley, G. T. (1969). Aortic disease with valvular insufficiency as the principal manifestation of systemic lupus erythematosus. *Ann. Intern. Med.,* **71**, 81–7
76. Bridgen, W., Bywaters, E. G., Lessof, M. H. and Ross, I. P. (1960). The heart in systemic lupus erythematosus. *Br. Heart J.,* **22**, 1–16
77. Bulkley, B. H. and Roberts, W. C. (1975). The heart in systemic lupus erythematosus and the changes induced in it by corticosteroid therapy: A study of 36 necropsy patients. *Am. J. Med.,* **58**, 243–64
78. Bidani, A. K., Roberts, J. L., Schwarz, M. M. and Lewis, E. H. J. (1980). Immunopathology of cardiac lesions in fatal systemic lupus erythematosus, *Am. J. Med.,* **69**, 849–58
79. Markenson, J. A. and Phillips, P. E. (1978). Type C viruses and systemic lupus erythematosus. *Arthr. Rheum.,* **21**, 266–70
80. Sakane, J., Steinberg, A. D. and Green, I. (1978). Failure of autologous mixed lymphocyte reactions between T and non-T cells in patients with systemic lupus erythematosus. *Proc. Natl. Acad. Sci. USA,* **75**, 3464–8
81. Asherson, R. A., Mackay, I. R. and Harris, E. N. (1986). Myocardial infarction in a young man with systemic lupus erythematosus, deep vein thrombosis, and antibodies to phospholipid. *Br. Heart J.,* **56**, 190–3
82. Olsen, E. G. J. (1985). Die endocarditis -- ein weltweites problem. *Deutsches Arzteblatt,* **51/52**, 3855–8
83. Williams, R. C. Jnr. and Kunkel, H. G. (1962). Rheumatoid factor complement and conglutinin aberration in patients with subacute bacterial endocarditis. *J. Clin. Invest.,* **41**, 666–74
84. Bayer, A. S., Theofilopoulos, A. N., Eisenberg, R., Dixon, F. J. and Guze, L. B. (1976). Circulating immune complexes in infective endocarditis. *New Engl. J. Med.,* **295**, 1500–5
85. Phair, J. P., Klippel, J. and MacKenzie, M. R. (1972). Antiglobulins in endocarditis. *Infect. Immun.,* **5**, 24–6
86. Bacon, P. A., Davidson, C. and Smith, B. (1974). Antibodies to candida and autoantibodies in sub-acute bacterial endocarditis. *Q. J. Med.,* **43**, 537–50
87. Keslin, M. H., Messner, R. P. and Williams, R. C. Jnr. (1973). Glomerulonephritis with subacute bacterial endocarditis. *Arch. Intern. Med.,* **132**, 578–81
88. Alpert, J. S., Krous, H. F., Dalen, J. E., O'Rourke, R. A. and Bloor, C. M. (1976). Pathogenesis of Osler's nodes. *Ann. Intern. Med.,* **85**, 471–3
89. Torp, A. (1981). Incidence of congestive cardiomyopathy. In Goodwin, J. F., Hjalmarson, A. and Olsen, E. G. J. (eds.). *Congestive Cardiomyopathy, Kiruna, Sweden 1980.* pp. 18–22. (Molndal, Sweden: AB Hassle)
90. Williams, D. G. and Olsen, E. G. J. (1985). Prevalence of overt dilated cardiomyopathy in two regions of England. *Br. Heart J.,* **54**, 153–5
91. Olsen, E. G. J. (1979). Pathology of cardiomyopathies. A critical analysis. *Am. Heart J.,* **98**, 385–92
92. Baandrup, U., Florio, R. A., Roters, F. and Olsen, E. G. J. (1981). Electron microscopic investigation of endomyocardial biopsies in hypertrophy and cardiomyopathy. A semiquantitive study in 48 patients. *Circulation,* **63**, 1289–98
93. Sakakibara, S. and Kono, S. (1962). Endomyocardial biopsy. *Jpn. Heart J.,* **3**, 537–43
94. Richardson, P. J. (1974). King's endomyocardial bioptome. *Lancet,* **1**, 660–1
95. Fowles, R. E. (1985). Treatment of myocarditis and cardiomyopathy in the USA. In Sekiguchi, M., Olsen, E. G. J. and Goodwin, J. F. (eds.). *Myocarditis and Related Disorders, Proceedings of the International Symposium on Cardiomyopathy and Myocarditis.* Tokyo, pp. 173–4 (Tokyo: Springer-Verlag)
96. Olsen, E. G. J. (1983). Myocarditis – a case of mistaken identity? *Br. Heart J.,* **50**, 303–11

97. Olsen, E. G. J. (1985). Histopathologic aspects of viral myocarditis and its diagnostic criteria. In Sekiguchi, M., Olsen, E. G. J. and Goodwin, J. F. (eds.). *Myocarditis and Related Disorders, Proceedings of the International Symposium on Cardiomyopathy and Myocarditis.* pp. 130–2. December 1984, Tokyo (Tokyo: Springer-Verlag)

98. Cambridge, G., MacArthur, C. G. C., Waterson, A. T., Goodwin, J. F. and Oakley, C. M. (1979). Antibodies to Coxsackie B viruses in congestive cardiomyopathy. *Br. Heart J.*, **41**, 692–6

99. Archard, L.C., Bowles, N.E., Olsen, E.G.J. and Richardson, P.J. (1987). Detection of persistent Coxsackie B virus RNA in dilated cardiomyopathy and myocarditis. *Eur. Heart J.*, **8** (Suppl J), 437–440

100. Schultheiss, H.-P. (ed.) (1988). *New Concepts in Viral Heart Disease. Virology, Immunology and Clinical Management*, pp. 504. (Berlin, Heidelberg: Springer)

101. Fallon, J.T., Stamenkovic, I., Frisman, D.M., Leary, C., Palacios, I. and Kurnick, J.T. (1988). Characterization of T-lymphocytes cultured from human endomyocardial biopsies. In: Schultheiss, H.-P. (ed.) *New Concepts in Viral Heart Disease*, pp. 274–281. (Berlin, Heidelberg: Springer)

102. Ulrich, G., Kuhl, U., Melzner, B., Janda, I., Schafer, B. and Schultheiss, H.-P. (1988). Antibodies against the adenosine di-/triphosphate carrier cross-react with the Ca channel – functional and biochemical data. In: Schultheiss, H.-P. (ed.) *New Concepts in Viral Heart Disease*, pp. 225–235. (Berlin, Heidelberg, Springer)

103. Kuhl, U., Toussaint, M., Ulrich, G., Wagner, D., Wolff, P. and Schultheiss, H.-P. (1988). Evaluation of immunohistological data for the diagnosis of myocarditis. In: Schultheiss, H.-P. (ed.) *New Concepts in Viral Heart Disease*, pp. 325–336. (Berlin, Heidelberg: Springer)

104. Amorim, D. S. and Olsen, E. G. J. (1982). Assessment of heart neurons in dilated (congestive) cardiomyopathy. *Br. Heart J.*, **47**, 11–18

105. WHO Expert Committee (1984). *Cardiomyopathies.* Technical Report series 697, p. 48

106. Sanderson, J. E., Olsen, E. G. J. and Gatei, D. (1986). Peripartum heart disease: an endomyocardial biopsy study. *Br. Heart J.*, **56**, 285–91

107. Abelman, W. (1978). In discussion: congestive cardiomyopathy, *Postgrad Med. J.*, **54**, 509

108. Bowles, N. E., Richardson, P. J., Olsen, E. G. J., Archard, L. C. (1986). Detection of Coxsackie-B-virus-specific RNA sequences in myocardial biopsy samples from patients with myocarditis and dilated cardiomyopathy. *Lancet*, **1**,1120–3

109. St. Geme, J. W., Davis, C. W. C. and Nuren, G. R. (1974). An overview of primary endocardial fibroelastosis and chronic viral cardiomyopathy. *Perspect. Biol. Med.*, **17**, 495–505

110. Hutchins, G. M. and Vie, S. A. (1972). The progression of interstitial myocarditis to idiopathic endocardial fibroelastosis. *Am. J. Pathol.*, **66**, 483–96

111. Factor, S. M. (1978). Endocardial fibroelastosis: Myocardial and vascular alterations associated with viral-like nuclear particles. *Am. Heart J.*, **96**, 791–801

112. St Geme, J. W., Peralta, H. and van Pelt, L. F. (1972). Intrauterine infection of the rhesus monkey with mumps virus. *J. Infect. Dis.*, **126**, 249–56

113. Engle, M. A., Gay, W. A. Jnr., Zabriskie, J. B. and Senterfit, L. B. (1981). Immunological aspects of postcardiac injury syndrome. In Lessof, M. H. (ed.). *Immunology of Cardiovascular Disease, Basic and Clinical Cardiology.* Vol. 1. pp. 267–307. (New York: Marcel Dekker)

114. Lessof, M. H. (1978). Editorial: Immunological reactions in heart diseases. *Br. Heart J.*, **40**, 211–14

115. Lawrence, M. T. S. A. and Wright, R. (1972). Tamponade in Dressler's syndrome with immunological studies. *Br. Med. J.*, **1**, 665–6

116. Lessof, M. H. (1976). Postcardiotomy syndrome: Pathogenesis and management. *Hosp. Pract.*, **11**, 81

5
Amyloid heart disease

C.M. OAKLEY

INTRODUCTION

Virchow gave amyloid its name because the material gives a colour reaction to iodine which is similar though not identical to that given by starch. Amyloidosis is a disorder of protein metabolism and amyloid is an abnormal eosinophilic fibrillar protein which is laid down inter-cellularly. The characteristic fibrillar deposits can be formed from a number of different precursor proteins which in all cases are bound to a normal non-fibrillar glycoprotein, amyloid P component. Different forms of amyloid fibrils are identified by distinctive light and electron microscopic appearances[1,2]. Amyloid can be deposited in almost any organ of the body and occurs in many characteristically distinct forms in different clinical conditions and by several different pathogenetic mechanisms.

CLASSIFICATION

(1)   Amyloidosis associatd with an immunocyte dyscrasia in which the amyloid AL fibrils are derived from monoclonal immunoglobulin light chains. This type of amyloid is seen in:

      (a)   Myeloma, less often Waldenstrom's macroglobulinaemia, malignant lymphomas (dyscrasias of cells of the B lymphocyte lineage).

      (b)   'Primary' amyloidosis in which the immunocyte dyscrasia cannot be identified. This type of amyloid may either be organ limited occurring in the heart, bone marrow, kidney, peripheral nerves or skeletal muscle (either in one or several sites) or generalized.

(2)   In the familial amyloidoses the major protein component of the amyloid varies but is not an immunoglobulin. The pre-albumin fibrils are derived from genetic variants of plasma pre-albumin in:

(a)   the predominantly neuropathic forms (e.g. Portuguese type) but also cardiopathic forms and in nephropathic (Balkan) forms

(b)   in familial Mediterranean fever in which the fibrils are the same as in reactive amyloidosis.

(3)   Reactive amyloidosis is associated with chronic suppuration (as in osteomyelitis), chronic infection (as in tuberculosis) or chronic inflammation (as in rheumatoid arthritis, ankylosing spondylitis and Reiter's syndrome). The heart is not usually involved. The AA fibrils are derived from serum amyloid A protein (SAA).

In organ-limited and endocrine-associated amyloid (such as medullary carcinoma of the thyroid) the heart is not involved.

(4)   In senile amyloid the pre-albumin ASc_1 fibrils are derived from a variant of plasma pre-albumin.

PATHOLOGY

Cardiac involvement is common both in primary amyloid and in amyloidosis associated with multiple myeloma. Patients with cardiac amyloidosis sometimes also have amyloid infiltration of skin and mucous membrane, tongue, skeletal muscle, peripheral nerves and gastrointestinal tract. Since the amyloid associated with multiple myeloma is similar to that seen in primary cardiac amyloid it has been supposed that in primary amyloidosis the monoclone producing the abnormal protein light chains may rarely be insufficient in size to be detected evey by careful marrow examination and immunocytochemical staining. In amyloidosis associated with overt myeloma the neoplastic clone is more advanced and some myeloma patients may present with serious cardiac amyloid at a time when the myeloma seems to be early[3].

The amyloid which is commonly found in the hearts of those dying in advanced old age differs both in substance and in amount from that found in AL cardiac amyloidosis[4] and is only rarely associated with any detectable clinical abnormality, although its presence along with other degenerative changes in the elderly heart may contribute to a diminished cardiac reserve in the elderly in whom heart failure may develop with seemingly little provocation. Cardiac failure and death have however been attributed to it[5,6].

Amyloid material is deposited in the walls of capillaries, small arteries and veins. Characteristically, amyloid stains apple green with congo red when viewed by polarized light and gives a metachromatic reaction to methyl violet. The staining reactions of AL amyloid fibrils may be atypical, the iodine reaction and even the histological stains may be negative. These stains may be negative therefore on cardiac biopsy specimens and light microscopic examination may fail to reveal the underlying amyloid unless electron microscopic sections are made in which the characteristic irregularly arranged fibrillary protein deposition is easily recognizable.

Years ago, intravenous injection of congo red was used as a diagnostic test for amyloid, the red pigment being removed from the plasma because of its physical affinity for the amyloid deposits. However, a positive test depended on massive amyloid deposits so that false negatives were common and, since allergic reactions as well as false negatives could occur, the test has long ago been abandoned. Recently a radionuclide imaging technique has been developed in which purified serum amyloid P component SAP is labelled with ^{123}I. Affected patients show specific uptake into the amyloid deposits and high resolution scintigrams reveal even small deposits. This diagnostic procedure will also provide information on the natural history of amyloidosis and has already revealed extremely slow degradation of the ^{123}I SAP in the deposits.

Pathology of the heart (Figure 5.1)

The heart is usually not enlarged but it is overweight and appears to show concentric hypertrophy involving both ventricles. The ventricular cavities are not dilated and may appear small. The heart is abnormally firm and rubbery and holds its shape on the post mortem table. The gross appearance of marked generalized hypertrophy with an exaggeration of the size of the papillary muscles and the trabecula architecture has often led to a mistaken preliminary diagnosis of hypertrophic cardiomyopathy and it is of interest that in a few older patients with hypertrophic cardiomyopathy clinical distinction from cardiac amyloid can also be difficult.

The amyloid heart may be surrounded by a pericardial effusion associated with focal deposits of amyloid in the pericardium. The outside of the heart may show petechiae and the cut surface may have a 'lardaceous' look. Typically the myocardium stains bluish black with iodine but a negative reaction is often seen in primary amyloidosis.

The endocardium is usually involved, there may be visible deposits and occasionally the valves are thickened. When mitral regurgitation occurs it is usually attributable to heavy infiltration of the papillary muscles. Irregularity of the endocardial surface may, rarely, predispose to thrombosis and embolism. Most of the amyloid mass is within the myocardium and is responsible for the gross thickening of the ventricular and even atrial walls. Microscopically the amyloid is found between the myocardial fibres in the interstitium separating and compressing them and extensively in the blood vessels[8]. The walls of the intramural coronary arteries may be so heavily infiltrated that the lumen is compromised. Amyloid deposits in the conducting tissue explain the frequency of sinoatrial disorders and fascicular block on electrocardiogram (ECG) as well, perhaps, as apparent increased sensitivity to digitalis[9-11].

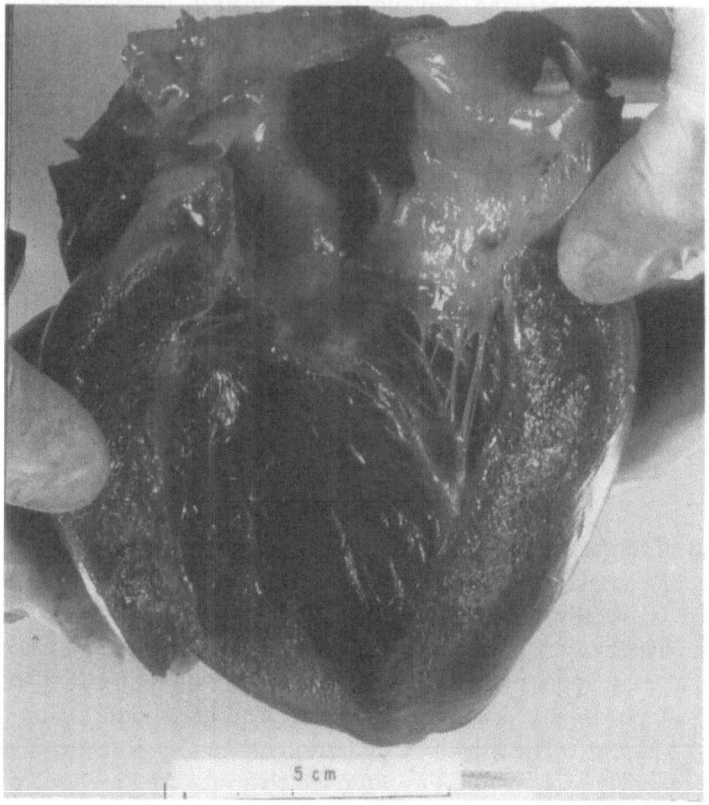

Figure 5.1 Macroscopic appearance of the amyloid heart showing thick walls, exaggerated internal architecture and glistening 'lardaceous' look

CLINICAL FEATURES

Amyloidosis is the most common infiltrative heart disease and has been extensively studied. It is infrequent below the age of 50 and most patients are in late, middle or old age. However, in a personal series of 25 cases two patients with primary amyloidosis were in their early 40s. Cardiac amyloidosis complicating familial Mediterranean fever may result in cardiac failure at a much younger age.

Patients with primary amyloidosis may show a petechial rash because of amyloid infiltration of the skin; this may be almost confluent in the periorbital tissues and it is most common on the face and neck. Macroglossia is rather uncommon in cardiac amyloidosis but when seen it can be very striking, causing dysarthria, and the tongue typically shows 'moulding' from pressure against the teeth. It feels abnormally firm and rubbery to the touch.

The patient usually looks chronically sick. He may have lost weight and may have thin wasted skeletal muscles. Rarely the skeletal muscles show a pseudohypertrophy on account of diffuse amyloid infiltration. Perineural involvement may lead to presentation with a carpal tunnel syndrome or a mononeuritis. The lymph nodes may be enlarged. Infiltration of the gastrointestinal tract may cause bleeding, diarrhoea or constipation. The liver may be very large on account of a high venous pressure even in the absence of amyloid infiltration. The spleen is not usually enlarged.

Examination of the heart usually reveals signs of a low output state, cool extremities, peripheral cyanosis and low blood pressure. There may be a bradycardia due to a conduction fault or atrial fibrillation. Digitalis has often been prescribed and toxicity is common.

The patient with cardiac amyloidosis usually presents with heart failure[12–14], but in the 10% or so who also have a nephrotic syndrome from renal amyloid cardiac involvement may be obscured by diuretics given for the hypoprotein-aemic oedema and resulting hypovolaemia. The cardiac output in amyloid is usually very low by the time of presentation, so non-specific complaints are common as well as fatigue and shortness of breath, oedema, syncope or angina. Syncope may result from orthostatic hypotension or from conduction defects sometimes induced by digitalis intoxication. Angina results from deposition in the walls of coronary arteries.

The systemic venous pressure is usually high with a small amplitude of pulsation, but tricuspid regurgitation sometimes occurs. The cardiac impulse is quiet and usually impalpable. Typically there are neither murmurs nor added sounds, but occasionally either mitral or tricuspid regurgitant murmurs are heard and a right ventricular third sound may be heard when the venous pressure is high but then disappears with diuretics. A left ventricular third sound is usually conspicuously absent despite evidence of left ventricular failure seen on the chest X-ray.

INVESTIGATIONS

Electrocardiogram

The electrocardiogram typically shows very low voltage and this low voltage may first suggest the diagnosis[15]. Repolarization abnormalities are not invariable. Fascicular blocks are frequent and by increasing the voltage may tend to obscure the diagnosis. Occasionally the abnormality in the ECG is inconspicuous.

Radiography

The chest radiograph usually shows little or no cardiac enlargement but marked changes of pulmonary venous congestion. The superior vena cava and azygous vein shadows may be prominent, reflecting a high systemic venous pressure. A pericardial effusion when present may be sufficiently large to mimic gross cardiomegaly. Echocardiography quickly reveals the true situation.

Echocardiography

The echocardiographic features of amyloidosis are characteristic and usually diagnostic[16,17]. The M-mode echo reveals reduced dimensions of the left ventricular cavity with increased thickness of the right ventricle, the ventricular septum and the left ventricular posterior wall. A pericardial effusion may be seen. Diminished systolic thickening of the left ventricular wall can be recognized. The valves usually appear normal or thickened and the valve movement may reveal the shortened ejection time and low stroke volume with a tendency for the aortic valve to drift towards closure during systole.

Cross-sectional echocardiography shows abnormal texture of the myocardium from which the amyloid reflects the echoes giving rise to a so-called granular sparkle. Unfortunately, this is not totally specific, being seen also in hypertrophic cardiomyopathy and in other storage diseases such as haemochromatosis. In hypertrophic cardiomyopathy the sparkle comes from fibrous tissue and is typically most marked in the upper ventricular septum. In primary haemochromatosis the ventricular walls are not thickened and there is left ventricular dilatation. The generalized thickening of the ventricular walls and small ventricular cavities in amyloid are well appreciated on cross-sectional Doppler echo studies (Figures 5.2 and 5.3) which also show thickening of the atrial septum and valves not seen in hypertrophic cardiomyopathy.

Haemodynamics

The echocardiographic findings, if typical, are diagnostic and in the presence of other evidence of amyloidosis no further investigations are required but amyloid is found in other organs in less than 60% of patients with amyloid heart disease. Endomyocardial biopsy is then needed. Cardiac catheterization is usually unnecessary but if carried out it confirms the low stroke volume and minute output. There may be moderate or, rarely, severe pulmonary hypertension. The diastolic pressures are high in both ventricles but unlike constrictive pericarditis the pressure is very much higher in the left ventricle than in the right ventricle. Although the diastolic contours may suggest a dip and plateau form, the form of the diastolic pressure also differs from that in constrictive pericarditis because

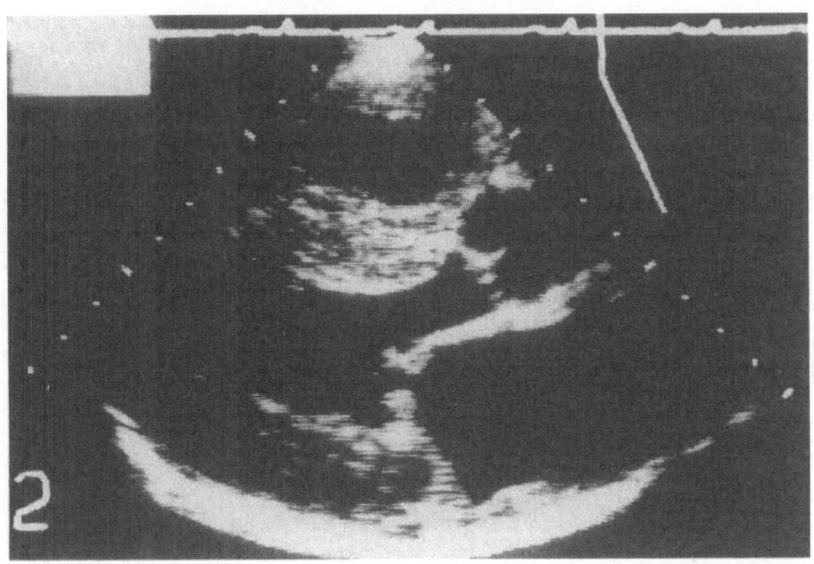

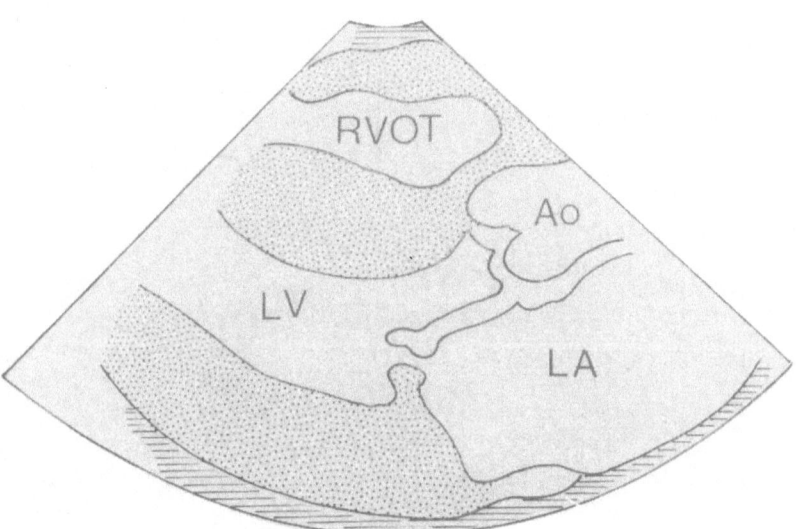

Figure 5.2 Cross-sectional echocardiographic frames showing thickened ventricular walls and small cavities, (a) long axis view, (b) apical four-chamber view. In the line drawings RVOT = right ventricular outflow tract; LV = left ventricle; AO = aorta; LA = left atrium; RV = right ventricle; RA = right atrium. (I am grateful to Dr Petros Nihoyannopoulos for this figure.)

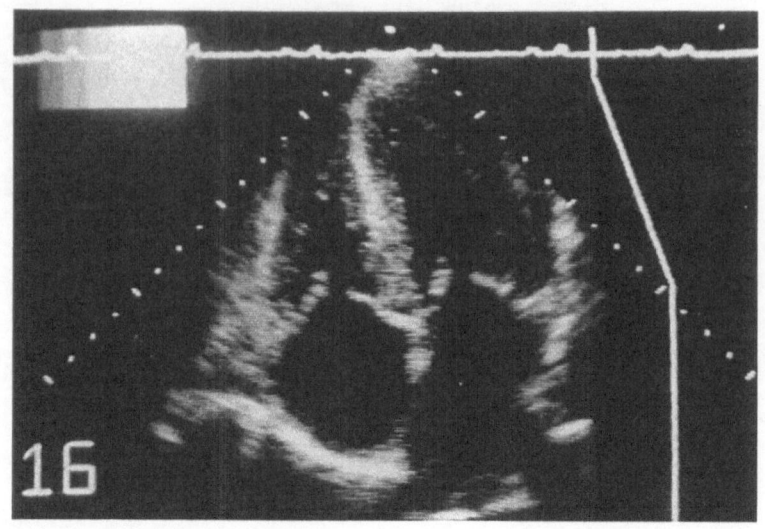

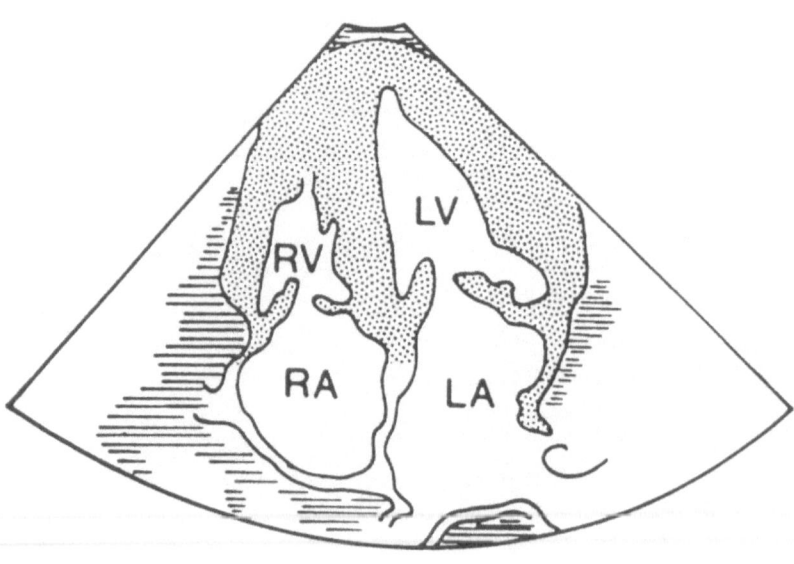

Figure 5.2 (b)

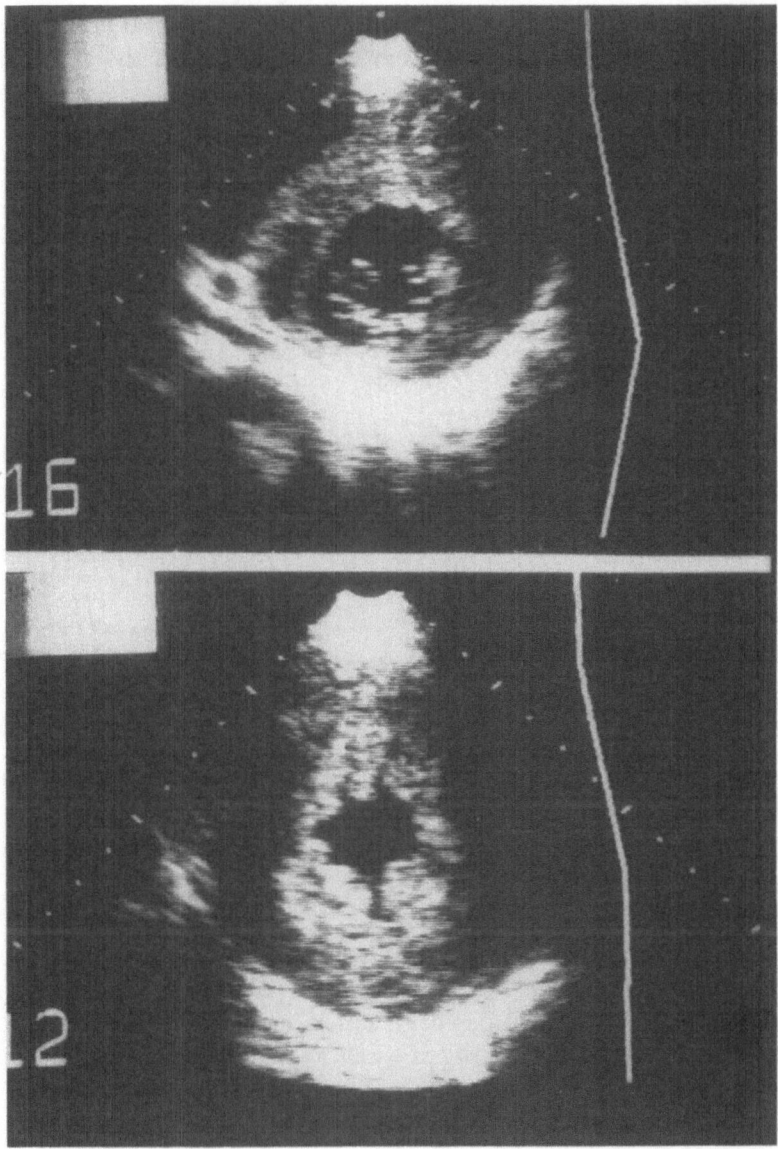

Figure 5.3 Short axis view of left ventricle, in diastole (*above*) and systole (*below*), showing the reduced size and movement of the greatly thickened LV and its markedly increased trabeculation. The increased echo reflectivity of the myocardium 'granular sparkle' is seen in each part of the figure. (I am grateful to Dr Petros Nihoyannopoulos for this figure.)

the beginning pressures are high and after an early rapid rise there tends to be a continued slow rise rather than a plateau, and there may also be a prominent a-wave (Figure 5.4). This difference may be missed unless the recording has been made on a fast paper speed.

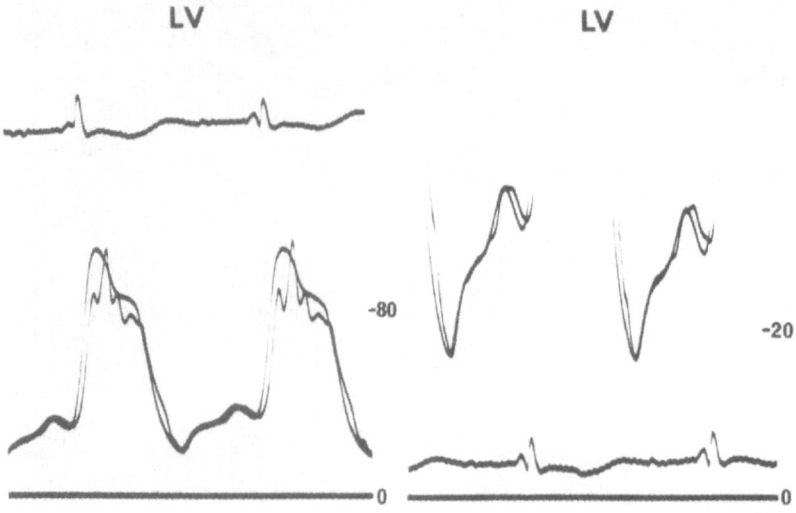

Figure 5.4 Left ventricle pressure contour (simultaneously recorded through fluid filled and manometer tipped catheter). On the left the low systolic pressure is seen and on the right at higher sensitivity the raised diastolic pressure, beginning at 15 mmHg and climbing through diastole to culminate in a prominent a-wave peaking at 40 mmHg with end-diastolic pressure 32 mmHg

Angiocardiography

The ventriculograms may look remarkably normal but on close inspection the left ventricle may display a rather shaggy internal outline due to coarsened trabeculation and exaggerated papillary muscle indentations (Figure 5.5). The 'grey zone' is widened. The cavity is small and the ejection fraction may be normal or low but the end-diastolic volume is usually below normal. This accounts for the very low stroke volume and spurious impression of systolic competence. Both peak positive and peak negative dp/dt max. are abnormally slow reflecting the splinting of the myocardium by the masses within it. Mitral regurgitation is occasionally seen and not being associated with ventribular dilatation adds greatly to the height of the left atrial pressure. There may be a pericardial effusion (Figure 5.5).

The advent of Doppler echocardiography has greatly added to our understanding of abnormalities in diastolic function and the differentiation of myocardial restriction and pericardial constriction. Furthermore, evolutionary changes in filling abnormality as amyloid infiltration progresses have been

(a)

(b)   (c)

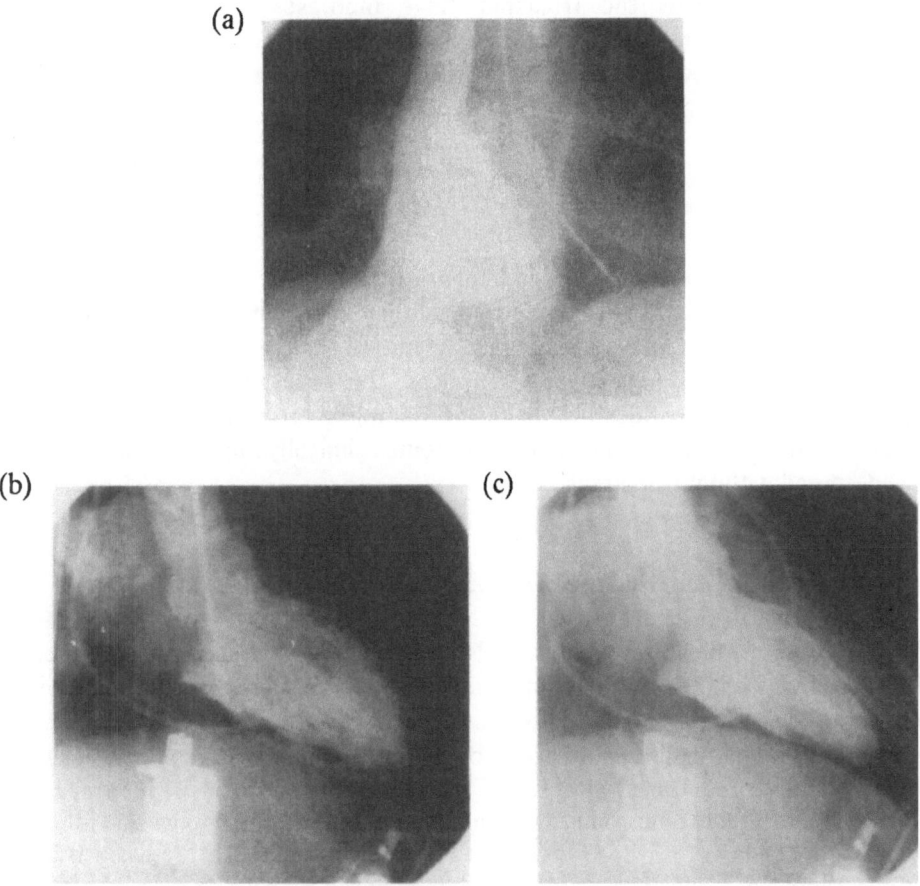

Figure 5.5 (a) Right atrial angiogram showing pericardial effusion, and **(b,c)** left ventricular angiograms showing normal size and contour apart from shaggy outline and reduced emptying

identified. The earliest change is a prolongation of active myocardial relaxation and this progresses to a restrictive phase due to abnormality in the viscoelastic properties of the myocardium and an increase in passive stiffness.

Hatle has recently analysed the differences between constriction and restriction. In constriction ventricular inter-dependence results in reciprocal changes in left and right ventricular filling with respiration which can be shown both on Doppler echocardiography and at catheterization. In constriction right ventricular systolic and diastolic pressures rise on inspiration but left-sided pressures fall because of the fixed cardiac volume whereas in restriction the pressure changes are concordant throughout the respiratory cycle. Similarly, with Doppler, patients with restrictive cardiac disease show minor and congruent changes in Doppler inflow velocities with respiration, whereas in constriction inflow velocity across the tricuspid valve increases on inspiration and simultaneously decreases across the mitral valve. Unfortunately, not all patients with constriction show a paradoxical arterial pulse or these phasic changes with respiration, so when absent constriction is not excluded[18].

Cardiac biopsy

The diagnosis can be made by endomyocardial biopsy. Biopsies of rectum, gingiva or other tissues may also be positive in patients with cardiac amyloidosis, but not invariably so. Percutaneous per femoral venous biopsy of the right ventricle can be carried out very simply at the time of diagnostic cardiac catheterization and provides the diagnosis. Sampling errors are not a problem, because by the time cardiac amyloidosis becomes clinically important the disease is widespread without skip areas.

CARDIAC AMYLOID IN FAMILIAL MEDITERRANEAN FEVER

Familial Mediterranean fever, known also as recurrent polyserositis, is a genetic disorder in which bouts of abdominal pain and fever occur together usually with pleurisy and arthritis[19]. The disease is particularly seen in Arabs, Jews, Armenians and Turks and is inherited by an autosomal recessive gene. Skeletal myalgia may occur and attacks of pericarditis together with transient electrocardiographic abnormalities. The most important complication of the disorder is amyloidosis whose incidence has been estimated at between 0 and 27% in reported series. The amyloid protein is of the reactive (AA) type seen in chronic inflammation. Renal amyloidosis is well known in this condition and may become complicated by renal vein thrombosis, renal failure and a need for haemodialysis and transplantation. Perivascular amyloid deposits are widespread in all the organs including the heart, but clinically important cardiac amyloidosis is uncommon. I have seen only one case, which occurred in a young boy in his early 20s. He was the only patient with cardiac amyloidosis that I have seen who also had systemic hypertension, and it was at first uncertain to what he owed his heart failure. He also had severe pulmonary hypertension. Cardiac investigations were typical of amyloidosis with all walls of the heart greatly thickened, with typical dense sparkling echoes seen on cross-sectional echocardiography, and with a positive cardiac biopsy.

The prognosis of familial Mediterranean fever has been greatly improved by the use of colchicine which prevents amyloidosis in this condition, although it is not yet known whether treatment with colchicine will lead to removal of already established deposits.

TREATMENT

There is still no effective treatment for primary AL cardiac amyloidosis. The disorder is relentlessly progressive[20] and most patients who present with symptomatic cardiac amyloidosis are dead within two years – and most of these within one year of the diagnosis being made. Digitalis should not be used because it does not help the functional disorder and because of the enhanced risk of inducing excessive bradycardia and conduction defects. Diuretics should be used sparingly because reduction of the high venous pressure tends to reduce forward input. Sufficient should be given only to relieve uncomfortable oedema. Arterial unloading is met by hypotension and even syncope because of inability to increase stroke volume. Venodilators working much as diuretics may be followed by some fall in systemic and pulmonary venous pressure although at the usual expense of some loss in output. Conduction system involvement may need a pacemaker.

References

1. Glenner, G.G. (1980). Amyloid deposits and amyloidosis. *N. Engl. J. Med.*, **302**, 1283–1333
2. Kyule, R.A. and Baynd, E.D. (1975). Amyloidosis: review of 236 cases. *Medicine*, **54**, 271
3. Isobe, T. and Osserman, E.F. (1974). Patterns of amyloidosis and their association with plasma cell dyscrasia monoclonal immunoglobulins and Bence-Jones proteins. *N. Engl. J. Med.*, **290**, 473
4. Pepys, M.B. (1988). Amyloidosis: some recent developments. *Q. J. Med.*, **67**, 283
5. Hodkinson, M. and Pomerance, A. (1977). The clinical significance of senile cardiac amyloidosis: A prospective clinico pathological study. *Q. J. Med.*, **46**, 677
6. Pitkanen, P., Westermark, P. and Cornwell, G.G. (1984). Senile systemic amyloidosis. *Am. J. Pathol.*, **117**, 391
7. Hawkins, P.N., Myers, M.J., Lavender, J.P. and Pepys, M.B. (1988). Diagnostic radionuclide imaging of amyloid: biological targeting by circulating human serum amyloid P component. *Lancet*, **1**, 1413
8. Buja, L.M., Khoi, N.B. and Roberts, W.C. (1970). Clinically significant cardiac amyloidosis. *Am. J. Cardiol.*, **26**, 394
9. James, T.N. (1965). Pathology of the cardiac conduction system in amyloidosis. *Ann. Intern. Med.*, **65**, 28
10. Ridolfi, R.L., Bulkley, S.H. and Hutchins, G.M. (1977). The conduction system in cardiac amyloidosis, clinical and pathological features of 23 patients. *Am. J. Med.*, **62**, 677
11. Cassidy, J.T. (1961). Cardiac amyloidosis: two cases with digitalis sensitivity. *Ann. Intern. Med.*, **55**, 989
12. Goodwin, J.F. (1964). Cardiac function in primary myocardial disease. *Br. Med. J.*, **1**, 1526
13. Chew, C., Ziady, G.M., Raphael, M.J. and Oakley, C.M. (1975). The functional defect in amyloid heart disease. *Am. J. Cardiol.*, **36**, 438–44
14. Oakley, C.M. (1983). Amyloid heart disease. In Symons, C., Evans, T. and Mitchell, A.G. (eds.). *Specific Heart Muscle Disease*, (Wright PSG) 13–23
15. Wessler, S. and Freedberg, A.S. (1948). Cardiac amyloidosis. Electrocardiographic and pathologic observations. *Arch. Intern. Med.*, **32**, 63
16. Child, J.S., Levisman, J.A., Abbas, A.S. and Macalpin, R.N. (1976). Echocardiographic manifestations of infiltrative cardiomyopathy. A report of seven cases due to amyloid. *Chest*, **70**, 726–31
17. Borer, J.S., Henry, W.L. and Epstein, S.E. (1977). Echocardiographic observations in patients with systemic infiltrative disease involving the heart. *Am. J. Cardiol.*, **39**, 184–8

18. Hatle, L.K., Appleton, C.P. and Popp, R.L. (1989). Differentiation of constrictive pericarditis and restrictive cardiomyopathy by Doppler echocardiography. *Circulation*, **79**, 357
19. Ehrenfeld, E.N., Eliakim, M. and Rachmilewitz, M. (1961). Recurrent polyserositis. *Am. J. Med.*, **31**, 107
20. Brandt, K., Cathcart, E.S. and Cohen, A.S. (1969). A clinical analysis of the course and diagnosis of 42 patients with amyloidosis. *Am. J. Med.*, **44**, 955

6
Fetal echocardiography

L.D. ALLAN

Recent developments in ultrasonic imaging techniques allow the visualization of fetal anatomy in extraordinarily fine detail. Cross-sectional imaging can display the connections of the fetal heart from as early as 14–16 weeks' gestation. M-mode echocardiography and Doppler interrogation can give additional information about the measurement and function of the fetal heart. Thus structural and functional anomalies of the heart can be explored in prenatal life.

Examination of the heart in intrauterine life is of interest for several reasons. Firstly, the normal anatomy and growth of the heart can be studied[1-6]. Study of the normal physiological function of the heart in utero has hitherto been confined to animal experiments but can now be directly evaluated in the human fetus by Doppler ultrasound. This can provide blood flow measurements of reasonable accuracy.[7] Secondly, when disordered cardiac anatomy is demonstrated in early pregnancy the parents have the option of termination where a major defect is present. Alternatively, preparation for the abnormality and delivery in a centre equipped for immediate paediatric cardiological care will optimize the infant's chance of survival. Delay in diagnosis and inter-hospital transfer of a sick neonate are significant factors contributing to the morbidity and mortality of congenital heart disease in infancy. If prenatal diagnosis can eliminate these factors, this should be reflected in improved infant survival. However, it should be noted that the nature of the technique and the pattern of referral will produce a predominance of major structural heart disease particularly associated with extracardiac anomalies, for whom the prognosis is unavoidably extremely poor. Doppler evaluation will increase the precision of the diagnosis of structural abnormalities. Lastly, once the normal cardiovascular physiology is thoroughly understood, the extension of flow investigation into disordered obstetric states promises interesting results[8,9]. Such measurements should give greater insight into some of the mechanisms controlling the fetal circulation.

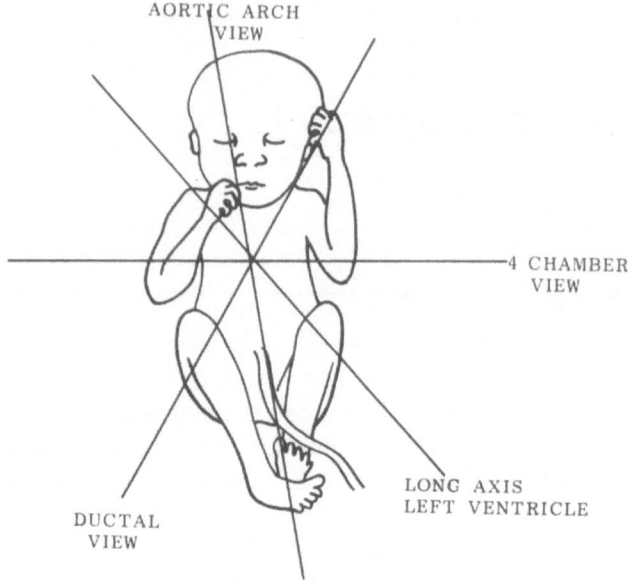

Figure 6.1 The transducer orientation, relative to the whole fetus, necessary to produce the described cardiac sections

TECHNIQUE OF CROSS-SECTIONAL SCANNING

Once experience in fetal heart scanning has been gained, no matter how the heart is approached at the start of the examination, structures can be readily recognized. However, when beginning fetal heart scanning, the fetal position should first of all be ascertained, so that the orientation of the heart within the fetal thorax can be understood. A four-chamber view of the fetal heart can then be seen by visualizing a transverse cross-section of the fetal thorax. Angling the transducer from this section can allow complete identification of all the venous, intracardiac and arterial connections ideally in a continuous sweep. Figure 6.1 illustrates the directions of the transducer beam, relative to the whole fetus, which are necessary to visualize the cardiac connections. Figure 6.2a and b shows the transducer orientation relative to the intracardiac structures to achieve each required section.

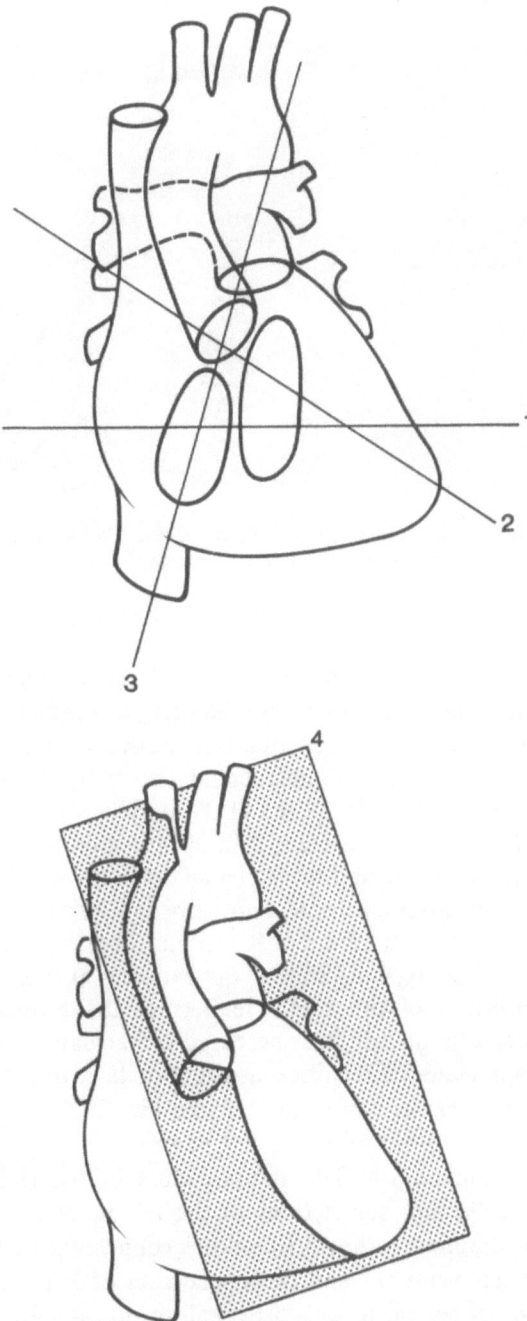

Figure 6.2a The transducer beam orientation as it cuts the heart in each of three in the sections: the four chamber (1); long axis left ventricle (2); right heart connections (3). The beam slices straight into the heart in these sections, unlike the angled direction necessary to visualize the aortic arch which is illustrated in Figure 6.2b

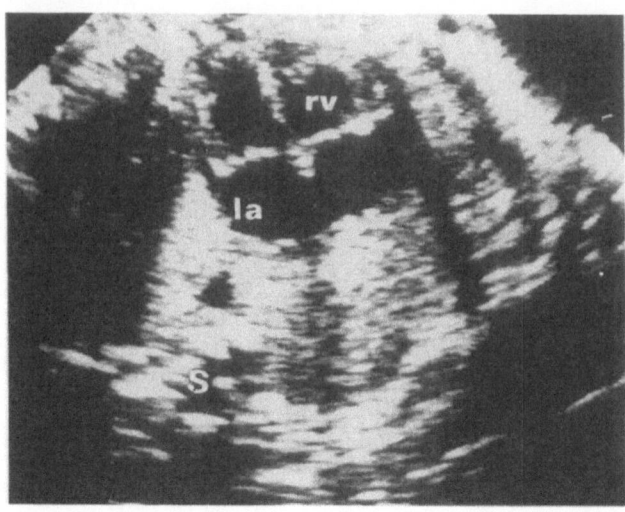

Figure 6.3 A transverse section of the fetal thorax allows the four chambers of the heart to be visualized. The spine is posterior, the sternum anterior. la = left atrium; rv = right ventricle; s = spine

Figure 6.3 shows a four-chamber view of the normal fetal heart. Many important features should be noted in examining this projection. The descending aorta is seen as a circle in cross-section lying between spine and left atrium. The two ventricles are of approximately equal size with the right ventricle lying beneath the sternum. The thicknesses of the posterior left ventricular wall, right ventricular wall and interventricular septum are approximately the same. The two atria are of similar size and there is a defect in the atrial septum which is the foramen ovale. The foramen ovale flap valve is a prominent moving structure which lies within the body of the left atrium. The two atrioventricular valves open normally. The typical 'offset' appearance at the crux of the heart representing insertion of the septal leaflets of the atrioventricular valves at different levels can be noted. The increased trabeculation of the right ventricle can often be appreciated. The differences in papillary muscle attachment of the two atrioventricular valves can sometimes be identifed. Angling the transducer from this projection to visualize the left ventricle in long axis will display the features seen in Figure 6.4. The infundibulum of the right ventricle is seen anteriorly. The following connections of the left heart can be seen: one right pulmonary vein draining to left atrium; the connection of left atrium through mitral valve to left ventricle and the connection of left ventricle to ascending aorta. Continuity of the posterior aortic wall to mitral valve and anterior aortic wall to septum can also be seen. Figure 6.5 illustrates the connections of the right heart. The inferior vena cava drains to right atrium, which in turn connects to right ventricle via a patent tricuspid valve. The muscular infundibulum can be seen 'wrapping around' the central aorta and supporting the pulmonary valve.

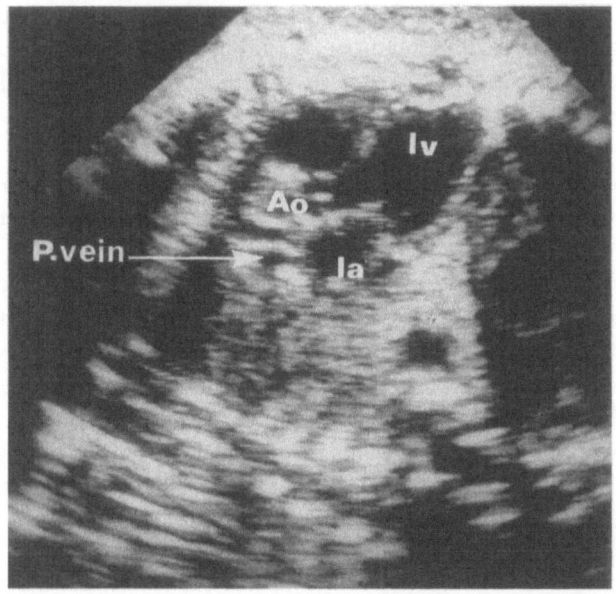

Figure 6.4 The left ventricle seen in long axis. The aorta arises from the left ventricle

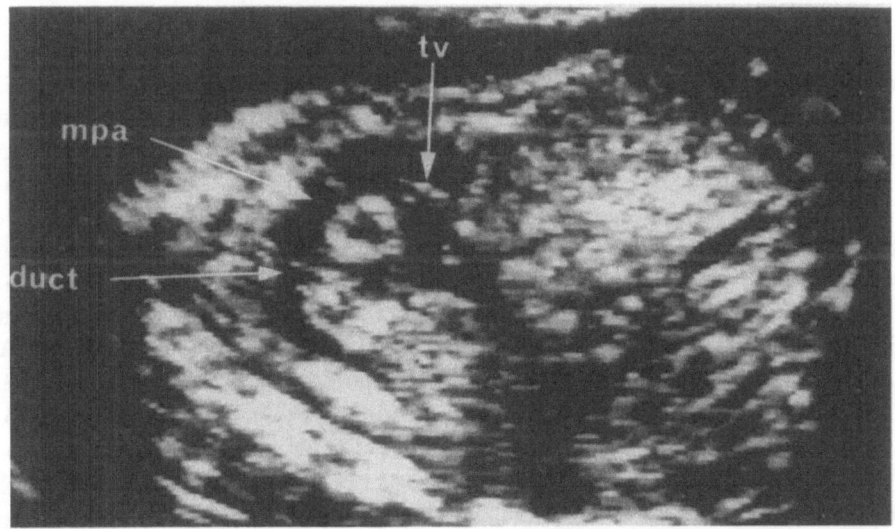

Figure 6.5 The inferior vena cava (IVC) can be seen to drain to right atrium. The right ventricular outflow 'wraps' around the central aorta. The main pulmonary artery (mpa) connects to the descending aorta via the ductus arteriosus at the site of entry of the subclavian artery

The main pulmonary artery can be seen in this projection to connect through the ductus arteriosus to the descending aorta. The arch of the aorta can be seen in the long axis of the fetus, giving rise to head and neck vessels. The right pulmonary artery is visible in cross-section in the centre of the hook-shaped aortic arch in Figure 6.6.

Examination of each of these sections to identify venous' intracardiac and arterial connections will exclude the vast majority of major congenital heart disease.

By 12 weeks of gestation it is possible to recognize four cardiac chambers and two great arteries. Figure 6.7 is a short axis view of the great arteries in a 10 week fetus. By 20 weeks all the connections described above can be recognized. In the last few weeks of pregnancy, penetration of the ultrasound beam is reduced by rib shadowing and the increased distance between the transducer and the fetal heart, making complete evaluation of cardiac connections more difficult although still possible. Oligohydramnios or maternal obesity will also limit image quality, rendering the study more difficult.

THE M-MODE ECHOCARDIOGRAM

M-mode echocardiography can provide accurate measurements of intracardiac structures. This method is preferred to the measuring of a frozen frame cross-sectional image as endocardial surfaces can be more precisely identified, and measurements can be timed within the cardiac cycle. Once the anatomy of the heart has been identified, the M-line can be directed in a standard and repeatable way. The aortic root and left atrium are identified in the projection seen in Figure 6.8a and the M-line directed across them: the tracing seen in Figure 6.8b will result. The aortic root is about two thirds of the size of the left atrium throughout pregnancy. Figures 6.9 and 6.10 chart the growth of these structures throughout pregnancy. The section shown in Figure 6.11 is sought in order to record left and right ventricular internal dimensions in systole and diastole, together with septal and posterior left ventricular wall thickness. A suitable tracing from which to make these measurements is seen in Figure 6.12. The growth of these measurements during pregnancy is seen in Figures 6.13, 6.14, 6.15 and 6.16. The growth charts are of particular value in the evaluation of structural cardiac anomalies. For example, if the ventricular chambers are of disparate sizes, it is not always obvious whether one is larger than appropriate for the gestational age or the other is too small. Reference to the growth charts will help clarify this. Doppler interrogation of all four cardiac valve orifices can be achieved in intrauterine life and blood flow characteristics observed. The traces achieved with spectral analysis are displayed in Figure 6.17. From these traces blood flow estimations can be made but results are still preliminary. It appears, however, that right heart flow is greater than left, becoming more equal to it towards term[10].

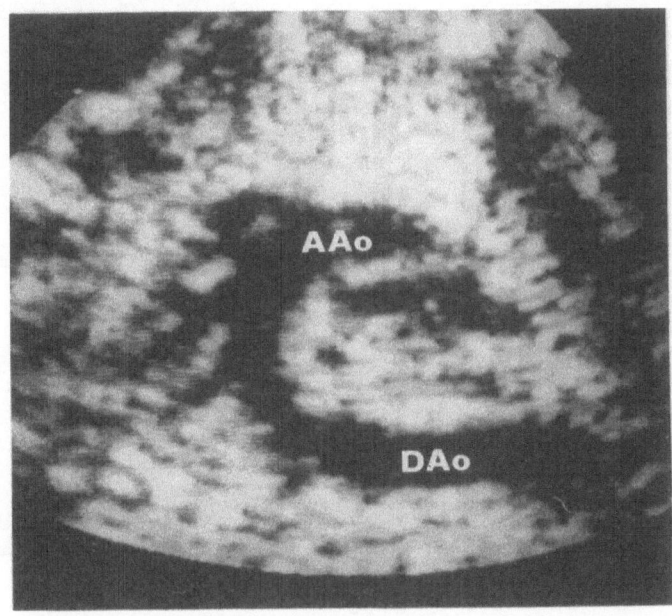

Figure 6.6 The arch of the aorta with the head and neck vessels arising from it. The right pulmonary artery lies within the 'hook' of the arch

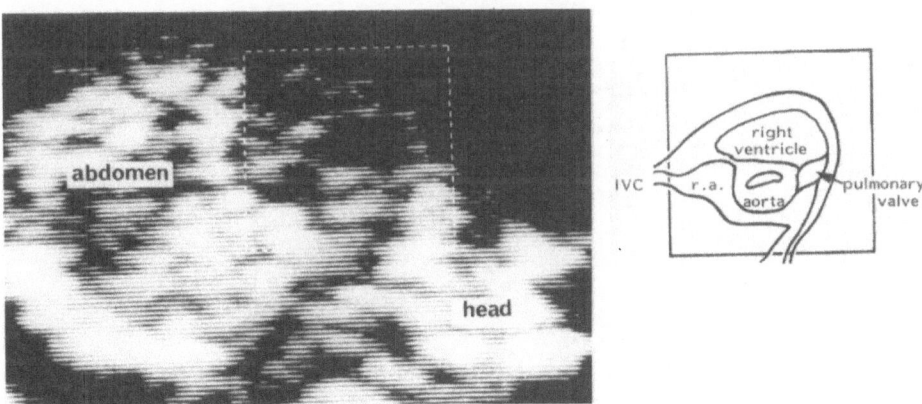

Figure 6.7 Two normally related great arteries in a section of a 10 week fetus

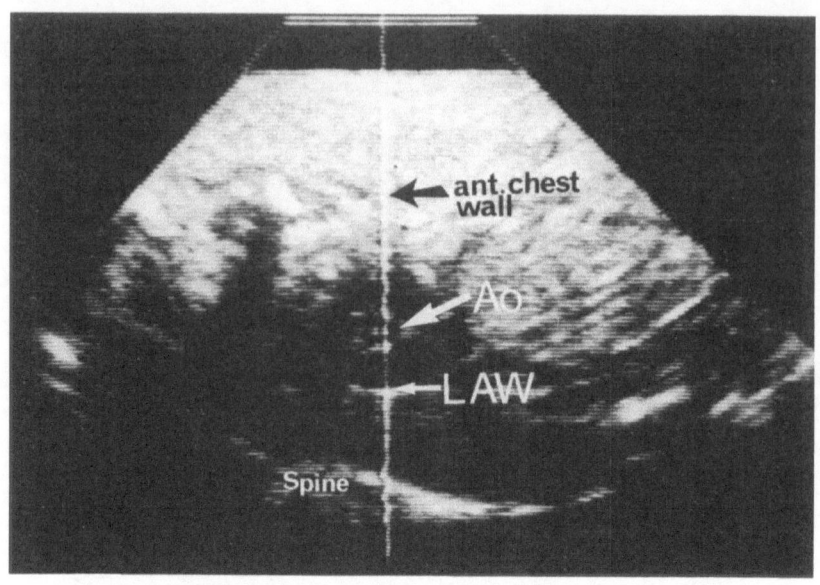

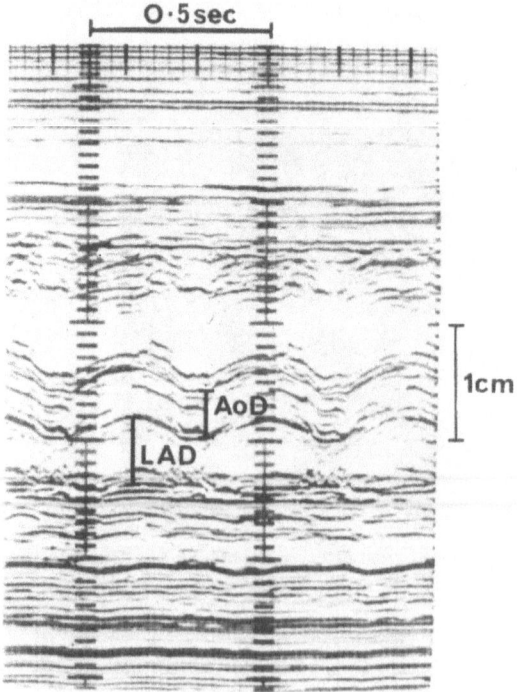

Figure 6.8 The M-line passing through the anterior chest wall to the aorta (Ao) and left atrium behind. The tracing achieved in this position is seen below

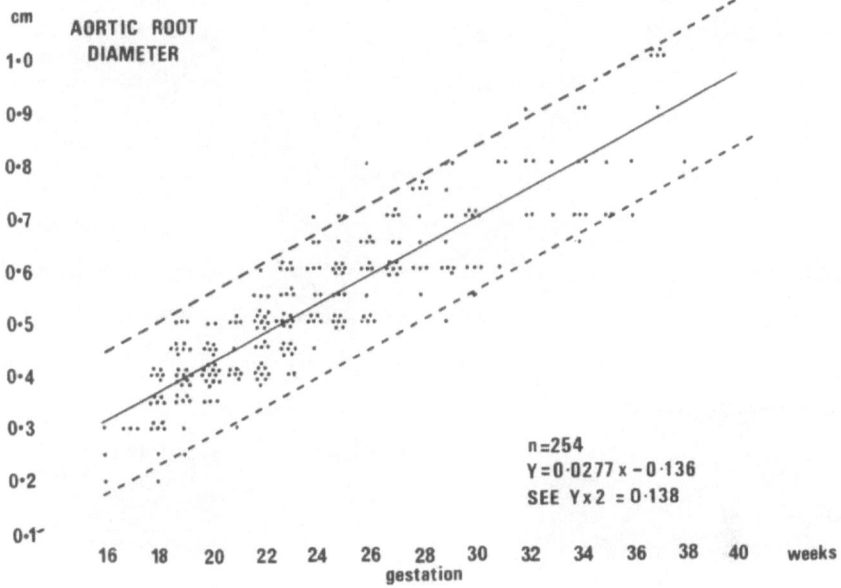

Figure 6.9 Aortic root growth with gestational age from 16 weeks to term

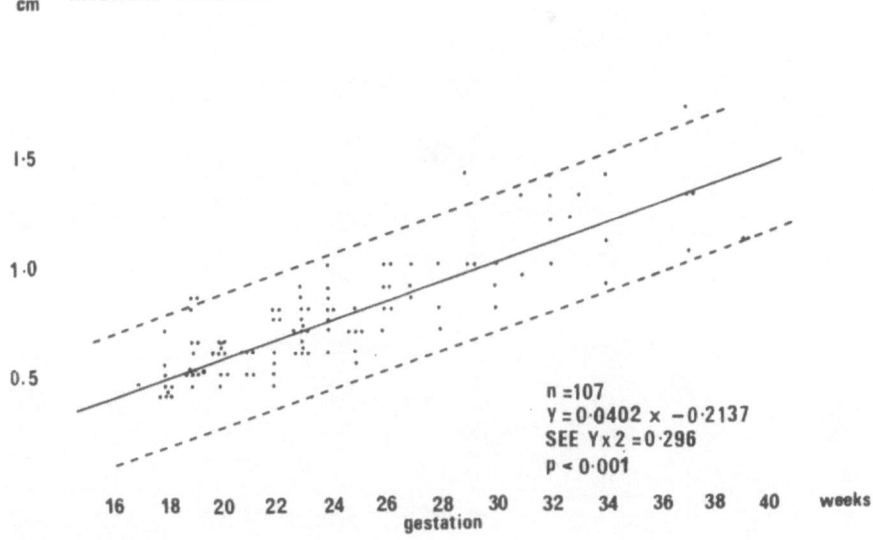

Figure 6.10 Left atrial dimensions between 16 weeks and term

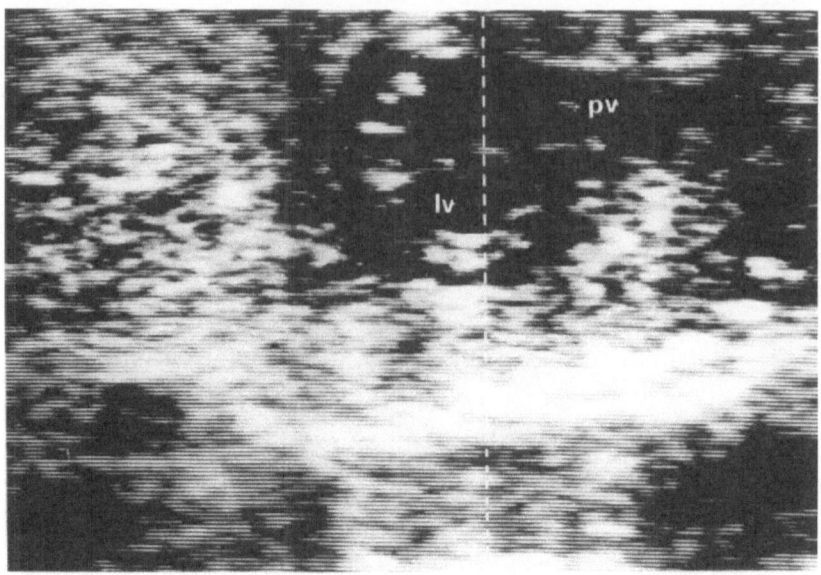

Figure 6.11 The heart sectioned to display the left ventricle in short axis. If the M-line is positioned through this plane the dimensions of two ventricles can be recorded

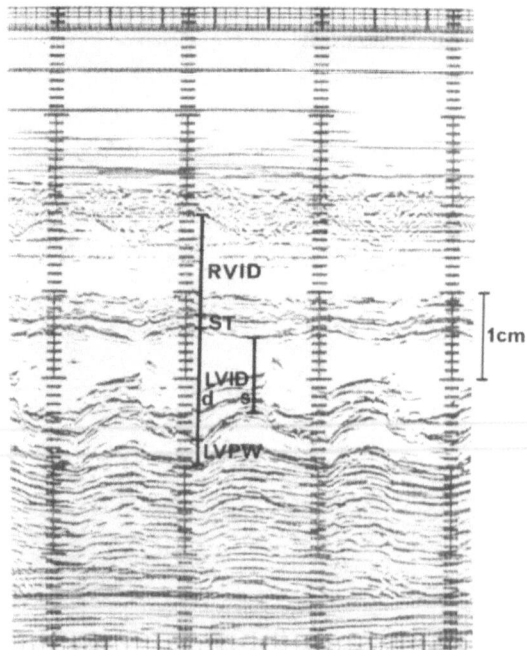

Figure 6.12 The M-mode and echocardiogram of the two ventricular chambers. The measurements which can be made from it are indicated

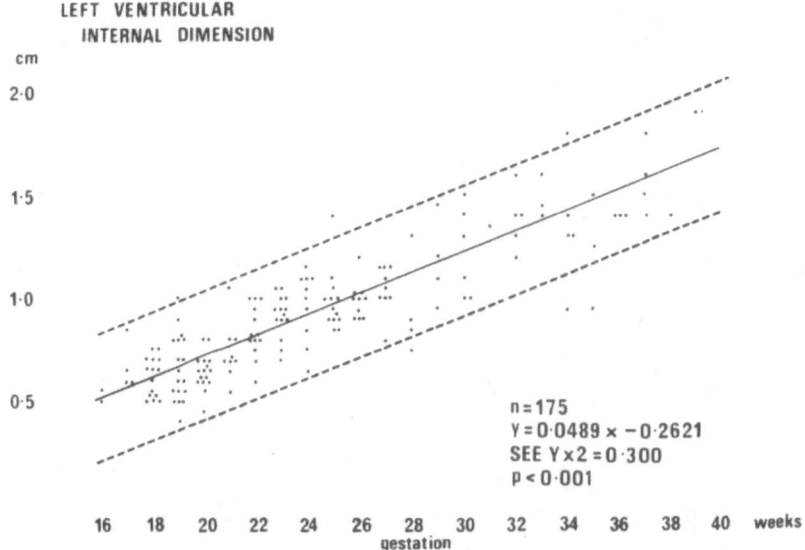

Figure 6.13 The growth of the left ventricular internal dimension in diastole throughout the second and third trimesters of pregnancy

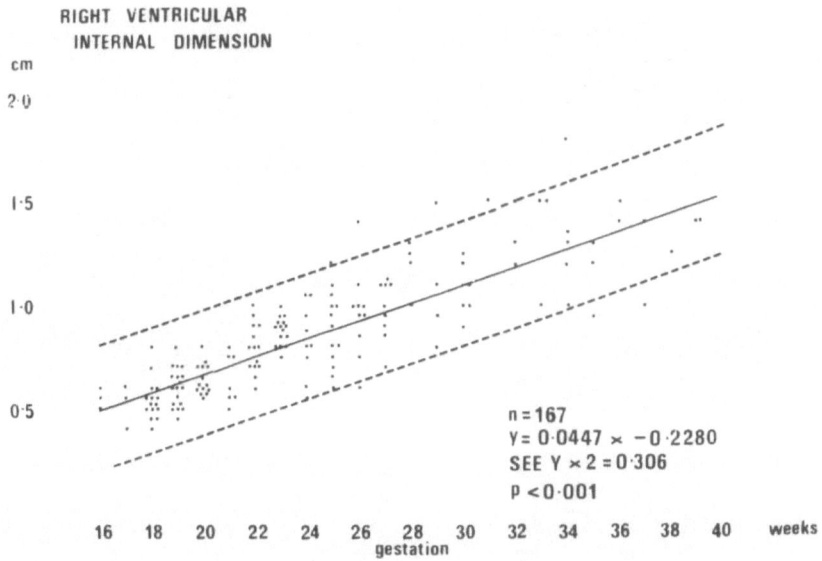

Figure 6.14 The growth of the right ventricular cavity

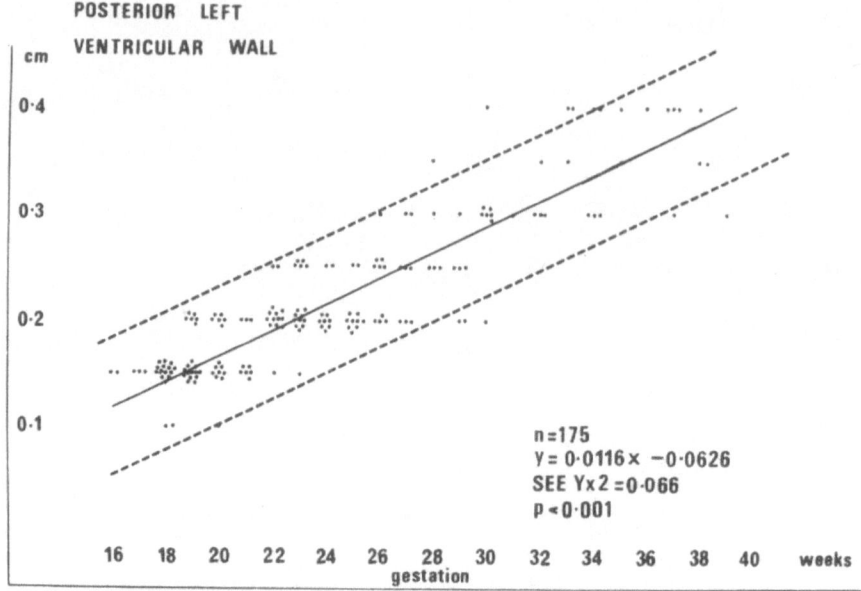

Figure 6.15 Left ventricular posterior wall thickness related to gestational age

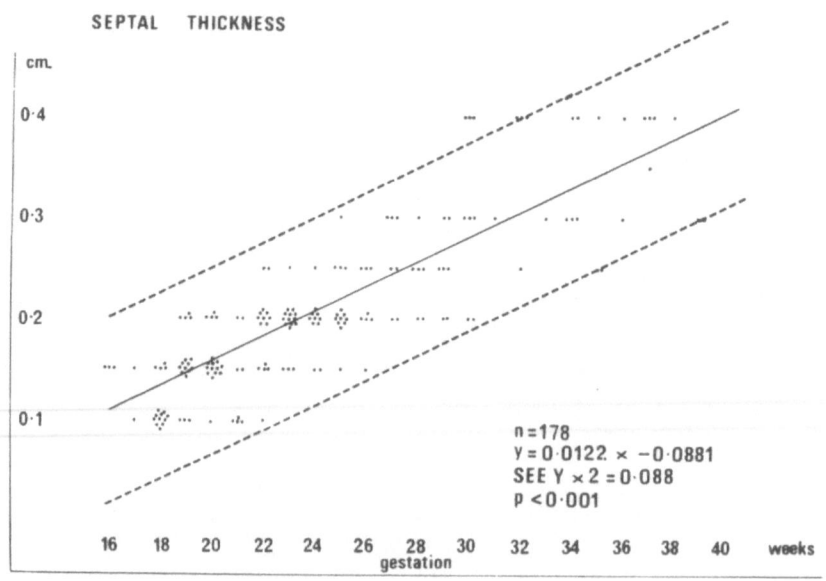

Figure 6.16 Septal thickness related to gestational age

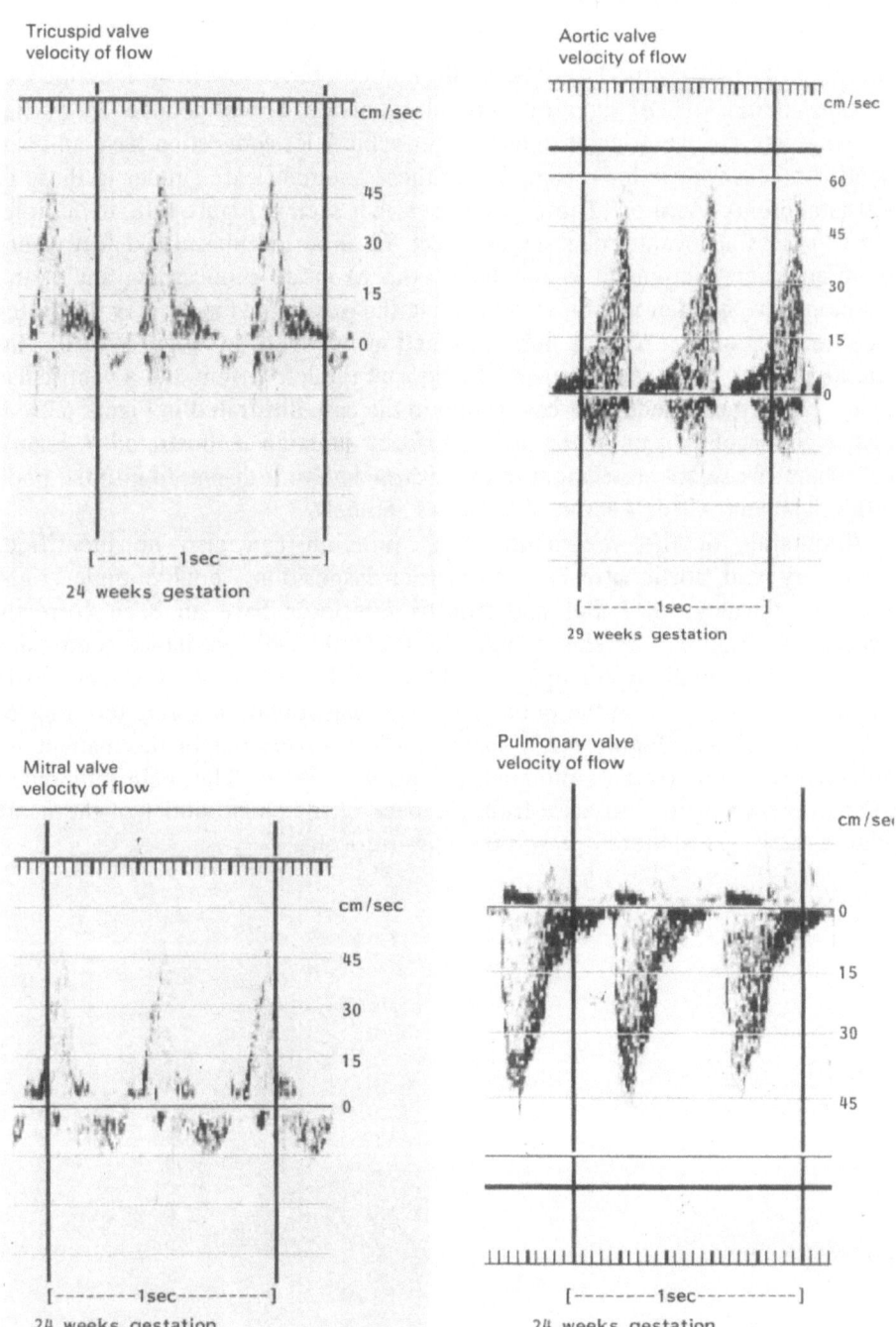

Figure 6.17 The Doppler tracings achieved across each cardiac valve

103

STRUCTURAL CARDIAC ANOMALIES

The majority of structural cardiac malformations have now been identified in intrauterine life[11-14]. At the atrioventricular junction, absent connection, partial and complete atrioventricular defects and double inlet connection have all been identified. The criteria for recognition of these anomalies are similar to those in postnatal life. A common atrioventricular valve is seen in Figure 6.18, in diastole, in a complete atrioventricular septal defect. In an atrioventricular defect where the ventricular component is not large, the M-mode echocardiogram of the common valve is often helpful in confirming the diagnosis. Figure 6.19 illustrates such an instance. Absent left connection is seen in Figure 6.20, no communication being seen between the floor of the left atrium and a ventricular cavity. There was absent right connection in the case illustrated in Figure 6.21. A further abnormality seen at the atrioventricular junction is illustrated in Figure 6.22 where the septal attachment of the tricuspid valve is displaced into the body of the right ventricle as a result of Ebstein's anomaly.

Anomalies of the ventriculoarterial junction can also be identified. Pulmonary and aortic atresia, complete transposition, double outlet right ventricle, tetralogy of Fallot and truncus arteriosus have all been correctly recognized. Figure 6.23 shows pulmonary atresia with an intact ventricular septum and a small hypertrophied right ventricle. Figure 6.24 shows aortic override in a heart where the pulmonary valve was found, denoting tetralogy of Fallot. In contrast, Figure 6.25a shows aortic override but in this patient no pulmonary outflow tract or pulmonary valve was found. The main pulmonary artery was seen instead to arise from the back of the single outlet of the heart (Figure 6.25b). This, therefore, was truncus arteriosus.

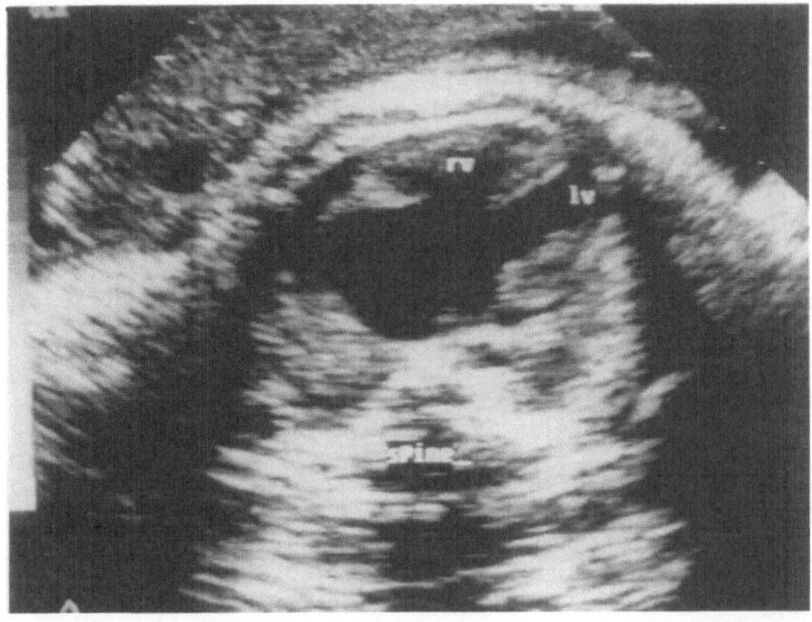

Figure 6.18 The heart in a four-chamber view. Only a small portion of atrial septum can be seen

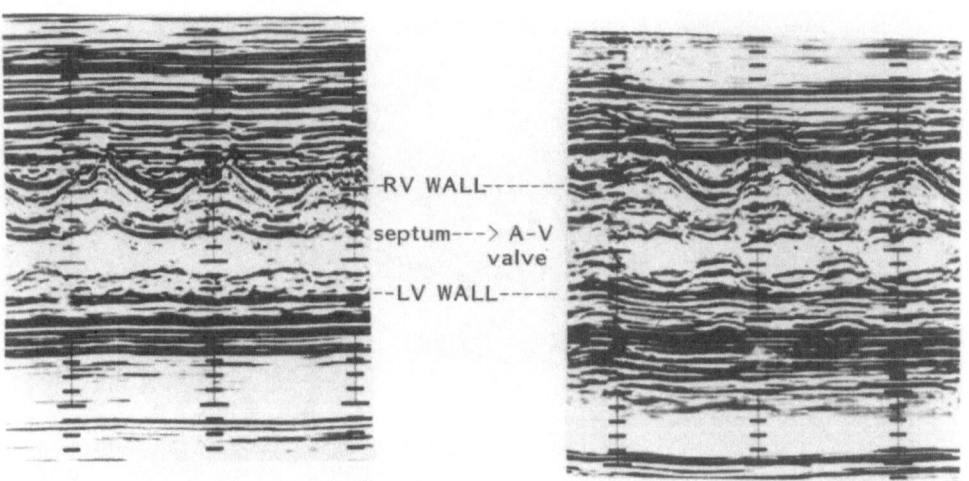

Figure 6.19 M-mode echocardiogram confirming the diagnosis of a common atrioventricular valve. Sweep from body of ventricle to A–V junction

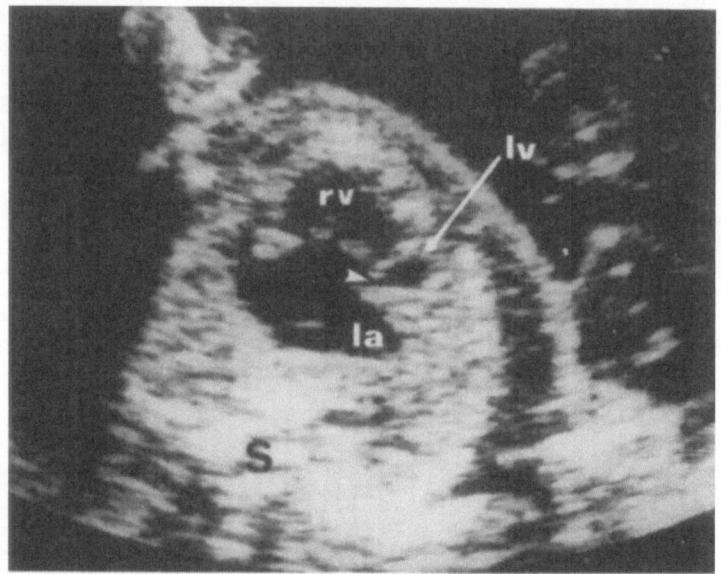

Figure 6.20 The heart seen in a cross-section of the thorax. There is only one ventricular chamber visible. There is no communication between left atrium (la) and a ventricular cavity

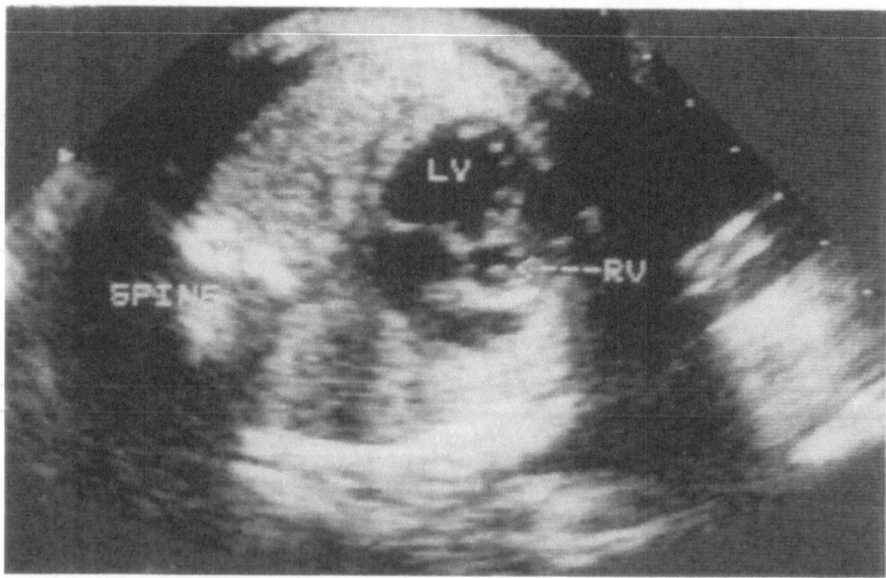

Figure 6.21 The aorta arising astride an outlet chamber and the main chamber. There is no patent right atrioventricular valve

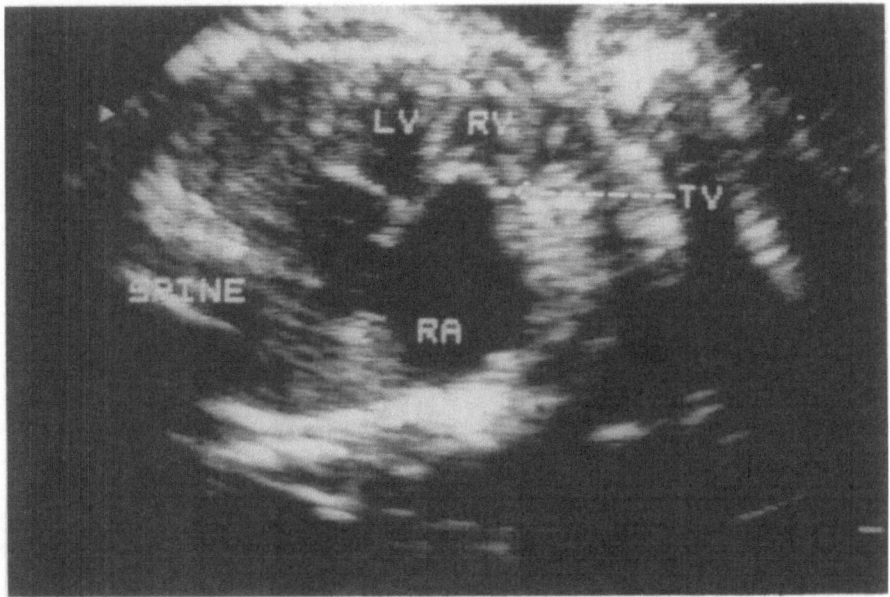

Figure 6.22 The heart filling most of the thorax. The tricuspid valve is displaced far down into the ventricular cavity producing a large 'atrialized' portion of right ventricle

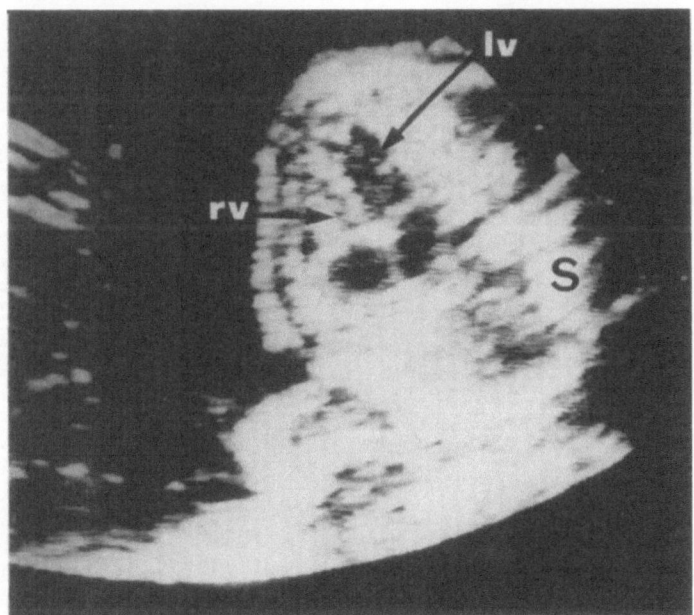

Figure 6.23 The heart sectioned to visualize right heart connections. The pulmonary valve did not open with ventricular systole

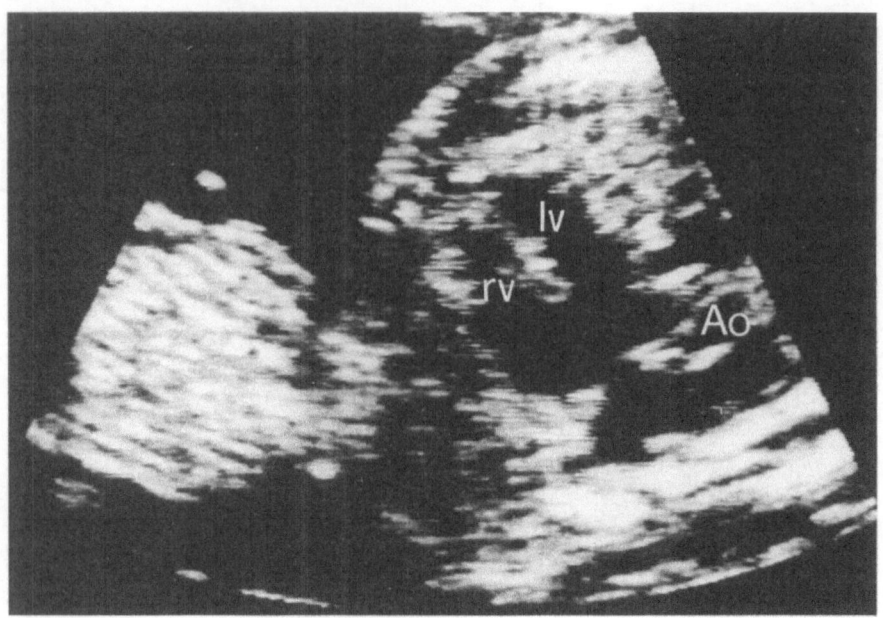

Figure 6.24 The aorta (Ao) arising astride a large ventricular septal defect

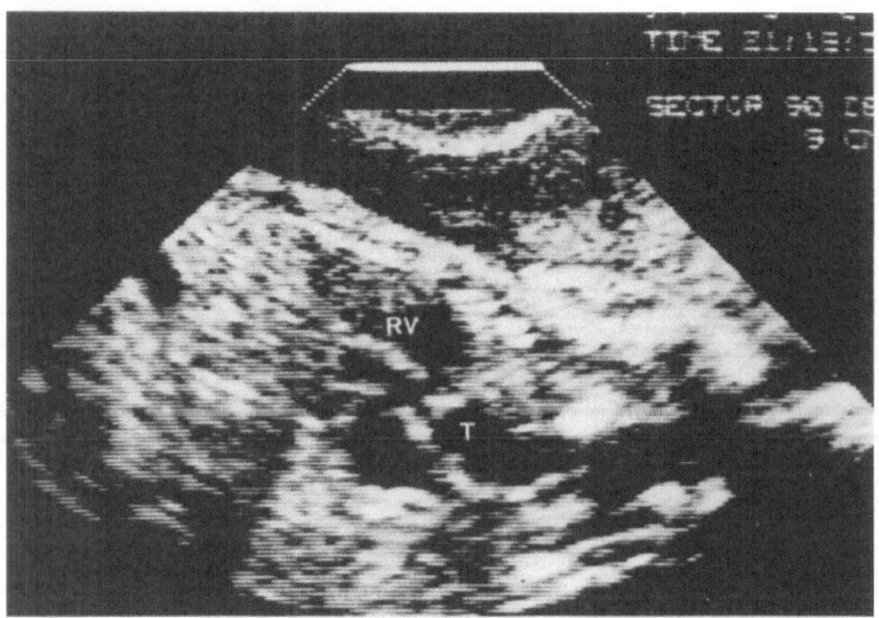

Figure 6.25a A single outlet of the heart seen to override the ventricular septum

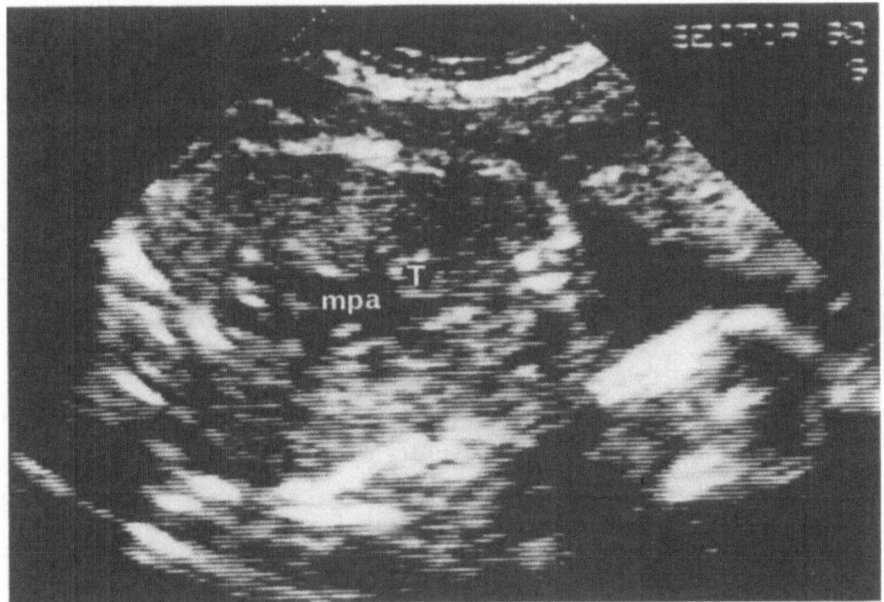

Figure 6.25b The main pulmonary artery seen to arise from the back of the artery shown in Figure 6.25b

Additional intracardiac defects which have been detected include ventricular septal defects, cardiac tumours and critical aortic stenosis. A trabecular ventricular septal defect was seen at 22 weeks' gestation (Figure 6.26). A cardiac tumour is illustrated in Figure 6.27. Histologically this was a rhabdomyoma. Critical aortic stenosis, seen in Figure 6.28, was associated with endocardial fibroelastosis affecting the left atrium and left ventricle. This produced a dilated poorly contracting left ventricle on echocardiography with a densely echogenic endocardial surface. The aortic root could be seen to be very small, only a pinhole orifice to the aortic valve being found at autopsy.

Aortic arch anomalies can also be seen. Figure 6.29 illustrates a very small aortic root which was found to stop and branch instead of forming an arch. This fetal heart was of only 18 weeks' gestation. Thus enlarging the echocardiogram does not give a good result. The anatomical specimen, in the same case, however, is cut in the same projection. In our experience direct examination of the aortic arch cannot exclude coarctation. Where the diagnosis of coarctation of the aorta has been made in intrauterine life, the clues have been from intracardiac findings, namely right ventricular dilatation and hypertrophy. The reasons for such findings are purely speculative[15], but probably relate to altered haemodynamics such that right ventricular output is increased in this situation.

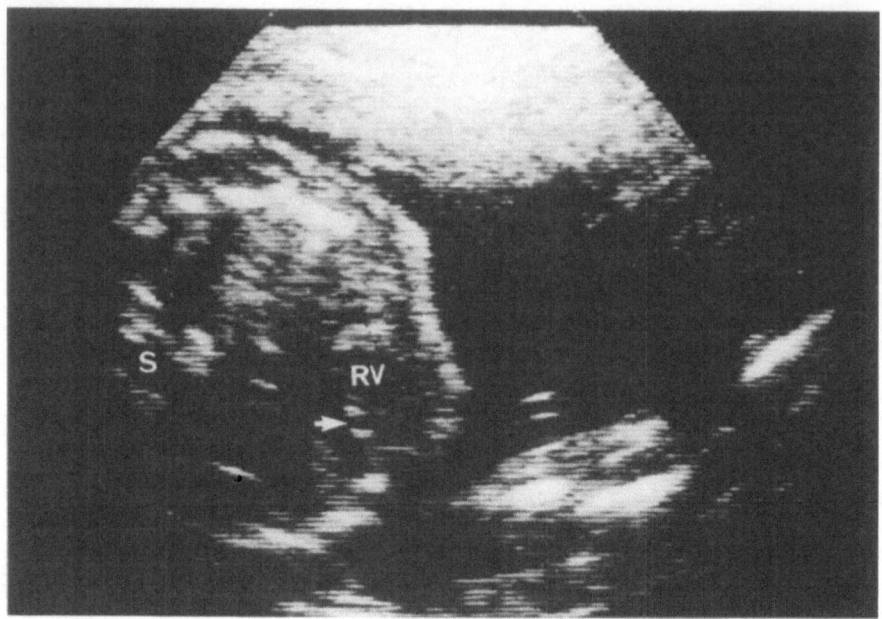

Figure 6.26 A well defined trabecular ventricular septal defect (arrowed) seen in a four-chamber view of the heart

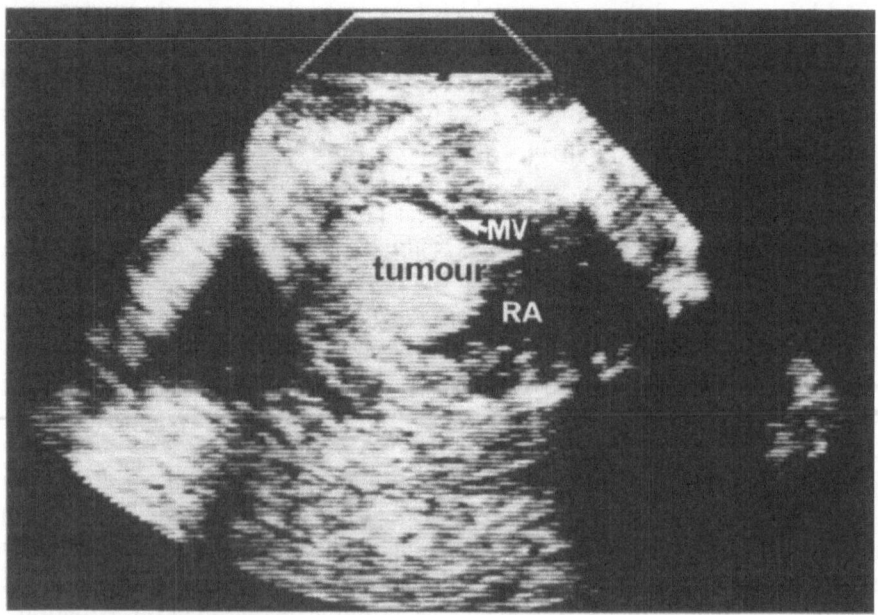

Figure 6.27 A large tumour seen in the ventricular septum causing obstruction to left and right ventricular inflow and outflow

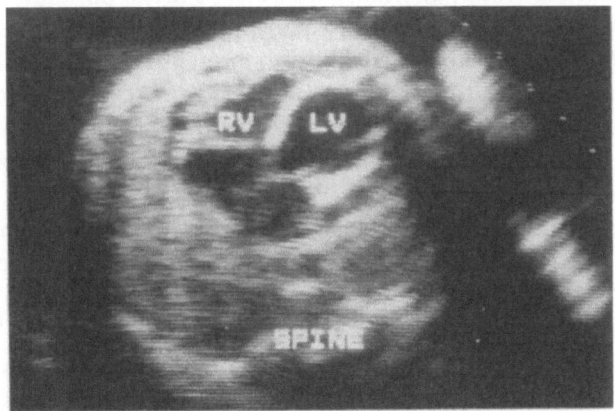

Figure 6.28 The left atrium and left ventricle were dilated and poorly contracting

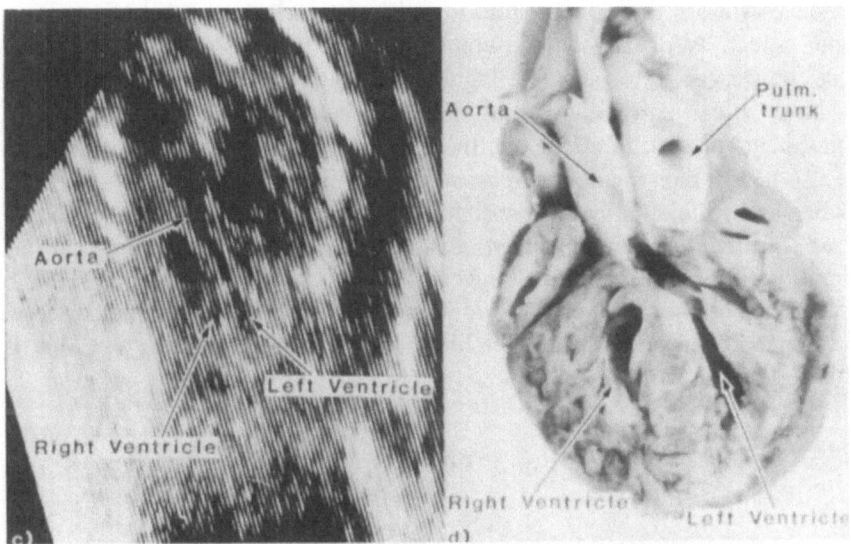

Figure 6.29 A small aorta which stopped and branched but did not form an arch

SELECTION OF HIGH RISK PREGNANCIES

The incidence of major structural heart disease of the kind readily detectable in intrauterine life is low, probably 4 per 1000 if unselected pregnancies are examined. However, population screening in the form of four chamber view scanning is possible as imaging equipment improves and an increasing number of centres include cardiac scanning as part of a routine obstetric scan. The ability to distinguish normal from abnormal cardiac structure is not difficult in general and an increasing source of our high yield referrals are pregnancies where the ultrasonographer is suspicious of cardiac abnormality. Alternatively, high risk pregnancies are selected for examination. They are scanned electively at 18 weeks' gestation and again at 26–28 weeks. These pregnancies are those with a family history of congenital heart disease, maternal diabetes or exposure to a cardiac teratogen in early pregnancy. Identification of a high risk factor appearing in an individual fetus, such as extracardiac fetal anomaly, cardiac arrhythmia or hydrops fetalis, is also an indication for specialized scanning. The recurrence rate of congenital heart disease where there has been an affected child in the family is approximately 1:50 in subsequent pregnancies[16], but where a parent has been affected the recurrence in offspring may be as high as 10-15%[17,18]. Maternal diabetes is said to double the risk of congenital heart disease[19]. Known cardiac teratogens, if the mother is exposed in early pregnancy, include lithium, phenytoin, steroids and rubella infection. Where an extracardiac anomaly is detected in fetal life, it is important also to scan the heart. Abnormality in more than one system may suggest a chromosomal anomaly or syndrome defect. Alternatively, the combination of two structural defects may influence the prognosis for surgery. Figure 6.30 illustrates a case of exomphalos with a large inlet ventricular septal defect. Exomphalos is associated with congenital heart disease in about one third of cases[20] but renal and intracranial defects also have a high incidence of associated cardiac anomaly.

Cardiac arrhythmias may be associated with structural heart disease. In our experience of fifty cases of tachyarrhythmia, only one was associated with cardiac malformation but some authors suggest an association as high as 11%[21]. However, complete heart block has a high incidence of associated heart disease. The incidence recorded in postnatal life is of the order of 25% but this is probably an underestimate[22].

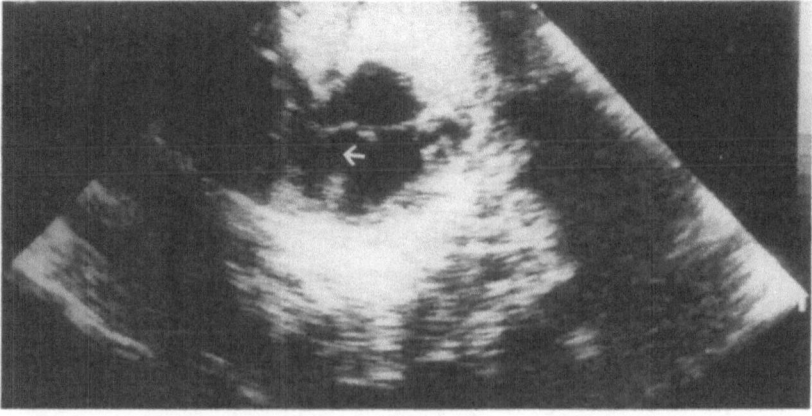

Figure 6.30 A large inlet ventricular septal defect (arrow)

The method of identification of arrhythmias involves the M-mode echocardiographic recording of atrial and ventricular contraction simultaneously. Normally atrial contraction precedes every ventricular contraction with a fixed time interval. Figure 6.31 illustrates this. Figure 6.32 illustrates atrial contraction occurring at approximately twice the rate of ventricular contraction and dissociated from it. This, therefore, is complete heart block. Figure 6.33 illustrates atrial contraction occurring at 480/min with a ventricular response to every second atrial contraction. This is atrial flutter with 2:1 conduction. We have not yet seen a ventricular tachycardia in utero but feel that it should be identifiable as such, unless it is very fast and there is retrograde conduction of every beat.

In our experience of cases of complete heart block, over 50% had structural heart disease[23]. Complete heart block with structural heart disease implies a very poor prognosis, and is commonly associated with atrial isomerism[24]. On the other hand, isolated complete heart block usually has a good prognosis. All our cases of isolated complete heart block had evidence of connective tissue disease in maternal serum[25]. This is an important association to seek, as the recurrence of complete heart block in such mothers is of the order of 30%[26].

Our current policy with supraventricular tachycardias is to treat the mother with flecainide or a combination of digoxin and verapamil. If there is intrauterine cardiac failure, it is important to achieve adequate blood levels of anti-arrhythmic drugs in the mother and the fetus. Placental transfer is less good if there is fetal hydrops. One should obtain therapeutic levels in maternal serum for at least a week to be sure that adequate quantities of the drugs are reaching the fetus. If there is no cardiac failure it is safe to start treatment with digoxin only and to add verapamil if control is not achieved with well-tolerated doses of digoxin.

Non-immune hydrops fetalis can be due to intrauterine cardiac failure as a result of structural heart disease. This therefore is an important high risk group of pregnancies to study.

CONFIDENCE LIMITS OF THE FETAL ECHOCARDIOGRAPHIC TECHNIQUE

To date we have not made a major false positive diagnosis in a series of over 7000 pregnancies. Extensive experience of the fetal echocardiographic technique must be gained before a diagnosis of normality or abnormality can be considered reliable. This is particularly true if intervention in a pregnancy is contemplated.

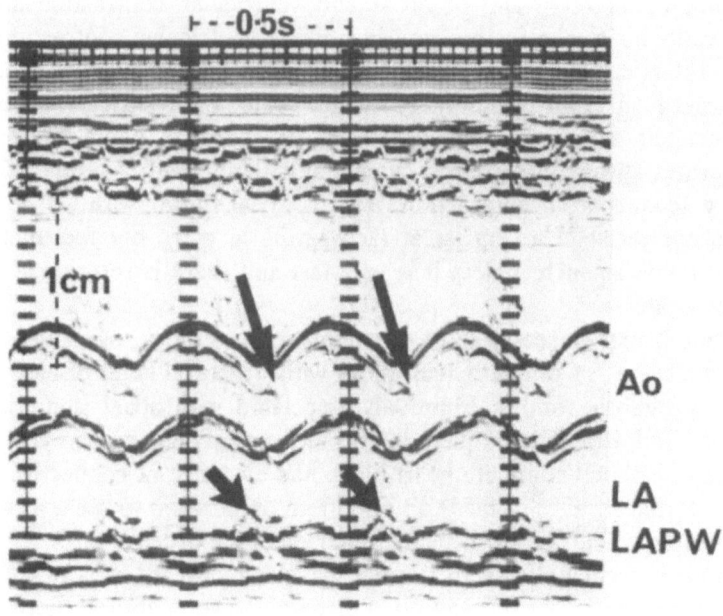

Figure 6.31 The normal sequence of atrioventricular contraction, atrial contraction occurring less than 80 ms prior to each ventricular contraction

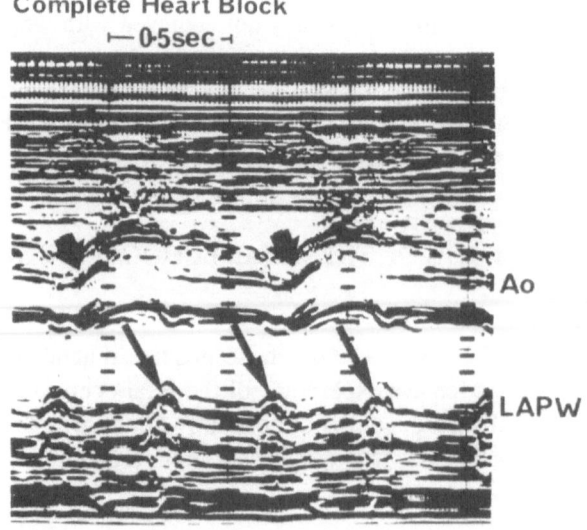

Figure 6.32 Atrial contraction occurring at approximately twice the rate of ventricular contraction (smaller arrows) and dissociated from it

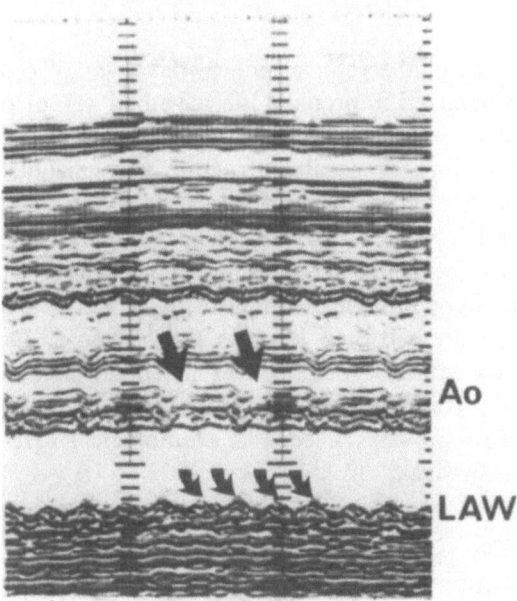

Figure 6.33 The posterior atrial wall is seen to flutter. Ventricular response is to every second contraction

Some cardiac malformations have been overlooked in intrauterine life. Three were major abnormalities of connection but were overlooked early in our experience. The scanning technique has been modified since then so that such errors should not be made in the future. Minor abnormalities have been overlooked: atrial septal defects; ventricular septal defects; and cases of mild coarctation of the aorta. In order to avoid overlooking ventricular septal defects of functional significance our current policy is to ensure cardiac connections at the initial visit at 18 weeks' gestation and to schedule the second visit for 24-26 weeks. The resolution capacity of current equipment will display a defect of greater than 2 mm in size. Such a defect is approaching half aortic root size at 24-26 weeks. If this proportion is maintained the defect will be of functional significance at birth[27]. Conversely, defects of less than 2 mm at this gestation will not be functionally important. It will remain, however, impossible to exclude all small defects, just as in postnatal life. Coarctation of the aorta may continue to be a weak spot of the fetal echocardiographic technique. Many cases have been recognized in utero, but some overlooked. The cases recognized were diagnosed from associated intracardiac features rather than directly from the appearance of the aortic arch, namely right ventricular dilatation and hypertrophy. A change in policy to re-scan patients with a history of coarctation at 32 weeks' gestation and the addition of a Doppler evaluation may improve our accuracy in this condition.

OUTCOME AND RESULTS

Largely as a result of the referral policy, the cases of congenital heart disease that have been detected in prenatal life have had a poor outcome. Many of the cardiac abnormalities seen had extracardiac anomalies occurring in association. The major distortions of cardiac structure recognizable by routine obstetric screening or causing intrauterine cardiac failure are also likely to have a poor prognosis. This is reflected in Figure 6.34 which tabulates the outcome of the first 320 cases of congenital heart disease recognized in utero. However, in the future it is to be hoped that less complex lesions will be detected; anticipation of the defect prenatally will then improve the outcome. Delay in diagnosis and transfer of a sick infant also influences morbidity and mortality in congenital heart disease. The transferring of antenatal care so that delivery takes place in a centre which also provides paediatric cardiological care should optimize the chance of infant survival.

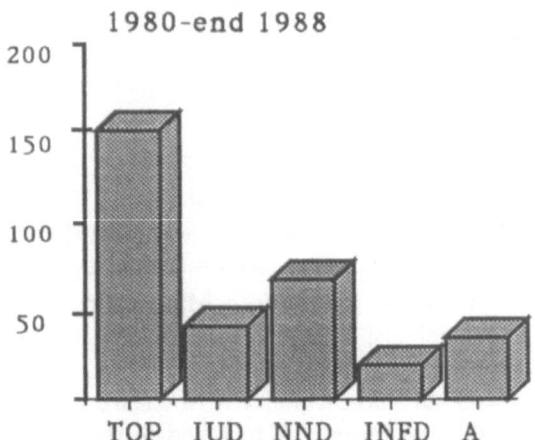

Figure 6.34 The outcome in the first 320 cases in which congenital heart disease (CHD) was predicted. Over half the cases had coexistent extracardiac anomalies

References

1. Allan, L.D., Tynan, M.J., Campbell, S., Wilkinson, J.L. and Anderson, R.H. (1980). Echocardiographic and anatomical correlates in the fetus. *Br. Heart J.*, **44**, 445–51
2. Devore, G.R., Donnerstein, R.L., Kleinman, C.S., Platt, L.D. and Hobbins, J.C. (1982). Fetal echocardiography. I Normal anatomy as determined by real-time directed M-mode ultrasound. *Am. J. Obstet. Gynecol.*, **144**, 249
3. Lange, L.W., Sahn, D.J., Allen, H.D., Goldberg, S.J., Anderson C.P. and Giles, H. (1980). Qualitative real-time cross-sectional echocardiographic imaging of the human fetus during the second half of pregnancy. *Circulation*, **62**, 799–806
4. Nisand, I., Spielmann, A. and Dellenbach, P. (1984). Fetal heart. present investigative means. *Ultrasound Med. Biol.*, **10**, 79–105

5. Allan, L.D., Joseph, M.C., Boyd, E.G.C.A., Campbell, S. and Tynan, M. (1982). M-mode echocardiography in the developing human fetus. *Br. Heart J.*, **47**, 573–83

6. Sahn, D.J., Lange, L.W., Allen, H.D., Goldberg, S.J., Anderson, S.J., Giles, H. and Haber, K. (1980). Quantitative real-time cross-sectional echocardiography in the developing human fetus and newborn. *Circulation*, **62**, 588–97

7. Maulik, D., Nanda, N.C. and Saini, V.D. (1984). Fetal Doppler echocardiography: methods and characterization of normal and abnormal hemodynamics. *Am. J. Cardiol.*, **53**, 572–8

8. Fitzgerald, D.E., Stuart, B., Drumm, J.E. and Duignam, N.M. (1984). The assessment of the feto-placental circulation with continuous wave Doppler ultrasound. *Ultrasound Med. Biol.*, **10**, 371–6

9. Griffin, D., Bilardo, K., Masini, L., Diag-Racoseus, J., Pearce, J.M., Willson, K.P. and Campbell, S. (1984). Doppler blood flow waveforms in the descending thoracic aorta of the human fetus. *Br. J. Obstet. Gynecol.*, **9**, 997–1006

10. Meijboom, E.J., de Smedt, M.C.H., Visser, G.H.A., Jager, W., Bossina, K.K. and Huisjes, H.J. (1985). Cross-sectional Doppler echocardiographic evaluation of the fetal cardiac output during IInd and IIIrd trimester of pregnancy. A longitudinal study. In Jones, C.T. and Nathaniels, P.W. (eds.) *The Physiological Development of the Fetus and Neonate.* (London: Academic Press)

11. Allan, L.D., Crawford, D.C., Anderson, R.H. and Tynan, M.J. (1984). Echocardiographic and anatomical correlates in fetal congenital heart disease. *Br. Heart J.*, **52**, 542

12. Kleinman, C.S., Donnerstein, R.L., Devore, G.R., Jaffe, C.C., Lynch, D.C., Berkowitz, R.L., Talner, N.S. and Hobbins, J.C. (1982). Fetal echocardiography for evaluation of in utero congestive heart failure. *N. Engl. J. Med.*, **10**, 568–75

13. Stewart, P.A., Wladimiroff, J.W. and Essed, C.E. (1983). Prenatal ultrasound diagnosis of congenital heart disease associated with intrauterine growth retardation. *Prenatal Diagn.*, **3**, 279–85

14. Sahn, D.J., Shenker, L., Reed, K.L., Valdes-Cruz, L.M., Sobonya, R. and Anderson, C. (1982). prenatal ultrasound diagnosis of hypoplastic left heart syndrome in utero associated with hydrops fetalis. *Am. Heart J.*, **104**, 1368–72

15. Allan, L.D., Crawford, D.C. and Tynan, M. (1983). Evolution of coarctation of the aorta in intrauterine life. *Br. Heart J.*, **52**, 471–3

16. Nora, J.J. (1968). Multifactorial inheritance hypothesis for the etiology of congenital heart disease. *Circulation*, **38**, 304–15

17. Emanuel, R.L., Somerville, J., Inns, A. and Withers, R. (1983). Evidence of congenital heart disease in the offspring of parents with atrioventricular defects. *Br. Heart J.*, **49**, 144–7

18. Whittemore, R., Hobbins, J.C. and Engle, M.A. (1982). Pregnancy and its outcome in women with and without surgical treatment of congenital heart disease. *Am. J. Cardiol.*, **40**, 641–51

19. Miller, H.C. (1946). The effect of diabetic and prediabetic pregnancies on the fetus and newborn infant. *J. Pediatr.*, **29**, 455–63

20. Crawford, D.C., Chapman, M.G. and Allan, L.D. (1985). The use of echocardiography in the investigation of anterior abdominal wall defects in the fetus. *Br. J. Obstet. Gynaecol.* (In press)

21. Newburger, J.W. and Keane, J.F. (1979). Intrauterine supraventricular tachycardia. *J. Paediatr.*, **95**, 780–3

22. Shenker, L. (1979). Fetal cardiac arrhythmias. *Obstet. Gynecol. Surv.*, **34**, 561–71

23. Machado, M.V.L., Tynan, M.J. and Allan, L.D. (1988). Complete heart block in prenatal life. *Br. Heart J.*, **60**, 512–15

24. Garcia, O.L., Mehta, A.V., Pickoff, A.S., Tamer, D.F., Ferrer, P.L., Wolff, G.S. and Gelband, H. (1981). Left isomerism and complete atrioventricular block: a report of six cases. *Am. J. Cardiol.*, **48**, 1103–7

25. McCue, C.M., Mantakas, M.E., Tingelstad, J.B. and Ruddy, S. (1977). Congenital heart block in newborns of mothers with connective tissue disease. *Circulation*, **56**, 82–9

26. Scott, J.S., Maddison, P.J., Taylor, P.V., Esscher, E., Scott, O. and Skinner, R.P. (1983). Connective tissue disease, antibodies to ribonucleoprotein and congenital heart block. *N. Engl. J. Med.*, **309**, 209–12

27. Canale, J.M., Sahn, D.J., Allen, H.D., Goldberg, S.J., Valdes-Cruz, L. M. and Ovitt, T.W. (1981). Factors affecting real-time cross-sectional echocardiographic imaging of perimembranous ventricular septal defects. *Circulation*, **63**, 689–97

7

The primary hyperlipidaemias – diagnosis and management

D.J. BETTERIDGE

INTRODUCTION

It is an opportune time to consider the management of hyperlipidaemia. Having accepted that there is sufficient evidence to attribute a causal role to plasma cholesterol in the development of atherosclerosis-related disease, particularly coronary heart disease (CHD), consensus committees on both sides of the Atlantic[1,2] have made recommendations with regard to optimal lipid and lipoprotein levels (Table 7.1). The British Hyperlipidaemia Association has accepted these guidelines and has published its own strategies for reducing coronary heart disease[3]. Furthermore, a study group of the European Atherosclerosis Society has published a policy statement on the recognition and management of hyperlipidaemia[4].

Table 7.1 Optimal lipid and lipoprotein levels[1,2]

Plasma cholesterol	< 5.2 mmol/l
Plasma triglyceride	< 2.3 mmol/l
LDL cholesterol	< 3.5 mmol/l
HDL cholesterol	> 0.9 mmol/l

This increasing awareness of the importance of hyperlipidaemia in relation to CHD reflects significant progress in many different research areas. Recent analysis of the huge data base of the men screened for the Multiple Risk Factor Intervention Trial (> 300,000 men) has demonstrated that CHD mortality increases continuously with increasing plasma cholesterol levels above 4.7 mmol/l[5]. The slope of this relationship is more steep when the plasma cholesterol is greater than 6.2 mmol/1. The conclusion of a causal link between plasma cholesterol and CHD has been strengthened by the publication of primary prevention trials of cholesterol-lowering such as the Lipid Research Clinics cholestyramine trial in the USA[6] and the Helsinki Heart Study of

119

gemfibrozil[7]. Both these trials show unequivocal benefits of cholesterol-lowering in reducing CHD events. In addition, the first report of the Cholesterol Lowering Atherosclerosis Study (CLAS) has shown that aggressive modulation of plasma lipoproteins can reduce progression of atheromatous plaques in coronary arteries and in some cases lead to regression as demonstrated by angiography[8].

In parallel with these major advances in epidemiological and clinical studies there have been advances in the understanding of lipoprotein metabolism and the importance of this work was recognized by the award of the Nobel Prize in 1985 to Drs Goldstein and Brown for their work on the low density lipoprotein (LDL) receptor and the regulation of LDL metabolism[9]. These advances, together with recognition of the role of blood monocyte/macrophage in foam cell formation, have enabled attractive hypotheses to be propounded for the interaction of lipoproteins with monocytes and the development of the fatty streak, the initial lesion of atherosclerosis[10,11].

In this chapter I will give a brief outline of plasma lipid and lipoprotein metabolism as a basis for a description of the primary hyperlipidaemias. In addition, the current management of hyperlipidaemias will be discussed, together with prospects for future developments.

PLASMA LIPID AND LIPOPROTEIN METABOLISM

The major plasma lipids, cholesterol ester and triglyceride, are transported in plasma in a family of lipoproteins. The insoluble lipids such as esterified cholesterol and triglyceride are contained in a hydrophobic core which is surrounded by a coat containing the more polar lipids, phospholipid and free cholesterol. The protein part of the lipoprotein complex known as apoprotein is also found in this outer coat. The apoproteins are important in stabilizing the lipoprotein particles, but have other actions in lipoprotein metabolism affecting the activity of enzymes and binding to cellular receptors. The lipoproteins are generally referred to by terminology derived from their separation by ultracentrifugation on the basis of their density (Table 7.2). Several useful reviews have appeared recently giving comprehensive accounts of lipoproteins and their metabolism[12,13].

Chylomicrons

Chylomicrons are the largest of the lipoprotein species and transport dietary fat, principally triglyceride, with a small amount of cholesterol, from the intestine via the lymphatics and thoracic duct into the circulation. The triglyceride component is hydrolysed by the enzyme lipoprotein lipase which is localized on the endothelial surface of capillary beds. Apoprotein C-II is an important activator of this enzyme. The relatively cholesterol-rich chylomicron remnant particle is removed by the liver through a process that recognizes apoprotein E.

Very low density lipoproteins

Very low density lipoproteins (VLDL) are secreted by the liver and to a lesser extent, the intestine. These particles transport endogenously synthesized triglyceride and cholesterol from the liver into the circulation. VLDL triglyceride is hydrolysed by lipoprotein lipase, the particles becoming progressively more cholesterol-rich and forming VLDL remnant particles (intermediate-density lipoproteins; IDL). IDL are either removed from the circulation directly by the liver or undergo further conversion to LDL. Hepatic IDL uptake involves the LDL receptor which recognizes apoprotein B and apoprotein E. VLDL size appears to be an important determinant of the metabolic fate of the particles. Large VLDL behave like chylomicrons in that the VLDL remnants are removed directly by the liver. On the other hand, small VLDL particles tend to be converted rapidly to LDL via IDL.

Low density lipoproteins

Approximately 70% of the total plasma cholesterol is transported on LDL, mainly as cholesterol ester. LDL particles result from the progressive delipidation of VLDL and serve to deliver cholesterol to the liver and peripheral cells. LDL are removed from the circulation principally by the liver through endocytosis following binding to specific high affinity receptors (LDL receptors) which recognize apoprotein B, the major apoprotein of LDL. The LDL receptor, a glycoprotein, which has been cloned and sequenced, and the gene localized to the short arm of chromosome 19, is of critical importance in the regulation of plasma LDL levels.

High density lipoproteins

High density lipoproteins (HDL), the smallest of the lipoprotein species, consist mainly of protein (apoprotein A-I and apoprotein A-II) and phospholipid with very little triglyceride. They carry 20–30% of plasma cholesterol. The lipoproteins separated in the HDL density range show considerable heterogeneity since the particles arise from different sources including direct hepatic and intestinal synthesis and as a product of the metabolism of triglyceride-rich lipoproteins. During hydrolysis of chylomicrons and VLDL by lipoprotein lipase, surface components, principally phospholipid and apoproteins, transfer to HDL.

Table 7.2 The plasma lipoproteins

	Chylomicrons	VLDL	IDL	LDL	HDL
Diameter nm	80–500	30–80	25–35	20	10
Electrophoresis	Origin	Pre-beta	Broad beta	Beta	Alpha
Principal core lipid	Exogenous triglyceride	Triglyceride Cholesterol esters	Cholesterol esters and triglyceride	Cholesterol esters Triglyceride	Cholesterol esters
Major apoproteins	AI and II B48 CII and III E	B100 CII and III E	B100 E	B100 E	AI and II CIII E(HDL$_1$ only)
Effect on atheroma	Nil	+	++	+++	Protects
Drug treatment	Diet Drugs ineffective	Fibrates Nicotinic acid Omega-3 fish oils	Fibrates Nicotinic acid HMG-CoA reductase inhibitors	Resins Nicotinic acid Fibrates Probucol HMG-CoA reductase inhibitors	Fibrates Nicotinic acid Omega-3 fish oil Resins Probucol (lowers)

Lipoproteins and atherosclerosis

It is the concentration of LDL which explains the relationship between plasma cholesterol and CHD, and LDL is the main source of cholesterol found in the arterial wall[14]. HDL is also strongly and independently related to the development of CHD but the association is inverse; low levels of HDL being an important risk factor and high levels appearing to protect[15,16]. The inverse relationship between HDL and CHD may be explained by the role of this lipoprotein in reverse cholesterol transport as an acceptor of cellular free cholesterol[17]. Lecithin cholesterol acyltransferase (LCAT), a key enzyme in cholesterol transport, circulates with HDL, and apoprotein A-I, the major apoprotein of HDL, is an important activator of the enzyme. The HDL/LCAT complex is able to act as an acceptor of cellular free cholesterol which is then esterified by LCAT and transferred to the core of the particle. Cholesterol ester can then transfer to other lipoproteins of lower density by a lipid transfer protein and ultimately reach the liver for excretion.

The relationship between plasma triglyceride and CHD is less clear. Many studies performed during the 1970s, both cross-sectional and prospective, pointed to plasma triglyceride as an important risk factor for CHD. However, when the statistical technique of multivariate analysis was applied to these studies, taking into account HDL cholesterol, cholesterol, obesity, etc., the 'independent' relationship disappeared[18]. More recently, reports from the Framingham group have suggested that triglyceride is an independent risk factor for CHD when HDL cholesterol levels are low[19]. It is likely that the relationship between triglyceride and CHD will depend on the nature of the triglyceride-rich lipoprotein involved. There is no doubt that IDL are strongly and independently related to CHD[20]. These particles accumulate in type III hyperlipidaemia or remnant-particle disease which is associated with severe and extensive premature vascular disease. On the other hand, excess chylomicrons do not confer excess cardiovascular risk but do predispose to pancreatitis. It remains to be seen whether VLDL particles are directly related to CHD.

ASSESSMENT OF HYPERLIPIDAEMIA

Based on the guidelines of the Consensus Conference statements there is a massive cholesterol education programme supported by all the major health agencies under way in the USA[21]. Every adult is being encouraged to have a cholesterol check. Although this approach is probably premature in the UK it will undoubtedly come as more resources are diverted to preventive medicine. In the meantime, lipid measurements should be part of the assessment of overall cardiovascular risk in those with premature vascular disease; a family history of premature CHD; a family history of hyperlipidaemia; the presence of other major risk factors such as hypertension or diabetes mellitus and those with the clinical stigmata of hyperlipidaemia. In the future a cholesterol measurement should become part of the general medical assessment and this will be facilitated by wider availability of desk technology for lipid measurement. For screening purposes a random cholesterol is convenient but if this test is not satisfactory a fasting sample with measurement of triglyceride as well as cholesterol and HDL cholesterol is required. The measurement of HDL cholesterol is assuming increasing importance; it enables calculation of LDL cholesterol concentrations by the Friedewald[22] calculation (Table 7.3). In addition, there is increasing evidence of the importance of low HDL concentration as a major risk factor for CHD[23] and preliminary evidence that increasing HDL concentrations by therapy may reduce the development of CHD[24].

Table 7.3 The Friedewald calculation for LDL cholesterol[22]

LDL cholesterol =

Total cholesterol − HDL cholesterol − $\dfrac{\text{triglyceride}}{2.19}$

PRIMARY HYPERLIPIDAEMIAS

The Frederickson classification of the hyperlipidaemias[25,26] is based on the laboratory measurement of plasma lipids and lipoproteins and does not differentiate between the pathological processes leading to the lipid abnormality. A high plasma cholesterol due to the accumulation of LDL, for instance, could be due to familial hypercholesterolaemia, familial combined hyperlipidaemia, i.e. primary genetic disorders of cholesterol metabolism or secondary to the endocrine abnormality myxoedema. Furthermore, plasma HDL concentrations do not feature in the Frederickson classification. For these reasons the primary hyperlipidaemias are considered as individual diseases bearing in mind that there is likely to be considerable heterogeneity in some disorders, particularly the hypertriglyceridaemias (Table 7.4).

Hyperlipidaemia is a common metabolic problem and as screening programmes are instigated more subjects will be identified. Attempts should be made to try and identify the particular hyperlipidaemia responsible for the plasma lipid abnormality as this has important implications for CHD risk and appropriate therapy. For instance, familial hypercholesterolaemia is associated with a much higher risk of CHD than polygenic hypercholesterolaemia and will respond less to dietary measures. Hypertriglyceridaemia due to familial combined hyperlipidaemia carries a higher risk than polygenic hypertriglyceridaemia.

Table 7.4 Classification and characteristics of primary hyperlipidaemias

	Frederickson lipoprotein phenotype	Typical lipid levels (mmol/l)	Lipo-proteins	IHD Risk	Pancreatitis	Clinical signs
Polygenic hypercholesterolaemia	IIa	Cholesterol 6.5–9 Triglyceride <2.3	LDL↑ HDL→↓	+	–	Xanthelasma, corneal arcus
Familial combined (mixed) hyperlipidaemia	IIa, IIb IV	Cholesterol 6.5–10 Triglyceride 2.5–12	VLDL↑→ LDL→↑ HDL→↓	++	–	Corneal arcus, xanthelasma
Familial hypercholesterolaemia	IIa or IIb	Cholesterol 7.5–16 Triglyceride <5.0	LDL↑ VLDL→↑ HDL→↓	+++	–	Tendon xanthomata, corneal arcus, xanthelasma
Remnant particle disease (dysbeta lipoproteinaemia)	III	Cholesterol 9–14 Triglyceride 9–14	IDL↑ HDL→↓	+++	+	Palmar tuberous and occasional tendon xanthomata
Chylomicronaemia syndrome (lipoprotein lipase deficiency) apoprotein C-II deficiency)	I	Triglyceride 10–30 Cholesterol <6.5	Chylo-microns↑	–	+++	Eruptive xanthomata Lipaemia retinalis Hepatosplenomegaly
Familial hypertriglyceridaemia	IV-V	Triglyceride 10–30 Cholesterol 6.5–12	VLDL↑ Chylo-microns→↑	?	++	Eruptive xanthomata Lipaemia retinalis Hepatosplenomegaly
HDL abnormalities						
Hypoalphalipoproteinaemia	–	HDL cholesterol <0.9	HDL↓	++	–	–
Hyperalphalipoproteinaemia	–	HDL cholesterol >2.0	HDL↑	–	–	–

Screening of family members as well as identifying affected individuals helps in the diagnostic process. In the future it is likely that molecular genetics will provide useful diagnostic markers.

FAMILIAL HYPERCHOLESTEROLAEMIA

Familial hypercholesterolaemia (FH) is characterized clinically by high plasma cholesterol concentrations due to accumulation of LDL particles, autosomal dominant inheritance and premature vascular disease[27]. Approximately half the affected male heterozygotes will be dead by the age of 60 years. FH women also develop premature CHD with a mean age of onset of 57 years compared to 42 years for men. Tendon xanthomata are the characteristic clinical stigmata of FH and are found most frequently in the Achilles, extensor tendons of the hands and patella tendons. Occasionally xanthomata may become inflamed and tender and this is particularly troublesome in the Achilles and patellar tendons. Xanthomata consist of nodular deposits of fibrous tissue and macrophage foam cells full of cholesterol ester. Although the majority of patients will have xanthomata by the age of 40 years, some patients do not develop xanthomata. Corneal arcus and xanthelasma may occur at a young age in FH but are not pathognomic for the disease. The frequency of the heterozygous state in the UK is about 1 in 57. Homozygous FH is thankfully rare (~1 per million) as the development of atherosclerosis is very rapid and few patients survive through teenage.

The genetic defect in FH has been well delineated by the Nobel Laureates, Brown and Goldstein. They have described several abnormalities of the LDL receptor in these patients, which lead to delayed clearance of LDL from the circulation and a doubling of plasma LDL concentrations[28].

FAMILIAL COMBINED (MIXED) HYPERLIPIDAEMIA

This condition, first described in the 1970s[29], is a well recognized clinical entity but the genetic defect remains to be determined. There is often a strong family history of CHD and affected individuals may have a raised cholesterol, a raised triglyceride or both. In fact the particular pattern of lipid abnormalities may vary in the same individual, particularly with respect to plasma triglyceride. Definitive diagnosis is difficult but family screening is very useful showing variable forms of hyperlipidaemia within affected members of a single family. The risk of CHD is high regardless of the particular lipid pattern seen. Tendon xanthomata are not present in this condition.

The metabolic abnormality in this type of hyperlipidaemia appears to be increased hepatic lipoprotein production with increased plasma apoprotein B concentrations[30]. The plasma lipid pattern will vary depending on the efficiency of the catabolism of the lipoproteins. The condition is inherited as an autosomal dominant but the genetic defect remains unknown.

POLYGENIC HYPERCHOLESTEROLAEMIA

The diagnosis of polygenic hypercholesterolaemia is made when other causes of hypercholesterolaemia have been excluded. It represents most likely a heterogeneous group of disorders with multiple genes interacting with environmental factors such as obesity and high saturated fat/high cholesterol diets. Corneal arcus and xanthelasma can occur in polygenic hypercholesterolaemia but tendon xanthomata are not seen. The genetic factors responsible for this condition (or conditions) remain to be elucidated fully but the common polymorphisms of apoprotein E account for approximately 7% of the variation in plasma cholesterol[31,32].

REMNANT PARTICLE DISEASE

This interesting condition, also known as dysbetalipoproteinaemia or type III hyperlipidaemia, is generally expressed in early adult life and is associated with a high risk of premature CHD[33]. The clinical hallmark is the presence of yellow streaking of the palmar creases with soft tissue nodules either side of the skin crease. In addition, tuberous xanthomata (soft tissue xanthomata) may be seen on the elbows and knees. Frequent clinical associations are obesity, glucose intolerance and hyperuricaemia.

Both plasma cholesterol and plasma triglyceride show marked elevation due to the accumulation of remnant particles manifest as cholesterol-rich VLDL. Lipoprotein electrophoresis may show the characteristic broad-beta band but better definition of the lipid abnormality is obtained with ultracentrifugation. VLDL isolated by this technique has a molar ratio of cholesterol to triglyceride exceeding 0.6 in remnant particle disease.

Remnant particles are normally rapidly removed by the liver following hydrolysis of chylomicrons and VLDL by the enzyme lipoprotein lipase. The recognition of remnant particles by the liver depends on apoprotein E. There are three major isoforms of this apoprotein, E_2, E_3 and E_4, and they differ with respect to their ability to be recognized by the liver. The great majority of patients with remnant particle disease are E_2 homozygotes. As this occurs in approximately one in a hundred people, and the frequency of the disease itself is only one in five thousand, it is apparent that a further metabolic abnormality is required in the E_2 homozygote for the development of hyperlipidaemia such as the coexistence of other primary hyperlipidaemias, particularly familial combined hyperlipidaemia and causes of secondary hyperlipidaemia, such as diabetes mellitus, hypothyroidism and renal disease.

CHYLOMICRONAEMIA SYNDROME

Accumulation of chylomicrons in the fasting state may occur in several rare conditions[34]. The autosomal recessive disorder, lipoprotein lipase deficiency (prevalence 1 per million) may be manifest in childhood as chylomicronaemia due to ineffective clearance of chylomicrons. The fasting plasma triglyceride level is about 10 mmol/l, but this may rise rapidly after a fatty meal. The plasma cholesterol tends to be normal. Of the other lipoproteins VLDL may be normal or slightly elevated, and LDL and HDL are low. Several families have been described with chylomicronaemia because of a genetic absence of apoprotein C-II which is required for normal activation of lipoprotein lipase.

Lipaemia retinalis, eruptive xanthomata and hepatosplenomegaly due to the accumulation of fatty macrophages are the clinical hallmarks of chylomicron-aemia. However, the most serious clinical feature is pancreatitis, possibly due to plugging of the pancreatic capillaries by chylomicrons. An important practical point is that lipaemic plasma may produce unreliable plasma amylase assays and therefore hinder the diagnosis of pancreatitis.

Chylomicronaemia in adults affects about 3 in a thousand subjects. It is accompanied by an elevated VLDL which explains the associated hypercholesterolaemia. Secondary causes are responsible for many cases of chylomicronaemia such as diabetes or alcohol excess but a minority appear to have a primary abnormality which has been termed familial hypertriglycerid-aemia. The metabolic defect in this condition is not yet known. The activity of the enzyme lipoprotein lipase is generally normal and apoprotein C-II concentrations are also normal. VLDL production is increased but whether VLDL accumulates in plasma (and in the more severe cases chylomicrons) will depend on the coexistence of impaired clearance due to unknown mechanisms. Autosomal dominant transmission is the most likely inheritance pattern and clinical features resemble those for lipoprotein lipase and apoprotein C-II deficiency.

PRIMARY HDL ABNORMALITIES

Moderate elevation of total plasma cholesterol may be due to a high HDL concentration. This condition is reported to be associated with increased life expectancy[35]. On the other hand, low plasma HDL concentrations have been found in association with a specific DNA polymorphism of the apoprotein A gene. This condition is associated with increased risk of CHD[36].

MANAGEMENT OF THE PRIMARY HYPERLIPIDAEMIAS

It is important to remember that the management of hyperlipidaemia should be a part of general modification of CHD risk factors including anti-smoking advice, the reduction of obesity, the detection and treatment of hypertension and the encouragement of appropriate exercise. Furthermore these other risk factors interrelate with lipid abnormalities; smoking is associated with low HDL concentrations, obesity predisposes to hyperlipidaemia, particularly hypertriglyceridaemia, and some anti-hypertensive drugs may affect lipid profiles adversely.

NUTRITIONAL COUNSELLING

Nutritional counselling is the cornerstone of management of all hyperlipidaemias. Strenuous attempts to achieve weight reduction should be pursued in overweight patients. This is more likely to be effective if there are frequent consultations and mutually agreed target weights with the dietician. Advice is also given on dietary modification with special emphasis on the reduction of total fat intake, particularly saturated fat. The recommendations of the European Atherosclerosis Society[4] covering the general principles of the fat-modified diet are shown in Table 7.5. An important addition to dietary measures is the reduction of alcohol intake. A reduction in total fat to 15% of calories may be necessary when hyperchylomicronaemia is present.

Table 7.5. Dietary principles of the European Atherosclerosis Society[4]

Reduce total fat and particularly saturated fat (10% daily calories)
Moderately increase mono- and polyunsaturated fat (10% calories each)
Decrease dietary cholesterol (<300 mg/day)
Increase high protein, low saturated fat foods
Increase complex carbohydrates, fruit, vegetables
Decrease sodium intake

Dietary measures alone are often sufficient to achieve satisfactory lipid-lowering in polygenic disorders of lipid metabolism. Drug therapy is only considered after a prolonged trial of dietary measures, at least three months. The decision to intervene with hypolipidaemic agents is an important one as therapy is life-long and the risk/benefit has to be considered for the individual.

In general terms a condition with high CHD risk (e.g. familial hypercholesterolaemia, familial combined hyperlipidaemia and remnant particle disease); a strong family history; the presence of other risk factors (e.g. hypertension and diabetes mellitus) and a young patient, particularly a man, are factors that argue for drug intervention. Patients with type V hyperlipidaemia may require drug treatment to reduce their risk of pancreatitis.

Available drugs for the treatment of hyperlipidaemia are most easily categorized into those that reduce cholesterol, those that reduce triglyceride and those that reduce both major plasma lipids. Lipid-lowering drugs have recently been reviewed[37].

HYPOCHOLESTEROLAEMIC AGENTS

The resins

These agents (cholestyramine and colestipol) bind bile acids in the intestine, interrupting the enterohepatic circulation and are generally regarded as the first-line drugs in the treatment of hypercholesterolaemia. This leads to stimulation of hepatic synthesis of bile acids from cholesterol and consequent increased expression of LDL receptors on the liver and increased plasma LDL catabolism. Some of the hepatic cholesterol used for new bile acid formation during resin therapy comes from *de novo* cholesterol synthesis which partly overcomes the effectiveness of resins in stimulating LDL receptor activity. However resin therapy is effective in reducing plasma LDL cholesterol by up to 30%. Sometimes plasma triglyceride rises during resin therapy because of increased hepatic synthesis of VLDL. This may be a problem when treating familial combined hyperlipidaemia and the addition of a second drug such as fibrate or nicotinic acid may be required to lower the triglyceride. A slight rise in HDL cholesterol is occasionally seen with resins, which is probably advantageous.

A major advantage of the resins is that they are not absorbed from the intestine. They may also be used in children without apparent adverse effects on growth or development. However compliance with resin therapy is sometimes a problem because of gastrointestinal side-effects, constipation, nausea and a bloating sensation, the incidences of which are dosage-related. Occasionally diarrhoea and colicky pains may occur. Some patients find the preparation of resins time-consuming and the texture gritty.

Resin therapy is started at low dosage and gradually built up. Pre-mixing the granules with water or juice and refrigerating overnight helps to improve the texture. The absorption of drugs may be affected and it is best to take other drugs at least an hour before the resins. Folic acid supplements may be needed in childhood and pregnancy.

Resins are the first choice therapy in heterozygous familial hypercholesterol-aemia and severe polygenic hypercholesterolaemia. Combination drug therapy is often required in familial hypercholesterolaemia and familial combined hyperlipidaemia with resins plus fibrates or nicotinic acid.

Probucol

Probucol therapy results in a moderate reduction in plasma cholesterol through reductions in HDL as well as LDL cholesterol. The mechanisms of action of the drug are not fully understood; however, it appears that the LDL reduction is independent of effects on the LDL receptor. It is possible that the incorporation of probucol in the lipid core of LDL leads to modification of LDL and subsequent increased hepatic catabolism through a receptor independent pathway.

Probucol has not been used as a first line drug because of its effect in lowering HDL. However, an overall beneficial effect of probucol is suggested by the clinical observations of mobilization of tissue and tendon xanthomata. Recently probucol, presumably through its antioxidant properties, has been shown to inhibit oxidative modification of LDL and its interaction with monocyte/ macrophages to form foam cells in vitro. Probucol may theoretically have anti-atherogenic potential and preliminary evidence from LDL receptor deficient rabbits indicates that probucol delays the appearance of atheroma independent of cholesterol-lowering.

Probucol therapy is generally well tolerated with only occasional gastrointestinal upsets. Prolongation of the QT interval has been described but the clinical significance of this is debatable.

DRUGS WITH BOTH HYPERCHOLESTEROLAEMIC AND HYPOTRIGLYCERIDAEMIC PROPERTIES

Fibric acid derivatives

Fibric acid derivatives have several effects on lipoprotein metabolism. The enzyme lipoprotein lipase is stimulated by fibrates resulting in increased catabolism of triglyceride-rich lipoprotein particles. They also reduce cholesterol synthesis through non-specific inhibition of HMG-CoA reductase, the rate-determining enzyme of cholesterol synthesis. Plasma cholesterol and triglyceride are reduced through reduction in VLDL, IDL and LDL. On the other hand HDL cholesterol is increased by fibrates. Clofibrate, the first of the fibrates, predisposes to gallstones through its effect in increasing cholesterol excretion in bile.

Currently there are three fibrates available in the UK but clofibrate has been superseded by bezafibrate and gemfibrozil. Other fibrates including fenofibrate and cipofibrate are available in Europe and may be introduced into the UK in the future. Side effects are few with this class of drugs but untoward effects occur including gastrointestinal upset, a reversible myopathy and impotence. Renal impairment is a relative contraindication to fibrate therapy.

Fibrates are the drugs of choice in type III hyperlipidaemia (remnant particle disease) and are useful in the mixed hyperlipidaemia of familial combined hyperlipidaemia. A resin drug may be needed in addition for the latter condition to reduce LDL levels to satisfactory levels.

NICOTINIC ACID AND DERIVATIVES

Nicotinic acid at high doses is effective in reducing LDL and VLDL levels and increasing HDL through actions unrelated to its role as a vitamin. Nicotinic acid inhibits the release of free fatty acids from adipose tissue and consequently the flow of this substrate for the synthesis of triglyceride in the liver. This action does not fully explain the effectiveness of nicotinic acid in altering plasma lipoprotein levels and there are probably other effects including stimulation of lipoprotein lipase.

Compliance is a problem with nicotinic acid because of flushing and gastrointestinal effects. Tachyphylaxis to the flushing does occur with prolonged therapy and can be reduced by concurrent aspirin therapy as it appears to be prostaglandin-mediated. If therapy is started in low dosage with meals side effects may be reduced.

If tolerated, nicotinic acid is effective in the treatment of familial combined hyperlipidaemia, remnant particle disease and in familial hypercholesterolaemia combined with a resin. However, large doses of nicotinic acid (3–6 g/day) are needed for effective lowering of LDL. At these high doses abnormalities of liver function are sometimes seen together with an increase in uric acid. The presence of peptic ulcer is a relative contraindication to nicotinic acid therapy. Derivatives of nicotinic acid are being developed and one of these, acipimox, has been licensed in the UK. These derivatives tend to be better tolerated.

HMG CoA REDUCTASE INHIBITORS

This exciting new class of hypocholesterolaemic agents are in trial and are licensed for clinical use in some countries including America and the United Kingdom[38]. These drugs are specific competitive inhibitors of the rate-determining step in cholesterol synthesis. By reducing cellular cholesterol synthesis the expression of LDL receptors is increased with a reduction of plasma LDL. Plasma triglycerides are also reduced by mechanisms which remain unclear, and HDL cholesterol increases slightly with these drugs. Reductions in LDL cholesterol of 35% are commonly observed even in the severest cases of hypercholesterolaemia and combined with a resin reductions of over 50% are observed. So far side effects with the HMG CoA reductase inhibitors appear to be few but cases of myopathy have been described. If in the majority of cases these drugs are safe long-term, they will be a very useful addition to the range of hyperlipidaemic agents. The first of the reductase inhibitors to be introduced into the United Kingdom (Zocor) has a licence for the treatment of marked hypercholesterolaemia (>7.8 mmol/l).

HYPOTRIGLYCERIDAEMIC AGENTS

Omega-3 fatty acids

Omega-3 fatty acids are found in fish oils, particularly deep sea oily fish. Experimental diets rich in these fatty acids reduce plasma triglycerides by reducing VLDL synthesis in the liver. There are also effects on prostaglandin metabolism in platelets which reduces platelet activation. MaxEpa, a preparation containing 18% eicosapentaenoic acid is licensed in the UK for the treatment of hypertriglyceridaemia. It is important to monitor LDL levels during therapy with omega-3 fatty acids as in some circumstances LDL may rise.

References

1. Consensus Conferences. (1985). Lowering blood cholesterol to prevent heart disease. *J. Am. Med. Assoc.*, **253**, 2080–6
2. Study Group of the European Atherosclerosis Society. (1987). Strategies for the prevention of coronary heart disease, a policy statement of the European Atherosclerosis Society. *Eur. Heart J.*, **8**, 77–88
3. Shepherd, J., Betteridge, D.J., Durrington, P., Laker, M., Lewis, B., Mann, J., Miller, J.P., Reckless, J.P.D. and Thompson, G.R. (1987). *Br. Med. J.*, **295**, 1245–6
4. Study Group of the European Atherosclerosis Society. (1988). The recognition and management of hyperlipidaemia in adults: a policy statement of the European Atherosclerosis Society. *Eur. Heart J.*, **9**, 571–600
5. Martin, M.J., Hulley, S.B., Browner, W.S., Kuller, L.H. and Wentworth, D. (1986). *Lancet*, **ii**, 933–6
6. Lipid Research Clinics Program. (1984). The Lipid Research Coronary Primary Prevention Trials Results I & II. *J. Am. Med. Assoc.*, **251**, 351–71
7. Frick, M.H., Elo, O., Haapa, *et al.* (1987). Helsinki Heart Study: Primary prevention trial with gemfibrozil in middle-aged men with dyslipidaemia. *N. Engl. J. Med.*, **317**, 1237–45
8. Blankenhorn, D.H., Nessum, S.A. and Johnson, R.L. (1987). *J. Am. Med. Assoc.*, **257**, 3233–40
9. Brown, M.S. and Goldstein, J.L. (1986). *Science*, **191**, 15–4
10. Brown, M.S. and Goldstein, L. (1983). *Ann. Rev. Biochem.*, **52**, 223–61
11. Fagiotto, A., Ross, R. and Harker, L. (1984). *Arteriosclerosis*, **4**, 323–40
12. Shepherd, J. (ed.). (1984). *Lipoprotein Metabolism. Clinical Endocrinology and Metabolism*, Vol. 1, No. 3 (London: Baillière Tindall)

13. Steinberg, D. and Olefsky, J.M. (eds). (1987). *Hypercholesterolaemia and Atherosclerosis, Pathogenesis and Prevention. Contemporary Issues in Endocrinology and Metabolism*, Vol. 3 (Edinburgh: Churchill Livingstone)
14. Castelli, W.P., Garrison, R.J., Wilson, P.W. *et al.* (1986). Incidence of coronary heart disease and lipoprotein cholesterol levels: the Framingham Study. *J. Am. Med.*, **256**, 2835–8
15. Gordon, T., Castelli, W.P., Hjortland, M.C. *et al.* (1987). *Am. J. Med.*, **62**, 707–14
16. Miller, N.E., Forde, O.H., Thelle, D.S. *et al.* (1987). The Tromso Heart Study. High density lipoprotein and coronary heart disease. A prospective case control study. *Lancet*, ii, 965–8
17. Reichl, D. and Miller, N.E. (1986). *Clin. Sci.*, **70**, 221–31
18. Hulley, S.B., Roseman, R.H., Bawal, R.D. *et al.* (1980). *N. Engl. J. Med.*, **302**, 1380–3
19. Castelli, W.P. (1986). *Am. Heart J.*, **112**, 432–7
20. Zilverzmit, D.B. (1978). *Adv. Exp. Med. Biol.*, **109**, 45–59
21. Report of the National Cholesterol Education Programme Expert Panel on detection, evaluation and treatment of high blood cholesterol in adults. (1988). *Arch. Intern. Med.*, **148**, 35–69
22. Friedewald, W.T., Levy, R.I. and Frederickson, D.S. (1972). Estimation of the concentration of low density lipoprotein cholesterol in plasma without use of the preparative ultracentrifuge. *Clin. Chem.*, **18**, 499–502
23. Miller, N.E. (1986). In: Fidge, N.H. and Nestel, P.J. (eds.) *Atherosclerosis VII*. (Amsterdam: Elsevier), 61–4
24. Manninen, V., Elo, M.O., Frick, M.H. *et al.* (1988). *J. Am. Med. Assoc.*, **260**, 641–51
25. Beaumont, J.L., Carlson, L.A., Cooper, G.R., Fejfar, Z., Frederickson, D.S. and Strasser, T. (1970). *The Bulletin of World Health Organisation*, **43**, 891–915
26. Frederickson, D.S., Levy, R.I. and Lees, R.S. (1967). *N. Engl. J. Med.*, **276**, 32–44, 94–103, 148–56, 215–24, 273–81
27. Goldstein, J.L. and Brown, M.S. (1983). In: Stanbury, J.B., Wyngaarden, J.B., Frederickson, D.S., Goldstein, J.L. and Brown, M.S. (eds) *The Metabolic Basis of Inherited Disease*. (New York: McGraw-Hill), 672–712
28. Russell, D.W., Lehrman, M.A., Südhof, T.C. *et al.* (1987). *Cold Spring Harbor Symp. Quant. Biol.*, **51**, 811–19
29. Goldstein, J.L., Schrott, H.G., Hazzard, W.R., Bierman, E.L. and Motulsky, A.G. (1973). *J. Clin. Invest.*, **52**, 1544–68
30. Chait, A., Albers, J.J. and Brunzell, J.D. (1980). *Eur. J. Clin. Invest.*, **10**, 17–22
31. Ehnholm, C., Lukka, M., Kuusi, T., Nikkila, E. and Utermann, G. (1986). *J. Lipid Res.*, **27**, 227–35
32. Sing, C.F. and Davignon, J. (1985). *Am. J. Hum. Gen.*, **37**, 268–85
33. Brown, M.S., Goldstein, J.L. and Frederickson, D.S. (1983). In: Stanbury J.B., Wyngaarden, J.B., Frederickson, D.S., Goldstein, J.L. and Brown, M.S. (eds) *The Metabolic Basis of Inherited Disease*. (New York: McGraw-Hill), 655–71
34. Nikkila, E.A. (1983). In: Stanbury J.B., Wyngaarden, J.B., Frederickson, D.S., Goldstein, J.L. and Brown, M.S. (eds.) *The Metabolic Basis of Inherited Disease*. (New York: McGraw-Hill), 622–42
35. Avogaro, P. (1984). In: Miller, N.E. and Miller, G.J. (eds.) *Clinical and Metabolic Aspects of High Density Lipoproteins*. (Amsterdam: Elsevier), 289–95
36. Ordovas, J.M., Schaefer, E.J., Salem, D. *et al.* (1986). *N. Engl. J. Med.*, **314**, 671–7
37. Illingworth, D.R. (1987). *Drugs*, **33**, 259–79
38. Grundy, S.M. (1988). *N. Engl. J. Med.*, **319**, 24–33

8
Investigation and management of unstable angina

P.A. CREAN

INTRODUCTION

Unstable angina is a clinical term used to describe a number of syndromes of varying aetiology[1]. The need to identify patients with unstable angina is obvious as it frequently leads to myocardial infarction and death[2,3]. The definition of unstable angina is angina pectoris that is increasing in either frequency, duration or intensity in the absence of myocardial necrosis. This definition includes rest angina, variant angina, and angina of recent onset in addition to increasing symptoms in patients whose angina was previously stable. Although by definition a patient who has stable angina and then gets one extra episode of angina per week may be said to have unstable angina, this is not what is meant in clinical practice. Similarly, by definition, every patient must go through an 'unstable' phase when their angina starts but if it only occurs on walking five miles it can hardly be said to be unstable. Thus the practical definition should include a modification, which requires a change in angina symptoms of significant severity to require hospital admission

The pathophysiology of unstable angina has been addressed in detail in an accompanying chapter. From a practical point of investigating and managing, it is necessary to highlight just a few points. Firstly, nearly all patients have significant fixed coronary artery disease. Secondly, the mechanism which leads to the instability of angina may be due to a worsening of the fixed coronary disease[4], to the fissuring of the atheromatous plaque with intra-coronary clot formation[5], or to the superimposition of an element of coronary spasm[6]. In a patient with a 90% coronary artery stenosis a minor further reduction in the coronary diameter due to alteration in coronary tone will lead to critical reduction in myocardial blood supply and angina; whereas, in a patient with only a minimal coronary stenosis it requires a major degree of change in coronary tone to affect myocardial perfusion. Although arguments in the literature would suggest that fixed coronary disease and coronary spasm are mutually exclusive conditions it appears likely that in unstable angina the spectrums overlap considerably. Some patients have a major component of fixed disease, while

135

others have a major variable element, and between these two extremes lie patients with a combination of both. From a practical point of view it is important to direct the investigations to determine where in each patient the balance between fixed and variable stenosis lies. The investigation of unstable angina must include tests to determine why the condition has become unstable and to establish the presence and severity of the underlying coronary artery disease. When these factors have been established, a rationalized treatment plan can be devised for each individual patient.

MANAGEMENT OF UNSTABLE ANGINA

The overall management of unstable angina should include: initial stabilization of the condition with medical therapy; search for the reversible or initiating factors; assessment of the functional coronary reserve; documentation of the state of the underlying coronary disease and left ventricular function by arteriography; and finally a decision regarding long term therapy, be it medical therapy, angioplasty or coronary artery bypass surgery.

INVESTIGATIONS IN UNSTABLE ANGINA

Tests on admission

On admission the patient must have at least a resting ECG, chest X-ray and blood tests. Whether the resting ECC is abnormal, confirming the clinical impression of coronary artery disease, or normal, as it frequently is once the pain has resolved, the initial recording must be obtained for comparison against subsequent recordings. The chest X-ray must be obtained to look for cardiac enlargement and signs of left ventricular failure, which indicate extensive damage to the left ventricle and hence a poor prognosis. To exclude a myocardial infarction a series of normal cardiac enzymes is mandatory. These investigations should be repeated if symptoms recur after treatment.

Search for reversible non-cardiac causes of unstable angina

In all cases, simple causes for a deterioration in the patient's symptoms should be sought. Thyrotoxicosis, arrhythmia and anaemia should be easily detected and treated as illustrated in Figure 8.1. A 73-year-old man with previously stable angina complained of progressively increasing chest pain over three months. His exercise test was stopped during the warm up stage with chest pain and 3 mm ST segment depression at a peak heart rate of 110 beats per minute. At this time the patient had a microcytic anaemia with a haemoglobin level of 8.5 g and when this

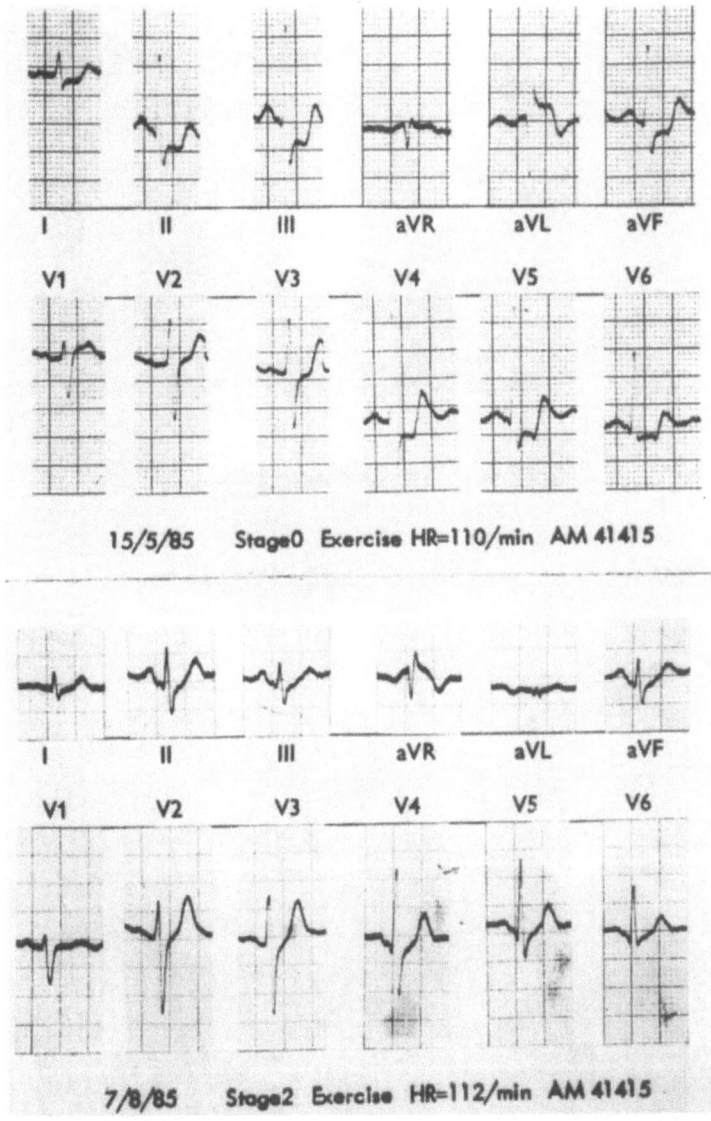

Figure 8.1 Twelve lead ECG at peak exercise, in a patient with significant left anterior descending coronary stenoses and anaemia. The exercise test in the top panel shows significant ST depression that accompanied chest pain at Stage 0 and at heart rate of 110 beats/min. Three months later, when the Hb increased from 8 to 15 g/dl, the patient reached Stage 3 of a modified Bruce protocol without chest pain and minimal ST change (bottom panel)

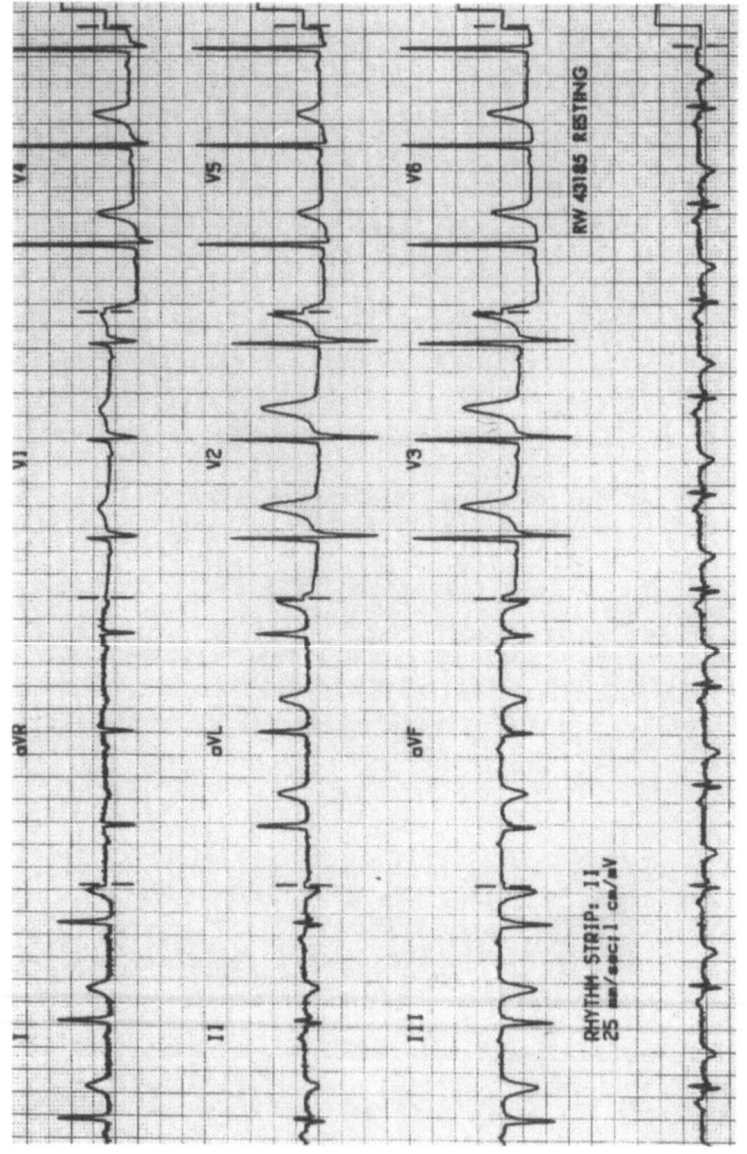

Figure 8.2 (a) The resting ECG of a patient with unstable angina and a previous inferior infarction

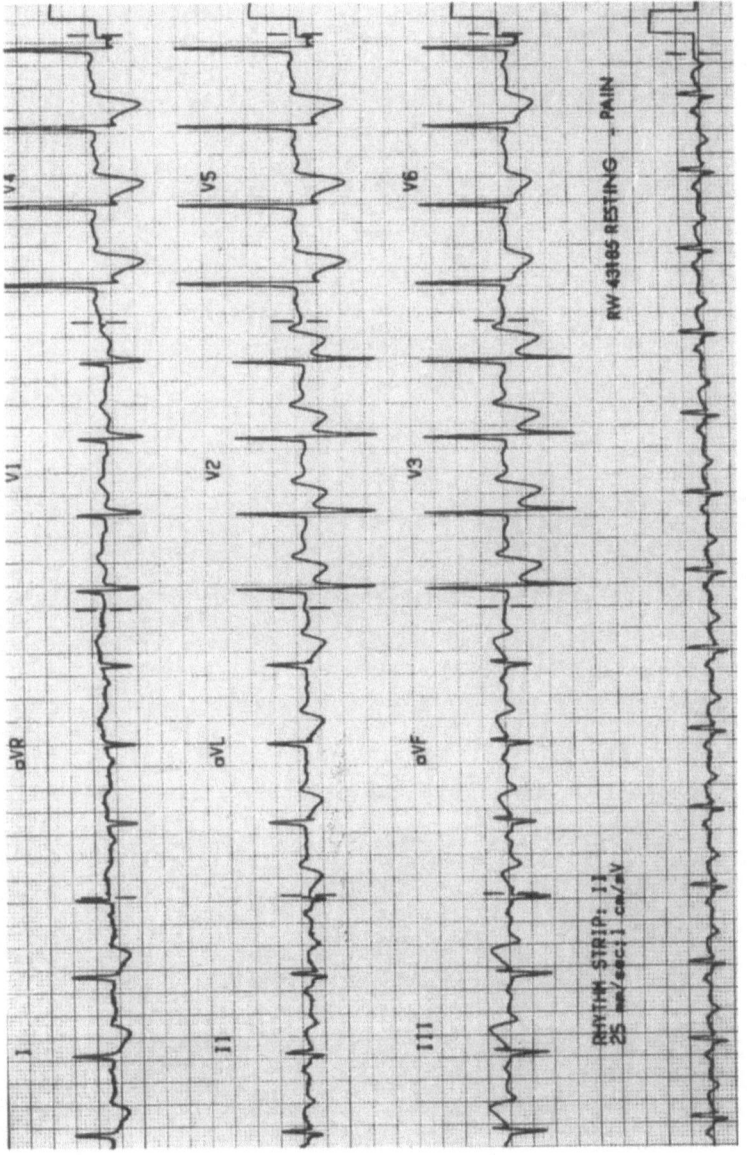

Figure 8.2 **(b)** The 12 lead ECG recording spontaneous chest pain in the same patient showing severe widespread ST segment depression. Coronary angiography demonstrated left main stem disease and a blocked right coronary artery

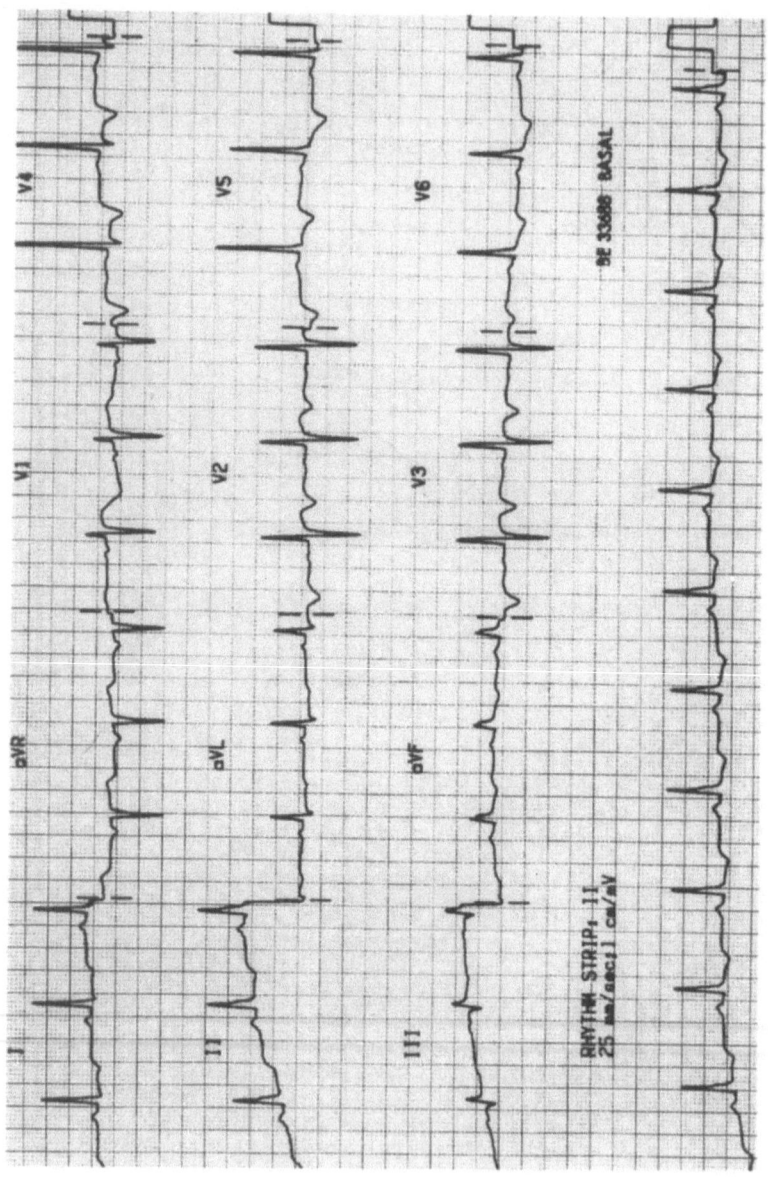

Figure 8.3 (a). Resting ECG in a patient with unstable angina and previous bypass surgery demonstrating widespread T wave depression

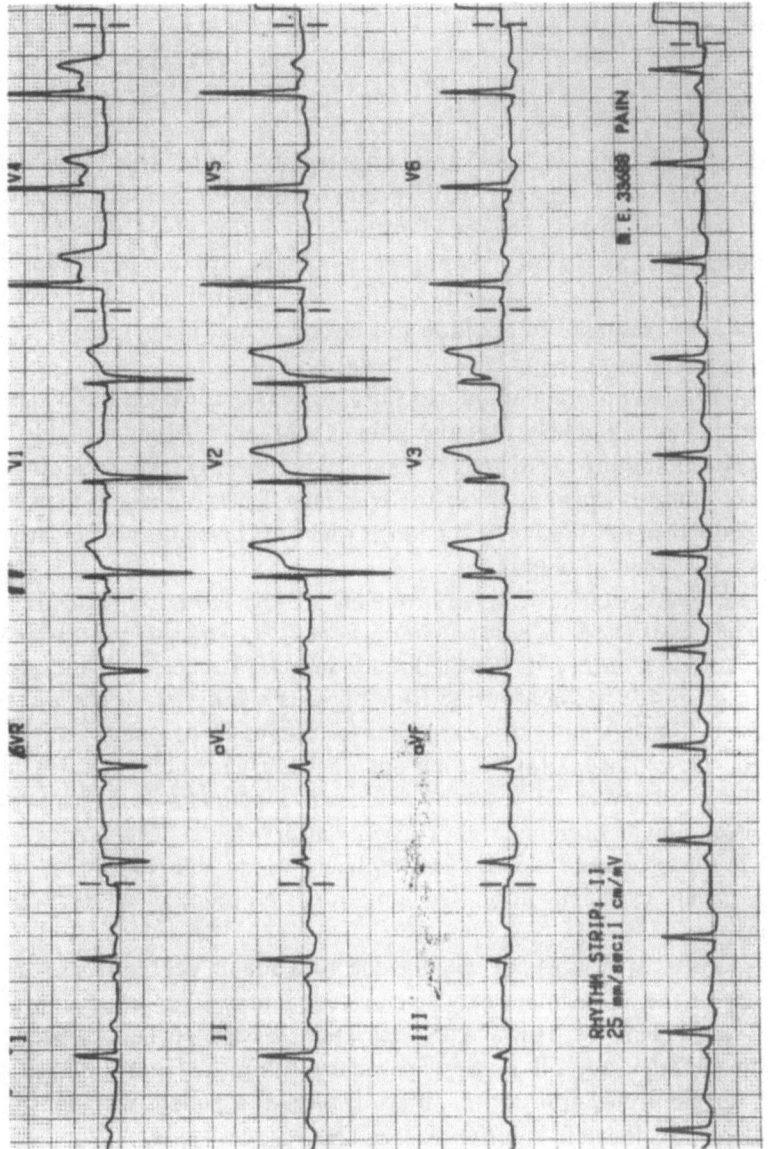

Figure 8.3 (b) During spontaneous chest pain there is new ST segment elevation in the anterior chest leads and pseudonormalization of previous inverted T waves

returned to his previously normal level of 15.3 g his angina settled and the corresponding exercise test to Stage 3 and a peak heart rate of 112 beats per minute shows minimal ST depression (lower panel).

Investigations during initial hospitalization

Electrocardiogram during pain

Patients with unstable angina should be monitored in a ward where a 12 lead ECG can be obtained once the pain occurs preferably before and after sublingual nitrates are given. The ECG recordings during chest pain provide valuable information as to the pathogenesis of the condition. Transient electrocardiographic changes may indicate the site and indeed the extent of underlying coronary disease. In addition the direction and magnitude of ECG changes during pain provide a guide to treatment.

If the basal ECG is normal and fails to show any changes during the patient's typical chest pain it is unlikely that the pain is cardiac in origin and further investigations including provocative tests should be pursued. Having stated this, particular care must be paid to look for transient T wave changes (such as peaking, pseudonormalization or inversion), which in unstable angina are as significant as ST segment changes.

ST segment depression or T wave inversion are the most frequent accompanying changes with chest pain. The sites where ECG changes are observed point to the coronary artery in which disease may be expected. Widespread anterior ST segment depression during pain suggests significant stenosis in the proximal part of the left anterior descending or left main coronary artery. In Figure 8.2 the electrocardiogram during spontaneous pain demonstrates new transient widespread severe ST segment changes in a patient who had a severe left main stenosis and an occluded right coronary artery. The mechanism causing pain with ST segment depression is more likely to be due to severe fixed coronary narrowings especially if the ischaemia is not preceded by an increase in the heart rate[7].

In those patients with unstable angina due to a major degree of coronary spasm during pain the ST segment may be elevated, depressed or associated with only minor T wave changes[8]. However, ST elevation, T wave peaking or pseudonormalization during pain all suggest coronary spasm[8]. Figure 8.3 shows transient ST segment elevation in the anterior leads in a patient with spasm in the proximal part of the left anterior descending coronary artery. Ventricular arrhythmias are a frequent accompaniment with spontaneous pain and ST segment changes[9]. These arrhythmias usually resolve with the relief of the pain, however. Figure 8.4 shows a 24 hour tape recording of a patient with angina ST segment depression and sudden death. The atrial fibrillation had been present for some time but new ST segment depression can be seen to precede the onset

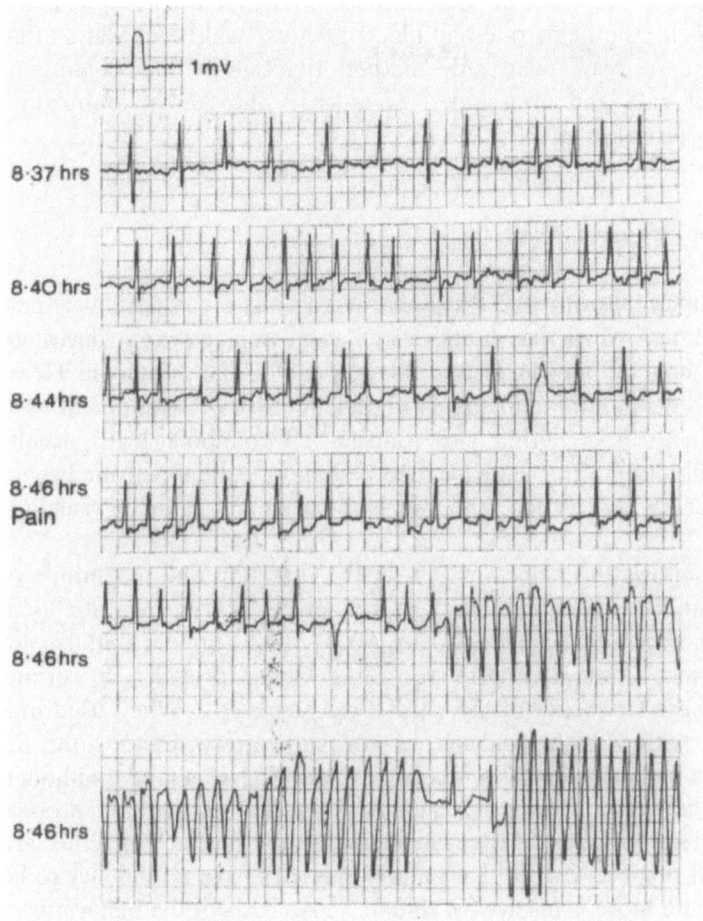

Figure 8.4. Continuous strip from a 24 hour recording in a patient with longstanding atrial fibrillation and unstable angina. ST segment depression and chest pain precede a number of ventricular ectopics, which initiated the onset of ventricular tachycardia

of chest pain, the rhythm then degenerated into ventricular tachycardia and later fibrillation.

The heart rate during chest pain has been used by some groups as a guide to treatment[10]. If ST segment depression is associated with an increase in heart rate or blood pressure (rate pressure product) it indicates that ischaemia is secondary to increased myocardial oxygen demand, which is therefore best treated with β-blocking agents. Should the pain and ECG changes not be associated with an increase in rate pressure product, then a primary reduction in coronary flow may be suspected and treated with calcium antagonist[6]. To implement this approach, continuous recordings of the heart rate must be obtained prior to and at the onset of pain; because if a single recording is made after the onset of pain, the heart rate and blood pressure will be elevated as an autonomic response to pain. The only method that allows this continuous evaluation of heart rate and even blood pressure is the use of ambulatory recording devices referred to later[11].

Ambulatory ST segment monitoring

Ambulatory 24 hour monitoring of ST segment changes is a comparatively new investigative technique, which has mainly been used as a research device to understand the pathogenic mechanisms of chest pain[12]. The American Heart Association has laid down minimum standard guidelines for the equipment used so that the ST segment can be faithfully reproduced[13]. Two bipolar leads, usually a modified CM5, and an inferior lead are recorded and a patient activated event marker and timer are also recorded. The tape is replayed and analysed visually[14] or by computer[11].

This technique allows the determination of the direction and magnitude of ST segment shifts and the estimation of their frequency. By studying patients in this way it has been shown that most episodes (80%) of ST segment shift are not associated with pain, thus symptom recording alone provides a serious underestimation of the frequency of myocardial ischaemia[12,15]. When used in a patient population with a high incidence of coronary artery disease, the ST segment shifts have been proven to be due to myocardial ischaemia[15]; although in each patient, the records must be examined carefully to exclude posture induced changes. The episodes of silent and painful myocardial ischaemia are similar in nearly all respects except that painful episodes have a tendency to be of longer duration and more extensive ST shifts[12,16]. Analysis of the behaviour of the heart rate response in association to the ST segment changes provides useful information as to the pathogenesis of angina (Figure 8.5).

In unstable angina the occurrence of silent ST segment depression in patients despite the use of conventional medical therapy has been shown to be associated with adverse outcome in the following two years[17]. In a study of 70 patients with unstable angina on medical treatment, 37 patients with ST segment changes had 10 infarcts and 11 required revascularization while in 33 patients with no ST changes only 2 had infarction and 5 required revascularization in the following two year period ($p < 0.05$)[17]. In this study, using a Cox hazard analysis, the best predictor of further problems in follow up was the finding of ST segment depression despite medical therapy. Thus in unstable angina continuous ST segment monitoring provides insight into the mechanisms causing unstable angina and useful clinical information.

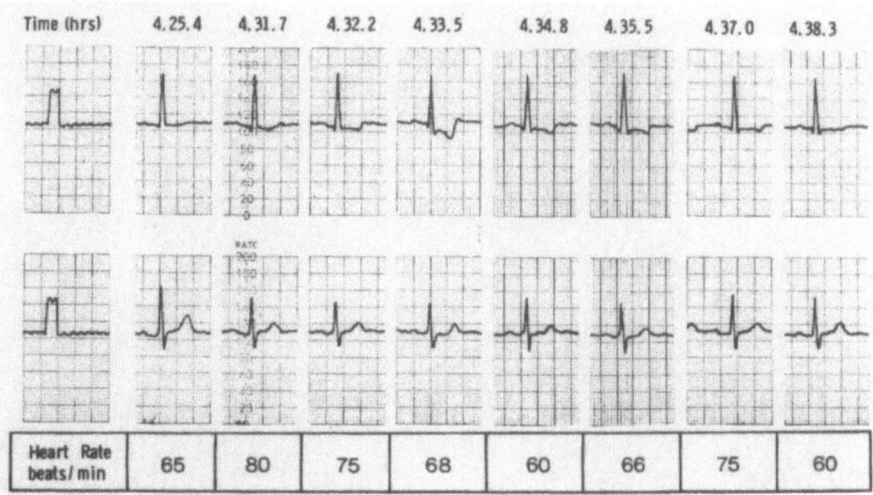

Time (hrs)	4.25.4	4.31.7	4.32.2	4.33.5	4.34.8	4.35.5	4.37.0	4.38.3

| Heart Rate beats/min | 65 | 80 | 75 | 68 | 60 | 66 | 75 | 60 |

Figure 8.5 Simultaneous ECG complexes from an anterior and inferior lead using FM 24 hour monitoring during an episode of painful ST segment depression. The top row shows the time of each complex and the lower row shows the heart rate at that time. This system provides useful information regarding the pathological mechanisms and treatment of the condition

Exercise testing

Stress testing electrocardiography in stable angina is a useful non-invasive test, which provides an important guide to the presence and severity of coronary artery stenosis[18] and also a guide to subsequent prognosis[19]. Exercise testing following myocardial infarction is also a safe test, which provides useful prognostic information[20]. Until recently, exercise tests were avoided in unstable angina as it was feared that infarction may be provoked by the stress. It has now been shown that patients may exercise safely some days following stabilization using a gentle protocol[21,22] with the exercise terminated by the onset of 1 mm ST change, a drop in blood pressure, angina, frequent ectopic beats or a heart rate of 70% of the age predicted maximal (Figure 8.6).

Early exercise tests performed 4 days after the last episode of chest pain in 72 patients provided a good long term guide to symptomatic status. Twenty nine of 32 patients (90%) with a positive test had severe angina (Grade 3–4 NYHA), while only 7 of 32 (21%) with a negative exercise test had severe angina at follow up one year later[23]. Similar findings with regard to the prediction of symptomatic status six months after discharge were also reported by Nixon *et al.* in a study of 55 patients[24]. Submaximal exercise testing also provided a guide to the severity of coronary disease present with 27/29 positive tests being in patients with multivessel disease[23]. The high incidence of false negative tests in that report further emphasizes the need for angiography in patients with unstable angina[23]. When combined with clinical findings and angiographic results, exercise tests

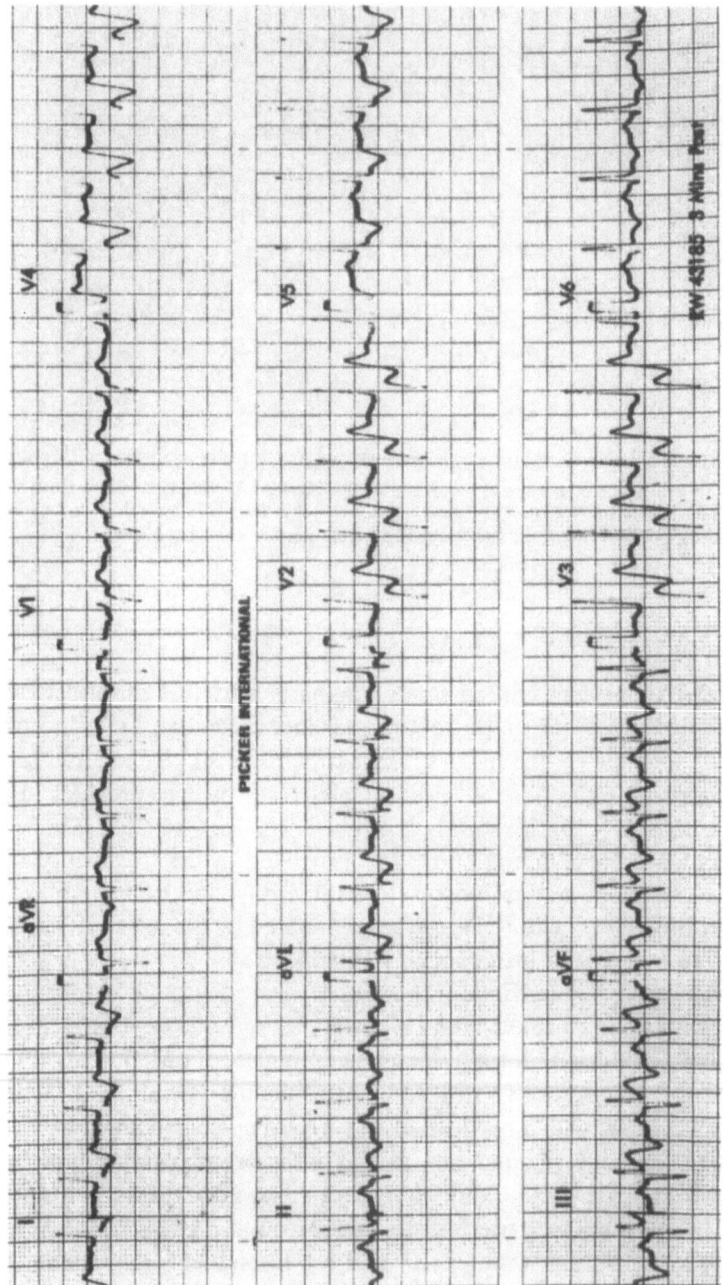

Figure 8.6 Twelve lead exercise ECG of the patient whose resting trace is shown in Figure 8.2 (a). This shows widespread ST depression exercise. This occurred with chest pain and a drop in the blood pressure during the warm up stage indicating an extensive area of myocardium subtended by a severe coronary stenosis

may be used to define a rational plan for those who may need early intervention by either coronary angioplasty or bypass surgery.

In patients with rest angina due to coronary artery spasm, stress testing may be used to induce myocardial ischaemia. The changes induced by exercise are also due to induced coronary spasm but do not give a reliable guide to the severity of the underlying coronary disease or prognosis. In a study of patients reported by Waters et al. one third of patients had ST segment elevation, one third ST segment depression, and the remainder no ST change. The results had very poor correlation with the extent of underlying coronary artery disease but related closely with the disease activity[25,26]. In a recent paper, however, when patients with variant angina were tested while on treatment with calcium antagonists to block any exercise induced spasm the results obtained were indicative of the severity of fixed underlying coronary stenoses. In 57 patients who exercised on treatment reported by Araki et al. 48 were negative and 9 positive. All 9 patients with a positive exercise test had significant stenoses, while only 2 of 48 patients with a negative test had significant disease (sensitivity 100%, specificity 96%)[27].

CORONARY ARTERIOGRAPHY

Coronary arteriography should be performed on all patients with unstable angina prior to hospital discharge. Ideally the angiographic examination should be performed some days after the patient has been rendered free of chest pain or earlier in those patients in whom spontaneous pain persists despite oral and parenteral therapy. Arteriography is only contraindicated when an intervention such as angioplasty or surgery is not a viable mode of treatment because of advanced age, systemic disease or known inoperable coronary disease. The examination may be performed via the femoral or brachial routes with adequate heparinization. In severe cases, a low ionic concentration contrast medium is preferable. Patients frequently experience pain during the procedure, which is best avoided by the continuous infusion of nitrates throughout the test.

The cause of unstable angina is multifactorial with a common element of fixed coronary arterial stenoses in over 90% of cases. Coronary arteriography in patients presenting with unstable angina reveals a high incidence of occluded or severely narrowed coronary arteries[28]. This high incidence of coronary disease has been confirmed by widespread intervention studies in patients with refractory chest pain and in the early stages of myocardial infarction[29]. The presence of multiple severe strictures alone does not explain the instability of unstable angina as a similar pattern of coronary arterial disease is observed in those patients undergoing elective investigation for the presence of chronic stable angina[30]. There are, however, a number of interesting angiographic observations to be noted. The incidence of normal coronary arteries in patients with unstable angina is approximately 10% and appears to be higher in those with recent-onset angina. Disease of a single vessel (usually the left anterior descending) was found in 31 of 75 patients with recent-onset angina[31], while triple vessel disease was present in only 10% of cases. In contrast to this a much higher incidence of multiple and/or multisegment vessel disease was found in those patients who had previous anginal symptoms[7]. Further interesting data come from a careful retrospective study from the Montreal Heart Institute. They demonstrated that progression of coronary artery disease was significantly more common in patients with unstable angina compared to those with stable angina, both groups being comparable for other variables[4].

Early angiographic studies in unstable angina have demonstrated the frequent occurrence of clot formation within the artery giving it a characteristic appearance of a filling defect or persistent dye staining[32]. This clot formation is usually associated with an excentric type lesion with irregular edges and suggests the recent worsening of an atherosclerotic plaque or the formation of a fissure in the plaque[33]. The irregular edges are in clear contrast of the findings of smooth borders of the stenotic lesions in patients with stable angina[34]. These findings have been supported by the intraoperative findings and by direct visualization with the use of angioscopy[5].

The prevalence of arterial spasm in patients with fixed coronary stenosis and unstable angina has been estimated at between 5 and 90% depending largely on the referral pattern to the reporting centres. Even in the presence of a large atherosclerotic plaque there is nearly always a non-diseased portion of the arterial wall, which can contract normally. This finding has been shown by Brown *et al.* in cases of both stable angina where there may be a critical reduction in the diameter in addition to an already tight stenosis[35]. An example of the latter is shown in Figure 8.7, which shows the angiograms of a patient with recent-onset unstable angina. The basal angiogram demonstrates a tight proximal left anterior descending artery stenosis. The patient's typical chest pain and anterior ST segment elevation were reproduced by hyperventilation and the stenosed artery was seen to occlude. All of these changes resolved with intra-coronary nitrates leaving a tight residual stenosis.

PROVOCATIVE TESTS IN UNSTABLE ANGINA

The provocative tests outlined below should only be performed with knowledge of the patient's coronary artery anatomy, and in patients in whom continuous observation has failed to yield a changing electrocardiogram during chest pain. Hence, the indications for such tests are (a) atypical chest pain with normal electrocardiogram, (b) a history suggestive of variant angina but no spontaneous episodes observed, and (c) as a research test to assess the effect of treatment in variant angina. No patient with left main, triple vessel disease or poor left ventricular function should undergo these tests.

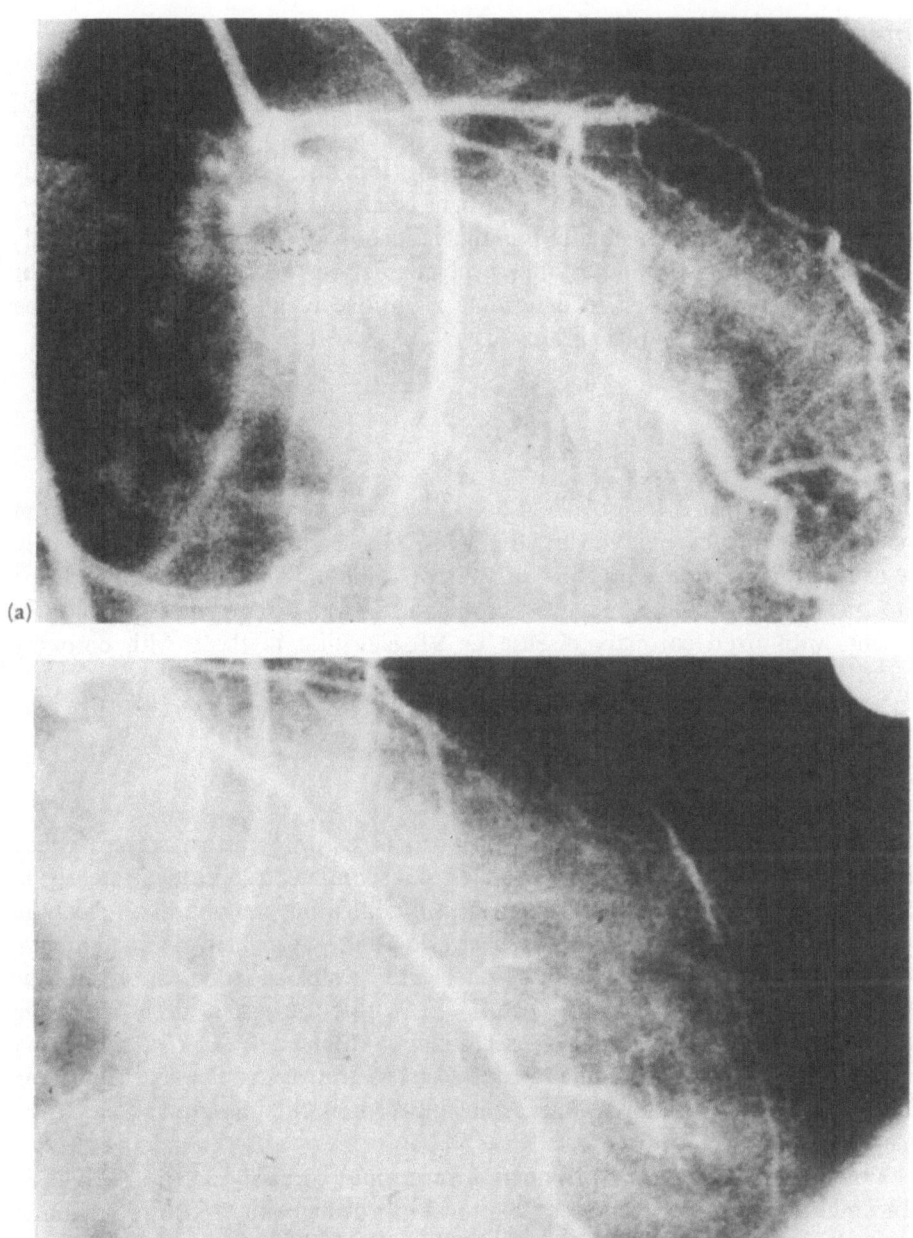

Figure 8.7 (a) Selective left coronary angiogram in the right anterior oblique projection with a significant proximal stenosis in the left anterior descending artery
(b) Repeat angiography in the same projection following hyperventilation which induced chest pain and ST elevation shows near total occlusion of the left anterior descending artery. The changes resolved completely following nitrate administration

Hyperventilation test

The patient is asked to breathe deeply and fast for at least two minutes and preferably five. Arterial samples may be taken before and after to ensure adequate shift of the pH to >7.5. During the test, the patient frequently experiences tingling in the fingers and light-headedness. As the test progresses, the heart rate increases slightly but the induction of coronary spasm usually occurs in the first two minutes after hyperventilation. The standard criteria for ST segment shift are used to determine a positive result. The test should be terminated with intravenous nitrates[36].

Cold pressor test

The aim of this test is to provoke a potent increase in alpha sympathetic output and hence reduce coronary artery diameter. One hand should be immersed in ice cold water to the level of the wrist for two minutes[37]. The alteration in heart rate and blood pressure may be accompanied by ST segment depression in patients with fixed coronary disease or ST elevation in those with coronary spasm.

Ergonovine test

This test is a sensitive test for the diagnosis of coronary artery spasm, which reproduces the chest pain and ST changes of a spontaneous episode in nearly all cases[38]. The test has been associated with fatalities but may be done safely in either the coronary care unit or at arteriography, provided an incremental dosage technique is used and nitrates are given as soon as diagnostic electrocardiographic changes are seen[38-40]. Whilst the test is performed, the patient should have his blood pressure and a 12 lead ECG recorded every minute during and for 10 minutes after the test. Nitrates, atropine and lignocaine should be drawn up ready to inject and full resuscitation equipment should be available.

Ergonovine causes a 20% reduction in normal coronary arteries, while an abnormal response is interpreted as a focal narrowing with >50% reduction in coronary diameter. The electrocardiographic changes most often observed are ST segment elevation in patients with variant angina which starts abruptly, while in patients with fixed severe lesions, segment depression is more likely due to the increase in left ventricular volume and minor reduction in coronary diameter rather than focal coronary spasm.

TREATMENT OF UNSTABLE ANGINA

Patients should be initially confined to bed and monitored in a coronary care unit. A simple step-wise approach to treatment in each case rather than the routine use of a large number of drugs in all cases is the best approach.

NITRATES

The first line of treatment in unstable angina must include a short acting nitrate preparation. Nitroglycerin will relieve the acute ischaemic episode irrespective of whether it occurs at rest or is exercise induced and whether it is associated with fixed or dynamic coronary obstruction. Nitrates when given by different routes exert the same haemodynamic effects but over a different time span and to a different magnitude.

The beneficial effects of nitrates are shown in Figure 8.8. The peripheral vasodilating effect results in a fall in systemic vascular resistance (afterload). The venous pooling effect decreases the ventricular end-diastolic volume (preload). Both effects are additive in reducing myocardial oxygen demand[41]. In unstable angina the direct coronary arterial dilating effect is probably the most important effect as most episodes occur at rest and are often not preceded by an increase in myocardial oxygen consumption. Nitrates dilate all the coronary arterial tree including the stenotic areas and indeed probably the stenoses to a greater degree than the normal artery[35].

Intravenous nitrates should be started at a low dose and increased as necessary. The dose should be titrated against the systolic blood pressure and symptoms. The maximal dose that can be administered is limited by the side effects of excessive vasodilators, i.e. headache and hypotension. In those patients in whom there are severe multiple coronary stenoses and little coronary reserve and in whom minimal exertion produces myocardial ischaemia, intravenous nitrates should be used with β-adrenergic blockers because the tachycardia and hypotensive effects of large doses of nitrates may be detrimental.

In variant angina, intravenous nitrates and placebo have been compared in a randomized double-blind cross-over study of 12 patients. The number of episodes of ST segment shift fell from a mean of 97 during placebo to 16 during a similar time interval with intravenous nitrates. Active treatment was as effective in reducing episodes of ischaemia, both silent and with pain, and equally in episodes that were associated with either ST elevation or depression[42]. In all 12 cases the authors reported an improvement in symptoms. Intravenous nitrates either on their own or as combined therapy can be expected to render over 60% of patients asymptomatic.

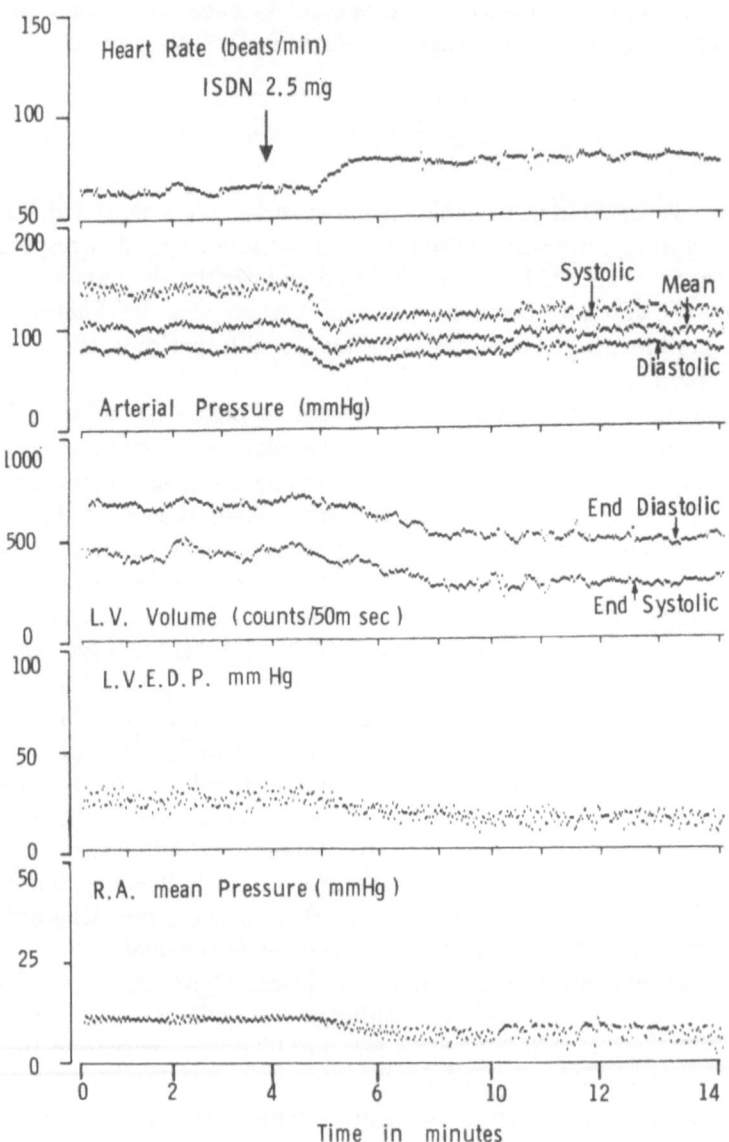

Figure 8.8 Continuous computer analysed recordings of heart rate, arterial pressure, left ventricular end diastolic pressure, LV volume using red cell labelling and right atrial pressure before, during and after the administration of nitrates. Following nitrate injection there is a decrease in left ventricular volume and filling pressure (preload) in association with a fall in blood pressure (afterload). There is a minimal rise in heart rate and fall in aortic diastolic pressure

CALCIUM ANTAGONISTS

The introduction of calcium antagonists has added a potent new regime for the treatment of angina[43]. The calcium channel agents presently available have similar basic properties but many differing effects that make one or other more suitable in certain conditions. Nifedipine is a potent vasodilator with little depressant effect on contractility and conduction, whereas verapamil potently depresses these two functions and diltiazem lies somewhere in between in its spectrum of effects. All three agents are given orally and are effective in improving exercise tolerance in patients with chronic stable angina[43].

In addition, calcium channel blocking drugs have been shown to block coronary artery spasm, either spontaneous or induced by ergonovine, with similar degrees of success both in the short term and during long term follow up[44]. Verapamil was reported as effective in controlling rest pain and has subsequently been demonstrated to be an effective treatment of angina in a randomized prospective trial by Parodi[45] in a double-blind cross-over trial of alternating placebo and verapamil 480 mg daily in 12 patients. The number of episodes of ST segment shift per 48 hour treatment period fell from a mean of 127 with placebo to 27 with verapamil, a highly significant effect. Metha reported a similar beneficial effect of verapamil in 15 patients with unstable angina studied in a further placebo controlled randomized trial[46]. Nifedipine has also been shown as effective in controlling symptoms in a randomized trial of 128 patients reported by Gerstenblith[47]. In this study, the addition of nifedipine to conventional medical therapy significantly reduced the incidence of death, surgery and infarction compared to placebo treatment. The three previous studies included patients with rest angina and both ST segment elevation and depression; whereas the overall effect of nifedipine and verapamil appears similar, it is important to note that verapamil was equally effective irrespective of the direction of the ST segment shift while nifedipine was only effective in those patients with elevation. Diltiazem in common with the other calcium antagonists is excellent in controlling spontaneous or ergonovine induced coronary artery spasm[44]. When patients with variant angina were excluded from a randomized trial in unstable angina diltiazem showed a significant reduction in the number of daily episodes of chest pain from 0.75 with placebo to 0.25 with therapy[43]. With long term follow up (4 to 5 months) diltiazem alone controlled symptoms in 42% of patients, while nifedipine in addition to propranolol, controlled 39% of patients satisfactorily[47,48].

Nifedipine should be started in a dosage of 10 mg t.d.s. and increased to 20 mg t.d.s. if necessary. Further increase in therapy is likely to result in side effects such as headache, hypotension and ankle swelling and other therapeutic regimes should be sought. Nifedipine has no effect on intra-cardiac conduction and thus may be safely combined with a β-adrenergic blocking effect. This combination is often effective as the β-blocker will prevent the reflex tachycardia induced by the potent vasodilator effect. Verapamil is an agent with many properties similar to β-blockers in its depressant effect on the atrioventricular node and on myocardial contractility. Thus, verapamil and β-blockers should not be combined except in carefully monitored situations. Verapamil should be avoided in patients with atrioventricular block or heart failure. The initial dosage of 40 mg t.d.s. may be augmented to 120 mg t.d.s. as required to gain symptomatic relief. Diltiazem has a spectrum of effects that lie somewhere between nifedipine and verapamil. It should be used in a dosage of 90 mg t.d.s. at least for effective control of unstable angina but this may be increased to 120 mg t.d.s.

β-ADRENERGIC BLOCKING AGENTS

β-adrenergic blocking drugs reduce the oxygen demands of the contracting myocardium by reducing the rate and force of myocardial contraction. At rest the heart rate and blood pressure are lowered, while on exercise the rate of increase of both of these indices is delayed. Hence they are effective in reducing exercise induced myocardial ischaemia, although it appears to be achieved by a more complicated mechanism than that which is simply outlined above[49]. Whatever their exact mode of action, they improve total exercise duration by approximately 30% in chronic stable angina and are equally effective in reducing episodes of ST segment depression and angina which are not preceded by an increase in heart rate as those episodes which occur following a rise in heart rate[49].

Since their introduction, β-blocking agents have been used either on their own or with nitrate preparations in order to treat unstable angina with good results. Indeed β-blockers have been accepted as effective therapy to such a degree that this type of treatment is the yardstick against which any new intervention (such as new drugs, surgery or coronary dilatation) must be evaluated[48,50]. With the realization that β-blockers may worsen symptoms in certain cases that have a vasospastic component, a number of studies have suggested that calcium antagonists are more effective than β-blockers in unstable angina. In the report by Gerstenblith, the addition of a calcium blocker to the already prescribed β-blocker resulted in improved success rate of medical therapy; however, this improvement was confined to those with ST elevation at rest[47]. In Parodi's study, the failure of propranolol to improve symptoms in unstable angina, as compared to the significant effect of verapamil, was due to the high percentage of patients with coronary spasm included in the study.

Given that clinicians now avoid β-blockers in variant angina, it is unfair to compare the results of treatment with calcium antagonists and β-blockers in unstable angina when a large proportion of the patients have variant angina. In the report by Theroux, in which treatment with propranolol was compared to diltiazem in patients with unstable angina specifically excluding patients with variant angina, the results of the two drug treatments were comparable. During hospital admission, the number of anginal attacks per day fell from 0.75 with placebo to 0.25 with diltiazem and 0.29 with propranolol. In the long term follow up of 5.1 months the control of symptoms, rates of myocardial infarction or death were similar in both groups[48]. Thus β-blocking agents are effective in controlling unstable angina when variant angina is excluded.

In unstable angina β-blockers should be started in a small dose. We prefer to use propranolol, which is a short acting agent that offers easy changes in dosage. A change to a cardiospecific agent or one which can be administered once daily may be carried out once the condition has been stabilized. β-Blocking agents are contraindicated in heart failure and heart block and should be used with caution in those patients with diabetes, obstructive airways disease and obviously variant angina. Worsening of symptoms in unstable angina after starting β-blockers should raise the possibility of coronary spasm.

Anticoagulants and antiplatelet agents in unstable angina

Antiplatelets

Evidence supporting a role of platelets in unstable angina is derived from the observation of an increase in biochemical markers of increased platelet activation during unstable compared to stable angina[51-53]. In addition, platelet activation could be the unifying event that leads to coronary vasospasm or thrombosis in the region of a ruptured atherosclerotic lesion.

Aspirin has been shown to be very effective in unstable angina. Lewis *et al.* reported a study randomizing 1266 men with unstable angina given 324 mg aspirin or placebo daily[54]. As early as three months following unstable angina mortality was reduced by 50% in the aspirin compared to the placebo group and this difference was highly significant at one year, being 5.5 and 9.6% in the respective groups ($p = 0.008$). The incidence of death and myocardial infarction was also significantly decreased by aspirin. In a subsequent trial in Canada 555 patients were randomised to aspirin, sulphinpyrazone, both or neither. No significant effect was observed with sulphinpyrazone, aspirin reduced the incidence of death by 71% ($p < 0.004$) and the incidence of deaths and myocardial infarctions by 51% ($p < 0.0008$)[55].

In variant angina there is convincing evidence to suggest that platelet activation is not the cause of coronary spasm. Firstly, in a series of observations increase in thromboxane B2 levels occurred at least 30 seconds after ST segment elevation suggesting platelet aggregation in a secondary rather than a primary event[56]. In two clinical trials, antiplatelet agents failed to reduce the incidence of spontaneous attacks as monitored by 24 hour ST segment analysis. Indomethacin, 50 mg eight hourly, prevents platelet aggregation but did not affect the frequency of angina – neither did low dose aspirin therapy or dipyridamole[57]. Prostacyclin given by intravenous infusion prevents platelet aggregation and reduces blood pressure by a direct vasodilating effect but again produced no improvement in spontaneous angina[58].

Anticoagulants

Nichol *et al.* reported impressive data in 318 patients suggesting a role for anti-coagulants in unstable angina[59]. A recent study, in 479 patients, with unstable compared the clinical outcome in three groups treated with aspirin 325 mg b.d., heparin 1000 units/hour or both together was compared to placebo treatment[60]. There was a significant reduction in the incidence of refractory angina and myocardial infarction in those patients receiving aspirin and/or heparin compared to placebo which was highly significant ($p < 0.01$). There was a trend favouring the use of heparin alone and the addition of aspirin to heparin did not improve the outcome but did not increase the risks of serious bleeding[60].

CORONARY ARTERY BYPASS SURGERY

In chronic stable angina coronary artery bypass surgery relieves angina and improves survival in certain subgroups of patients with specific coronary stenoses, while having a low mortality and morbidity[61]. Emergency bypass surgery in unstable angina was initially performed with a high mortality rate but this has now been reduced to less than 2%, thus rendering it a possible option for the treatment of unstable angina[62].

There have been a number of randomized prospective studies comparing surgical and medical therapy in unstable angina, the largest of which, the National Cooperative Unstable Angina Study, randomized 288 patients[50]. This trial excluded patients with left main stenosis, severe triple vessel disease and poor left ventricular function. The results of the study demonstrated an in hospital mortality of 3% in the medical group and 5% in the surgical group and a late mortality (68 months) of 16% and 15% for the respective groups ($p =$ ns). The incidence of infarction was higher in the surgical group compared to the medical group for both early 17% vs 8% and late results 33% vs 18% ($p < 0.05$). These results of no significant improvement in mortality with surgery in unstable angina are supported by similar findings from Seldon *et al.* and Pugh *et al.*[63,64]. One study from Bertolasi suggested that what they classified as an intermediate syndrome showed better results when managed surgically, but this may have been due to the inclusion of left main stem and other subgroups known to require surgery[65].

Although these studies showed no overall mortality benefit of surgery in unstable angina, they demonstrated that if necessary surgery may be performed with low mortality. They also showed a clear long term improvement in symptoms for those undergoing early surgery and also a high cross-over from the medical to surgical group during follow up; a finding supported by a later five-year follow up study in patients having surgery for unstable angina[66].

In a review of 14 reports of coronary artery bypass surgery in unstable angina from 1978 to 1988 Kaiser *et al.* studied the outcome, both short and long-term in

6136 patients. They found a mean operative mortality of 3.7%, the perioperative infarction rate was 9.9%. They concluded that although the incidence of perioperative problems was slightly higher the outcome in terms of angina relief, improved survival, and reduction in late nonfatal infarctions is similar in unstable compared to stable angina[67].

The overall policy in unstable angina should include urgent surgery in the early stages for angina, which fails to settle on maximal medical therapy (approximately 3%). In the remaining patients who settle, a high risk group may be combined with angiographic findings of left main stem, triple vessel or proximal left anterior descending and right coronary stenoses. These high risk patients should be operated upon, preferably during that hospital admission. In those patients in whom the symptoms settle and do not appear to be a high risk, surgery may be performed at any time in the future for prognostic or symptomatic reasons.

CORONARY ANGIOPLASTY

The initial limited clinical indications and narrow spectrum of suitable coronary anatomy for percutaneous balloon dilatation has been expanded because of the impressive initial and long term success[68]. Double or triple vessel stenoses may be dilated and total occlusions reopened. Unstable angina was considered a contraindication to angioplasty but except in a limited number of cases with variant angina, it now appears an attractive and effective form of treatment. This is particularly so in the case of recent-onset angina or worsening angina without a long preceding history – in these cases, angiography is likely to show severe single vessel stenoses. Angioplasty is indicated in patients with unstable angina and proximal stenoses in one or two of the major coronary arteries.

Because of the existence of plaque fissuring and the potential for coronary spasm, certain precautions should be followed. All patients should be treated with calcium antagonists before the procedure and β-blockers should be withdrawn. The patient should be stabilized and symptom free for a few days, if at all possible. Intravenous nitrates should be given by infusion throughout the procedure and full heparinization during and following the dilatation. The control angiogram should be repeated after intracoronary nitrates to ensure the stenosis is not due to reversible coronary spasm before dilatation is contemplated.

The results of coronary angioplasty in unstable angina show a high primary success rate in excess of 90% and a low incidence of emergency surgery for complications[69]. In the large series reported by Bentivoglio the results are similar in unstable and stable angina with regard to early and long term success and complications including infarction, emergency surgery and mortality[70-72]. The improved results have resulted from the development of low profile balloon dilatation catheters and steerable guide wires. In Figure 8.9 (a) the coronary

157

arteriogram from a 60-year-old man with a two week history of unstable angina shows a severe proximal left anterior descending coronary artery stenosis. Following dilatation the artery looks normal (Figure 8.9 (b)). The patient became asymptomatic and angiography six months later demonstrated no recurrence of the stenosis. Suryapranata et al. have recently advocated the use of intra-coronary streptokinase in patients who develop total artery occlusion, presumably due to clot formation, at the time of angioplasty, with improved, outcome[69].

A particularly cautionary note must be made with respect to patients with variant angina. The experience of the Montreal Heart Institute suggests that although a good angiographic result may be obtained at the time of dilatation, there is a 70% recurrence rate. Indeed their results of dilatation in this setting do not improve either the morbidity or mortality of the condition compared to its medical treated outcome with calcium antagonists[73].

ROLE OF THROMBOLYSIS IN UNSTABLE ANGINA

In recent years there has been considerable interest in the administration of thrombolytic agents in acute myocardial infarction. As angiographic studies have shown a high incidence of intra-coronary clot formation it appears logical that the use of thrombolytic agents in unstable angina should improve outcome. In a small randomized trial of rTPA in patients with unstable angina Gold et al. reported improved outcome with thrombolytic therapy[74]. In 24 patients randomized to receive rTPA or placebo there was a reduction in persistent chest pain and a reduction in intra-coronary thrombosis in those patients treated with rTPA. Ambrose et al. reviewed a series of 9 small studies with 5 to 41 patients treated with thrombolytic therapy in unstable angina[75]. They concluded that thrombolysis was associated with a reduction of pain but were cautious as to whether this form of treatment would reduce subsequent adverse coronary events or need for revascularization. The overall impression is that the results are not as dramatic as those seen with thrombolysis in acute infarction but a large scale study is awaited.

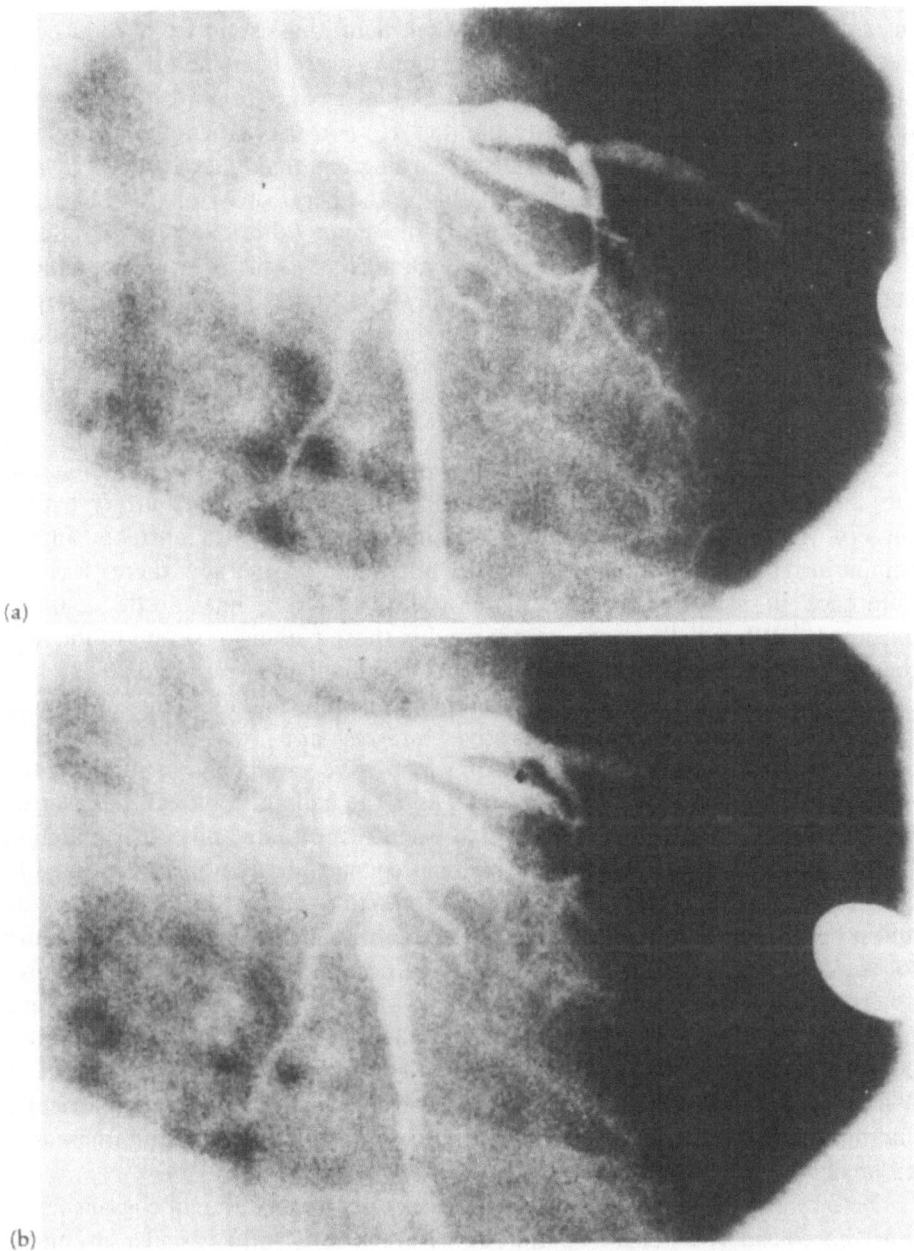

(a)

(b)

Figure 8.9. (a) Selective left coronary angiograms in the right anterior oblique view of a patient with unstable angina. A severe stenosis in the proximal portion of the left anterior descending artery is clearly visualized.
(b) Control angiogram in the same projection immediately following uncomplicated angioplasty with relief of the coronary stenosis

INTRA-AORTIC BALLOON PUMPING

Intra-aortic balloon counterpulsation is a mechanical assist device introduced in the early 1960s for the support of patients with severe heart failure. The 30 ml balloon is introduced either at an open surgical procedure or percutaneously into the femoral artery and advanced to the thoracic aorta. The balloon is triggered by the patient's R wave on the electrocardiogram to inflate in diastole and deflate at the onset of systole. By deflating at the onset of systole the heart can contract against reduced systemic vascular resistance (afterload), which reduces the work the heart must perform. The peak aortic systolic pressure is reduced but the mean arterial pressure is usually elevated, thus improving organ perfusion. When the balloon inflates in diastole it raises the aortic diastolic pressure and as 80% of coronary perfusion occurs in diastole, the coronary blood flow is augmented.

In patients with unstable angina who are refractory to medical therapy, the use of the intra-aortic pump frequently allows stabilization of the condition and the safer performance of cardiac catheterization and coronary artery bypass surgery. In a prospective randomized trial in patients with unstable angina comparing balloon pumping to intravenous nitrate therapy there was no difference in symptom control or mortality by using intra-aortic counter-pulsation[76]. When balloon pumping is used in those patients resistant to medical therapy it appears to offer a clear benefit. Weintaub et al. reported 60 cases of refractory angina pectoris treated with balloon counterpulsation and emergency surgery with only five perioperative infarcts and two deaths[77]. In a non-randomized study of 130 patients in whom 75 received balloon pumping, the results were compared to 55 patients in whom the balloon could not be inserted (control group). Langou et al. reported a 5.6% mortality and 5.1% infarction rate in those patients treated by balloon counterpulsation prior to surgery compared to a 14.5% mortality and 29% infarction rate for those with surgery and no prior counterpulsation[78]. The selection of patients as controls by failure to insert a balloon pump means that these patients had more extensive atherosclerosis and thus were more likely to be older and with a worse prognosis; however, this selection bias is unlikely to explain the large difference between the treated and untreated groups. The major haemodynamic effect of balloon counterpulsation in unstable angina is a reduction of the left ventricular end-diastolic pressure with a decrease in aortic systolic pressure and increased aortic diastolic pressure.

Before an intra-aortic balloon pump is inserted the high rate of complications must be considered. These complications are mostly local vascular problems with thrombus, embolic formation or ischaemia of the lower limb. The serious complications of aortic dissection and rupture are rare events. In all cases systemic heparinization with its attendant coagulation problems must be performed. In balance, intra-aortic balloon counterpulsation in medically refractory angina pectoris often allows stabilization of the condition prior to coronary arteriography and coronary artery bypass surgery.

CONCLUSION

Unstable angina is a serious clinical condition that requires a careful approach in order to achieve the best outcome. A rational plan to stabilise the patient with aspirin/or heparin, nitrates, calcium antagonists or β-blocker should be started at once. The recourse to revascularization, be it angioplasty or surgery, requires close liaison betweem medical and surgical teams to optimize the benefit for the patient.

References

1. Braunwald, E. (1989). Unstable angina: A classification. *Circulation*, **80**, 410–14
2. Conti, C.R., Brawley, R.K., Griffith, L S.C., Pitt, B., Humphries, J., Gott, V.L. and Ross, J.R. (1973). Unstable angina pectoris. Morbidity and mortality in 57 consecutive patients evaluated angiographically. *Am. J. Cardiol.*, **32**, 745–50
3. Mulcahy, R., Daly, L., Graham, I., Hickey, N., O'Donoghue, S., Owens, A., Ruane, P., and Tobin, G. (1981). Unstable angina natural history and determinants of prognosis. *Am. J. Cardiol.*, **48**, 525–82
4. Moise, A., Theroux, P., Taeymans, Y., Descoins, B., Lesperance, J., Waters, D.D., Pelletier, G.B. and Bourassa, M.G. (1983). Unstable angina and progression of coronary atherosclerosis. *N. Engl. J. Med.*, **309**, 685–9
5. Sherman, C.T., Litvack, F., Grundfest, W. *et al.* (1986). Coronary angioscopy in patients with unstable angina. *N. Engl. J. Med.*, **315**, 913–19
6. Chierchia, S., Brunelli, C., Simonetti, I., Lazzari, M. and Maseri, A. (1980). Sequence of events in angina at rest. Primary reduction in flow. *Circulation*, **61**, 759–68
7. Quyyumi, A.A., Wright, C.A., Mockus, L.T., and Fox, K.M. (1984). Mechanisms of nocturnal angina: Importance of increased myocardial oxygen demand in patients with severe coronary artery disease. *Lancet*, **1**, 1207–9
8. Maseri, A., Severi, S., De Nes, M., L'Abbate, A., Chierchia, S., Marzilli, M., *et al.* (1978). Variant angina: one aspect of a continuous spectrum of vasospastic myocardial ischaemia. Pathogenic mechanisms, estimated incidence and clinical and coronary arteriographic findings in 138 patients. *Am. J. Cardiol.*, **42**, 1019–35
9. Araki, H., Koiwaya, Y., Nakagaki, O. and Nakamura, N. (1983). Diurnal distribution of ST-segment elevation and related arrhythmias in patients with variant angina. A study by ambulatory ECG monitoring. *Circulation*, **67**, 995–1000
10. Conti, R., Hall, J.A., Feldman, F.L., Metha, J.L. and Pepine, C.J. (1983). Nitrates for treatment of unstable angina pectoris and coronary vasospasm. *Am. J. Med.*, **74**, 40–4
11. Gallino, A., Chierchia, S., Smith, G., Croom, M., Morgan, M., Marchesi, C. and Maseri, A. (1984). Computer system for the analysis of ST segment changes on 24-hour Holter monitor tapes: Comparison with other available systems. *J. Am. Coll. Cardiol.*, **4**, 245–52
12. Chierchia, S., Davies, G., Berkenboom, G., Crea, F., Crean, P. and Maseri, A. (1984). Alpha adrenergic receptors and coronary spasm: an elusive link. *Circulation*, **69**, 8–14
13. Bragg-Remschel, D.A., Anderson, C.H. and Winkle, R.A. (1982). Frequency response characteristics of ambulatory ECG monitoring systems and their implication for ST segment analysis. *Am. Heart J.*, **103**, 20–31
14. Crean, P.A., Ribeiro, P., Crea, F., Davies, G.J., Ratcliffe, D. and Maseri, A. (1984). Failure of transdermal nitroglycerin to improve chronic stable angina: A randomized placebo-controlled, double-blind, double cross trial. *Am. Heart J.*, **108**, 1494–1500
15. Deanfield, J.E., Selwyn, A.P., Chierchia, S., Maseri, A., Ribeiro, P., Krikler, S. and Morgan, M. (1983). Myocardial ischaemia during daily life in patients with stable angina: its relation to symptoms and heart rate changes. *Lancet*, **1**, 753–8
16. Deanfield, J. E., Shea, M., Ribeiro, P., Landsheere, C.M., Wilson, R.A., Horlock, ? and Selwyn, A.P. (1984). Transient ST segment depression as a marker of myocardial ischaemia during daily life. *Am. J. Cardiol.*, **54**, 1195–1200

17. Gottlieb, S.O., Weisfeldt, M.L., Ouyang, P., Mellits, E.D. and Gerstenblith, G. (1987). Silent myocardial ischaemia predicts infarction and death during 2 years follow-up of unstable angina. *J. Am. Coll. Cardiol.*, **10**, 756–61

18. Goldschlaher, N., Selzer, A. and Cohn, K. (1976). Treadmill stress tests as indicators of presence and severity of coronary artery disease. *Ann. Intern. Med.*, **85**, 277–86

19. Dagenais, G.R. (1982). Survival of patients with a strongly positive exercise electrocardiogram. *Circulation*, **65**(3), 452–6

20. Theroux, P., Waters, D.D., Halpen, C., Debaisieux, J.C. and Mizgala, H.F. (1979). Prognostic value of exercise testing soon after myocardial infarction. *N. Engl. J. Med.*, **301**, 341–5

21. National Exercise and Heart Disease Project: (1975). Common protocol. (Washington DC: George Washington Medical Center)

22. Fox, S.M., Naughton, J.P. and Haskell, W.L. (1971). Physical activity and the prevention of coronary heart disease. *Ann. Clin. Res.*, **3**, 304–10

23. Butman, S., Piters, K.M., Olson, H.G., Schiff, S.M. and Gardin, J.M. (1983). Early exercise testing in unstable angina: angiographic correlation and prognostic value. *J. Am. Coll. Cardiol.*, **1**, 638

24. Nixon, J.V., Hillert, M.C., Shapiro, W. and Smitherman, T.C. (1980). Submaximal exercise testing after unstable angina. *Am. Heart J.*, **99**, 772–8

25. Waters, D.D., Szlachicic, J., Bourassa, M.G., Scholl, J.M. and Theroux, P. (1982). Exercise testing in patients with variant angina: results, correlation and angiographic features and prognostic significance. *Circulation*, **65**, 265–74

26. Crean, P.A. and Waters, D.D. (1984). Interpreting the exercise ECG in the patient with variant angina. *Pract. Cardiol.*, **10**, 107–13

27. Araki, H., Hayata, N., Matsuguchi, T., Takeshita, A. and Nakamura, M. (1986). Value of exercise tests with calcium antagonist to diagnose significant fixed coronary stenosis in patients with variant angina. *Br. Heart J.* (in press)

28. Alison, H. W., Russell, R.O. Jr., Mantle, J.A., Kouchoukos, N.T., Moraski, R.E. and Rackley, C.E. (1978). Coronary anatomy and arteriography in patients with unstable angina pectoris. *Am. J. Cardiol.*, **41**, 204–9

29. Holmes, D.R, Jr., Hartzler, G.O., Smith, H.C. and Foster, V. (1981). Coronary artery thrombosis in patients with unstable angina. *Br. Heart J.*, **49**, 1146–51

30. Balcon, R., Brooks, N., Warnes, C. and Cattell, M. (1980). Clinical spectrum of unstable angina. In Raffenbeul, W., Lichteln, P.R. and Balcon, R. (eds.) *Unstable Angina Pectoris*, International Symposium. Hanover, pp. 42–44 (New York: Thieme-Stratton)

31. Victor, M.F., Likoff, M.J., Mintz, G.S. and Likoff, W. (1981). Unstable angina pectoris of new onset: A prospective clinical and arteriographic study of 75 patients. *Am. J. Cardiol.*, **47**, 228–32

32. Sherman, C.T., Litvack, F., Grundfest, W., Lee, M., Hickey, A., Chaux, A., Kass, R., Blanche, C., Matloff, J., Morgenstern, L., Ganz, W., Swan, H.J.C. and Forrester, J. (1986). Coronary angioscopy in patients with unstable angina pectoris. *N. Engl. J. Med.*, **315**, 913–19

33. Ambrose, J.A., Winters, S.L., Arora, R.R., Haft, J.I., Goldstine, J., Rentrop, K.P., Gorlin, R. and Fuster, V. (1985). Coronary angiographic morphology in myocardial infarction: A link between the pathogenesis of unstable angina and myocardial infarction. *J. Am. Coll. Cardiol.*, **6**, 1233–8

34. Ambrose, J.A., Winters, S.L., Arora, R.R., Eng, A., Riccio, A., Gorlin, R. and Fuster, V. (1986). Angiographic evolution of coronary artery morphology in unstable angina. *J. Am. Coll. Cardiol.*, **7**, 472–8

35. Brown, G.B., Lee, A.B., Bolson, E.L. and Dodge, H.T. (1984). Reflex constriction of significant coronary stenosis as a mechanism contributing to ischemic left ventricular dysfunction during isometric exercise. *Circulation*, **70**, 18–25

36. Yasue, H., Nagao, M., Omote, S., Takizawa, A., Miwa, K. and Tanaka, S. (1978). Coronary arterial spasm and Prinzmetals variant form of angina induced by hyperventilation and tris-buffer infusion. *Circulation*, **58**, 56–62

37. Raizner, A.E., Chahine, R.A., Ishimore, T., Verani, M.S., Zacca, N., Jamal, N., Mil, R. and Luchi, R.J. (1980), Provocation of coronary artery spasm by the cold pressor test. Hemodynamic, arteriographic and quantitative angiographic observation. *Circulation*, **62**, 925–32

38. Waters, D.D., Theroux, P., Szlachcic, J., Dauwe, F., Crittin, J., Bonan, R. and Mizgala, H.F. (1980). Ergonovine testing in a coronary care unit. *Am. J. Cardiol.*, **46**, 922–30

39. Bertrand, M.E., La Blanche, J.M., Tilmant, P.Y., Thieuleux, F.A., Deforge, M.R.A.G., Asseman, P., Berzin, B., Libersa, C. and Laurent, J.M. (1982). Frequency of provoked coronary spasm in 1089 consecutive patients undergoing coronary arteriography. *Circulation*, **65**, 1299–1306

40. Crean, P.A., Waters, D.D., Roy, D., Pelletier, G.B., Bonan, R. and Theroux, P. (1985). Sensitivity and safety of ergonovine testing inside and outside the catheterisation laboratory. *J. Am. Coll. Cardiol.*, **5**(2), 431

41. Crean, P.A., Crow, J. and Davies, G.J. (1984). Sequential changes in ventricular function following intravenous isosorbide dinitrate. *Vasc. Med.*, **2**, 205–9

42. Distante, A., Maseri, A., Severi, S., Biagini, A. and Chierchia, S. (1979). Management of vasospastic angina at rest with continuous infusion of isosorbide dinitrate. *Am. J. Cardiol.*, **44**, 533–9

43. Theroux, P. and Waters, D.D. (1983). Calcium antagonists. Clinical use in the treatment of angina. *Drugs*, **25**(2), 178–95

44. Waters, D.D., Theroux, P., Szlachcic, J. and Dauwe, F. (1981). Provocative testing to assess the efficacy of treatment with nifedipine, diltazem and verapamil in variant angina. *Am. J. Cardiol.*, **48**, 123–30

45. Parodi, O., Maseri, A. and Simonetti, I. (1979). Management of unstable angina by verapamil: a double blind cross over study in the CCU. *Br. Heart J.*, **41**, 167–74

46. Mehta, J., Pepine, C.J., Day, M., Guerrero, J.R. and Conti, C.R. (1981). Short term efficacy of oral verapamil in rest angina. A double blind placebo controlled trial in CCU patients. *Am. J. Med.*, **71**, 977–82

47. Gerstenblith, G., Ouyang, P., Achuff, S.C., Buckley, B.H., Becker, L.C., Mellits, D. *et al.* (1982). Nifedipine in unstable angina. *N. Engl. J. Med.*, **306**, 885–9

48. Theroux, P., Taeymans, Y., Morissette, D., Bosch, Z., Pelletier, G. and Waters, D. (1985). A randomised study comparing propranolol and diltiazem in the treatment of unstable angina. *J. Am. Coll. Cardiol.*, **5**, 717–22

49. Glazier, J.J., Chierchia, S., Smith, G.C., Berkenboom, G., Crean, P.A., Gerosa, S. and Maseri, A. (1986). β-Blockers for angina pectoris: how do they really work? (abstract). *Clin. Sci.*, **70**, 1

50. Co-operative Unstable Angina Study Group (1978). Unstable angina pectoris: National co-operative study group to compare medical and surgical therapy. In hospital experience and initial follow up results in patients with one, two and three vessel disease. *Am. J. Cardiol.*, **42**, 839–48

51. Irie, T., Imaizumi, T., Matugushi, T., Koyanagi, S., Kanaide, H., Takeshita, A. and Nakamura, ? (1989). Increased fibrinopeptide A during anginal attacks in patients with variant angina. *J. Am. Coll. Cardiol.*, **14**, 589–595

52. Hamm, C.W., Lorenz, R.L., Bleifeld, W., Kupper, W., Wober, W. and Weber, P.C. (1987). Biochemical evidence of platelet activation in patients with persistent unstable angina. *J. Am. Coll. Cardiol.*, **10**, 998–1005

53. Chesboro, J. and Fuster, V. (1987). The therapeutic challenge of plaque rupture: value of biochemical markers. *J. Am. Coll. Cardiol.*, **10**, 1005–7

54. Lewis, H.D., Davis, J.W., Archibald, D.A., Steinke, W.E., Smitherman, T.C., Dohert, J.E. *et al.* (1983). Protective effect of aspirin against acute myocardial infarction and death in men with unstable angina. *N. Engl. J. Med.*, **309**, 396–405

55. Cairns, J.A., Gent, M., Singer, J. *et al.* (1984). A study of aspirin and sulphinpyrazone in unstable angina pectoris. *Circulation*, **70**, 415

56. Robertson, R.M., Robertson, D., Friesinger, G.C., Timmons, S. and Hawiger, J. (1980). Platelets aggregates in peripheral and coronary sinus blood in patients with spontaneous coronary artery spasm. *Lancet*, **2**, 829–31

57. Robertson, D., Mass, R.L. and Roberts, L.J. (1980). Antiplatelet agents in vasospastic angina: a double blind cross-over study. *Clin. Res.*, **28**, 242A

58. Chierchia, S., Patrono, C., Crea, F., Giabattoni, G., de Caterina, R., Cinotti, G.A. *et al.* (1982). Effects of intravenous prostacyclin in variant angina. *Circulation*, **65**, 470–7

59. Nichol E.S., Phillips, W.C. and Casten, C.G. (1959). Virtue of prompt anti-coagulation therapy in impending myocardial infarction: experience with 318 patients during a 10 year period. *Ann. Intern. Med.*, **50**, 1158

60. Theroux, P., Quimet, H., McCans, J., Latour, J.G., Joly, P., Levy, G., Pelletier, E., Juneau, M., Stasik, J., DeGuise, P., Pelletier, G.B., Rinzel, D. and Waters, D.D. (1988). Aspirin, heparin, or both to treat acute unstable angina. *N. Engl. J. Med.*, **319**, 1105–11

61. European Coronary Surgery Study Group (1982). Long term results of prospective randomized study of coronary artery bypass surgery in stable angina pectoris. *Lancet*, **11**, 1173–80

62. Conti, R., Becker, L., Biddle, T., Hutter, A. and Resnekov, L. (1982). Unstable angina. NHLBI co-operative study group to compare medical and surgical therapy: long term morbidity and mortality. *Am. J. Cardiol.* (abstract), **49**, 1007

63. Selden, R., Neill, W.A. and Ritzman, L.W. (1975). Medical versus surgical therapy for acute coronary insufficiency. A randomised study. *N. Engl. J. Med.*, **293**, 1329–33

64. Pugh, B., Platt, M.R. and Mills, L.J. (1978). Unstable angina pectoris: a randomized study of patients treated medically and surgically. *Am. J. Cardiol.*, **41**, 1291–9

65. Bertolasi, C.A., Tronge, J.E. and Riccitelli, M.A. (1976). Natural history of unstable angina with medical or surgical therapy. *Chest*, **70**, 596–605

66. Parisi, F., Khuri, S., Deupree, R.H., Sharma, G.V.R.K., Scott, S.M. and Luchi, R.J. (1989). Medical compared with surgical management of unstable angina. *Circulation*, **80**, 1176–89

67. Kaiser, G.C., Schaff, H.V. and Killip, T. (1989). Myocardial revascularization for unstable angina pectoris. *Circulation*, **79** (Suppl. 1), 60–7

68. Bourassa, M.G., David, P.R. and Guiteras, V.P. Percutaneous transluminal coronary angioplasty. In Rowalds, D.J. (ed.). *Recent Advances in Cardiology*, Vol. 9, pp. 193–213 (Edinburgh: Churchill Livingstone)

69. Suryapranata, H., De Feyter, P.J. and Serruys, P.W. (1988). Coronary angioplasty in patients with unstable angina pectoris: Is there a role for thrombolysis? *J. Am. Coll. Cardiol.*, **12**, 69A–78A

70. Williams, D.O., Riley, R.S., Singh, A.K., Genirtz, H. and Most, A.S. (1981). Evaluation of the role of coronary angioplasty in patients with unstable angina. *Am. Heart J.*, **102**, 1–9

71. De Feyter, P.J., Serruys, P.W., Van der Brand, M., Balakumaran, K., Mocht Soward, A.L., Arnold, A.E.R. and Hugenholtz, P.G. (1985). Emergency coronary angioplasty in unstable angina. *N. Engl. J. Med.*, **313**, 342–6

72. Bentivoglio, L.G. (1983). Personal communication: Data from the NHLBI registry presented at the 1983 Bethesda workshop on PTCA. Bethesda, Maryland.

73. Corcos, T., David, P.R., Bourassa, M.G., Guiteras, P.V., Robert, J., Mata, L.A. and Waters, D.D. (1985). Percutanous transluminal angioplasty for the treatment of variant angina. *J. Am. Coll. Cardiol.*, **5**, 1046–54

74. Gold, H.K., Johns, J.A., Leinbach, R.C., Yasuda, T., Grossbard, E., Zusman, R. and Collen, D. (1987). A randomized, blinded, placebo-controlled trial of recombinant human tissue-type plasminogen activator in patients with unstable angina. *Circulation*, **75**, 1192–9

75. Ambrose, A. and Alexopoulos, D. (1989). Thrombolysis in unstable angina: will the beneficial effect of thrombolytic therapy in myocardial infarction apply to patients with unstable angina. *J. Am. Coll. Cardiol.*, **13**, 1666–72

76. Flaherty, J.T., Becker, L.C., Weiss, J.L., Brinker, J.A., Buckley, B.H., Gerstenbli, G., Kallman, C.H. and Weisfeld, M.L. (1985). Results of a randomised trial of intraaortic balloon counterpulsation and intravenous nitroglycerin in patients with acute myocardial infarction. *J. Am. Coll. Cardiol.*, **6**, 434–46

77. Weintaub, R.M., Voukydis, P.C., Aroesty, J.M., Cohen, S.I., Ford, P., Kurland, G.S., Raia, P.J., Morkin, E. and Paulin, S. (1974). Treatment of preinfarction angina with intraaortic balloon counterpulsation and surgery. *Am. J. Cardiol.*, **34**, 809–14

78. Langou, R.A., Geha, A.S., Hammond, G.L. and Cohen, L.S. (1978). Surgical approach for patients with unstable angina pectoris: Role of the response to initial medical therapy and intraaortic balloon pumping in perioperative complications after aortocoronary bypass graft. *Am. J. Cardiol.*, **42**, 629–33

9
Pathophysiology of angina pectoris

A.A. QUYYUMI

One of the earliest and best descriptions of the syndrome of angina pectoris was by William Heberden in 1772[1].

> They who are afflicted with it, are seized while they are walking, more especially if it be uphill, and soon after eating, with a painful and most disagreeable sensation in the breast, which seems as if it would extinguish life, if it were to increase or to continue; but the moment they stand still, all this uneasiness vanishes.

The link between coronary atherosclerosis and angina was established almost a century later by pathologic studies of Herrick and others[2,3]. This led to the current hypothesis that angina pectoris was a result of myocardial ischemia, which was a consequence of myocardial oxygen demand exceeding supply. Ischemia itself is a result of a combination of hypoxia, accumulation of ions and metabolites such as hydrogen, potassium and lactate, and reduction of substrate[4]. Myocardial ischemia can thus be more accurately defined as a state in which consumption of ATP exceeds its production, resulting in anaerobic cellular metabolism with consequent impairment of myocardial contractile function[5]. This state of affairs exists because of the inability of coronary blood flow to deliver oxygen for the given demand. When this imbalance is transient, ischemia is limited and is sometimes evident clinically as angina pectoris. If, however, it is prolonged, then myocardial necrosis occurs and is clinically evident as myocardial infarction.

DETERMINANTS OF MYOCARDIAL OXYGEN DEMAND

The major determinants of myocardial oxygen demand are heart rate, blood pressure, wall stress and contractility[5-7]. Wall stress is defined by Laplace's formula, wall stress = (radius × pressure) ÷ twice wall thickness. Thus wall stress is directly related to volume and pressure of the left ventricle and inversely related to wall thickness; therefore in the event of ventricular dilatation,

165

myocardial oxygen demand will increase because of increasing wall stress[8]. Interactions between these indices may be complex; for example, sympathetic stimulation not only increases oxygen consumption by increasing contractility and heart rate, but also reduces the ventricular volume and thereby wall stress. It is estimated that these two combined effects increase oxygen demand by 25% per unit of systolic pressure time index at maximal sympathetic stimulation[9].

DETERMINANTS OF MYOCARDIAL BLOOD FLOW

The two basic determinants of coronary blood flow are the perfusion pressure and coronary vascular resistance[10]. Perfusion pressure is defined as aortic–intramyocardial pressure. The intramyocardial pressure, which is responsible for compression on collapsible intramyocardial vasculature, also changes during the cardiac cycle and determines the phasic flow in the left coronary artery. Coronary blood flow is impeded during systole by both the direct contraction of muscle fibers around the intramyocardial vessels and by indirect compression from transmission of the ventricular chamber pressure[11]. Although the driving pressure in the coronary arteries remains constant in the epicardial vessels, the opposing tissue pressure in different areas of the myocardium is uneven[12]. Therefore, during systole, subendocardial blood flow virtually ceases although subepicardial blood flow continues. The endocardial to epicardial flow ratio varies between 0.8 and 1.2[8].

According to Poseuille's theorem, in the presence of normal coronary arteries, coronary vascular resistance is determined by blood viscosity and the diameter and length of the coronary arteries. Thus, the smaller the vessels the greater their contribution to resistance. As viscosity and vessel length do not normally change, the main determinant of vascular resistance is the cross-sectional area of the coronary vessels. The large epicardial conductance coronary vessels contribute relatively little to the total resistance of the coronary tree and the major determinants of coronary vascular resistance are the smaller intramyocardial vessels. These intramyocardial resistance vessels are autoregulated in the heart[11,13]. As myocardial oxygen demand increases, only a relatively small amount of oxygen can be made available by increasing oxygen extraction. This is because the heart extracts a relatively high percentage of oxygen even under resting conditions, and further demand has to be met by net increases in coronary blood flow. This is achieved by coronary vascular dilatation, which if the circumstances require, can cause coronary blood flow to increase by up to 4 to 5 fold. Autoregulation also ensures that change in perfusion pressure over a substantial physiologic range (60 to 110 mmHg) does not lead to any change in coronary blood flow if myocardial oxygen demands remain constant. It is postulated that a work-dependent increase of a metabolite is responsible for changes in coronary vascular resistance[14]. Adenosine, a metabolite of adenosine triphosphate, and a powerful vasodilator, has been hypothesized as being responsible for increasing blood flow during periods of increased myocardial work. The importance of coronary vascular smooth muscle and endothelium in determining coronary blood flow will be discussed further.

In the presence of epicardial coronary atherosclerosis, it is the cross-sectional reduction of the lumen and the consequent drop in pressure and flow distal to the stenosis that determines the degree of ischemia. When the pressure beyond the stenosis drops below 55 mmHg, subendocardial ischemia may develop[15]. The more severe the stenotic lesion, the greater is the pressure drop and reduction in flow. The relationship between stenosis resistance and degree of stenosis is nonlinear, in that the resistance changes rapidly once the stenosis exceeds 50% in internal diameter[16]. Thus a reduction from 80 to 90% in diameter results in a 3-fold increase in resistance and consequently a dramatic reduction in blood flow (Figure 9.1). It can therefore be appreciated why small reductions in the size of already stenosed atherosclerotic segments of coronary arteries could produce dramatic increases in symptoms and ischemia[17].

Although the severity of the epicardial stenosis at the narrowest point in the coronary artery is the most important determinant of resistance, the number of obstructions in series and the length of the narrowing also contribute to the reduction in flow[18]. In vitro experiments have demonstrated that flow reduction across a 6 mm long and 50% narrowed lesion was 8%; however three serial 50% diameter narrowings of 2 mm each resulted in a flow reduction of 19%. This is presumed to be due to turbulence at each stenotic segment before blood reaches the next segment.

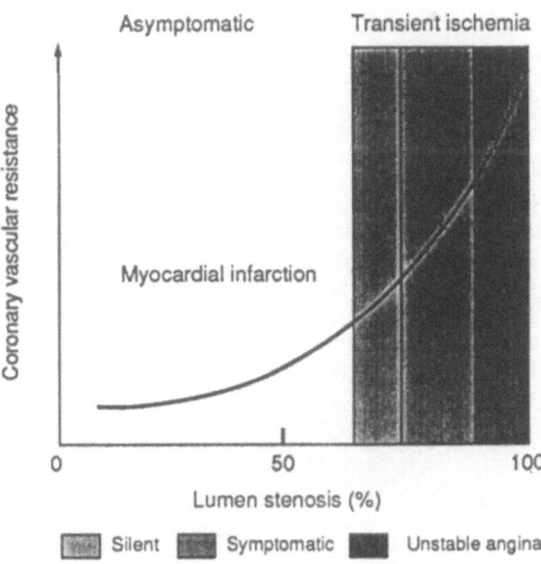

Figure 9.1 Relationship between lumen stenosis, coronary vascular resistance symptoms. Adapted from *Postgraduate Medicine*, 1989, **86**, 62–75

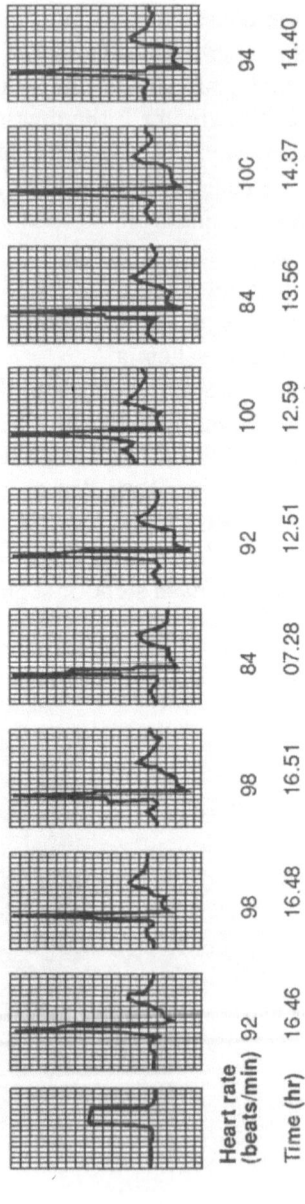

Figure 9.2. Heart rate at onset of episodes of ST-segment depression recorded during normal daily activities in 24-hour period. (Adapted from ref. 22)

STABLE ANGINA PECTORIS

Stable angina is defined as chest pain precipitated by exertion, emotion or after meals which occurs fairly reproducibly and is often exacerbated by cold and relieved by alleviation of precipitating factors. Although some patients give a fairly reproducible history of angina occurring with exertion (fixed threshold), others have symptoms at variable workload ranging from moderately intense exercise to rest or sleep (mixed angina). Sometimes the character and location of pain may be atypical, but the precipitating factors are typical, which allows the diagnosis to be made.

Precipitating factors

With the advent of ambulatory ST segment monitoring, it has become feasible to record episodes of myocardial ischemia during daily life[19,20]. Analysis of heart rate and blood pressure at the onset of spontaneous episodes of myocardial ischemia recorded as ST segment changes during daily activities, has revealed that the ischemic threshold (heart rate × blood pressure) varied considerably from episode to episode in the same individual, and is often considerably lower than the ischemic threshold during graded treadmill exercise testing (Figure 9.2)[21,22]. Thus, it became clear that myocardial ischemia could be precipitated by diverse stimuli during daily life, which not only included strenuous or moderately strenuous activities, but also less intense activities such as driving, eating and mental stress, and also occasionally during rest and sleep (Figure 9.3)[23].

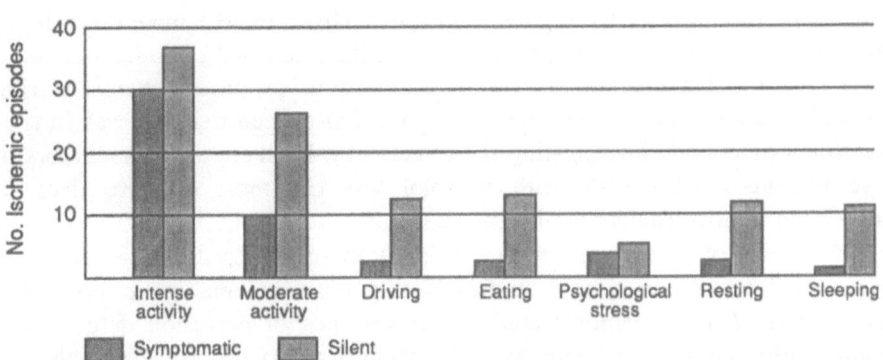

Figure 9.3 Occurrence of symptomatic and silent ischemic episodes with different activities during ambulatory ST-segment monitoring (total symptomatic episodes, 54; total silent episodes, 116). Adapted from Cecchi *et al.*, ref. 23

MECHANISMS FOR THE VARIABLE THRESHOLD IN STABLE ANGINA PECTORIS

Earlier studies in patients with rest angina had highlighted the frequent lack of change in heart rate and blood pressure before the onset of ST segment depression or elevation. Often these hemodynamic changes followed the onset of ST segment change[24,25]. It was proposed that these ischemic episodes were precipitated primarily by a sudden reduction in coronary blood flow, due to coronary vasospasm. However, in a study of 1089 consecutive patients with stable coronary artery disease, coronary spasm could not be provoked in the majority of patients after ergonovine administration during coronary arteriography[26]. Intravenous ergonovine produced coronary spasm in 85% of patients presenting with variant angina.

Other studies have also demonstrated that coronary spasm alone is probably not the sole mechanism for angina and ischemia occurring at rest or with minimal activity in patients with stable coronary artery disease. A series of studies were undertaken by Quyyumi *et al.* to investigate the precipitating factors for nocturnal ischemia in patients with chronic stable coronary artery disease[27,28]. An analysis of beat-to-beat changes in heart rate before the onset of ST segment depression was conducted in patients who had both daytime exertional and nocturnal resting episodes of ST segment change. There was invariably an increase in heart rate before the onset of ST segment change in these patients (Figures 9.4, 9.5)[27]. During sleep studies in these patients, careful analysis of heart rate, ST segment change, electroencephalogram, electromyogram and oxygen saturations were made. The vast majority of episodes of ST segment change were preceded by arousal and awakening from sleep and bodily movements. These events resulted in increases in heart rate, and were then followed by the onset of ST segment change[28]. However, the increase in heart rate before the onset of ST depression during the nocturnal episodes was often lower than the increase in heart rate required to produce ischemia during treadmill exercise. The importance of myocardial oxygen demand was further underlined by a study investigating the effects of β-blockers and vasodilators in these patients. β-Blockade with atenolol was the most effective drug in suppression of nocturnal ischemic episodes[29].

The effects of mental stress on precipitation of myocardial ischemia have been well described in several studies. Using positron emission tomography, Deanfield *et al.* have demonstrated the appearance of perfusion defects with mental arithmetic in some patients with coronary artery disease. Not only was blood flow to the ischemic region lower compared with the non-ischemic region, but the regional defect was identical in location to the defect produced by exercise[30]. Rozanski *et al.* investigated the effect of mental stress tasks on myocardial ischemia, measured as wall motion worsening during radionuclide ventriculography. Performance of speech in some patients precipitated ischemia, which was indistinguishable in magnitude from ischemia produced during exercise. The heart rate – blood pressure product during mental stress tasks was lower than during bicycle exercise[31].

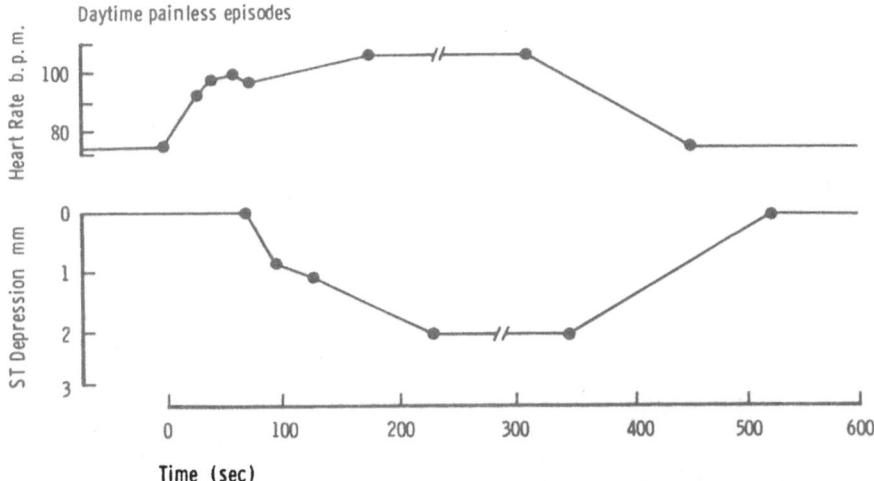

Figure 9.4 Relationship between the heart rate and the development of ST segment depression during the day in the absence of chest pain. The pattern of development is identical with the painful daytime episodes with an increase in heart rate preceding the development of ST segment depression with resolution of the heart rate before the ST segment changes returned to normal. Again these painfree episodes of ST segment depression tended to be shorter than the painful episodes. Reproduced with permission from the *Lancet* (ref. 27)

Thus, studies in stable patients in whom ischemia can be precipitated by either exercise, mental stress or sleep, clearly demonstrate the role of both increases in myocardial oxygen demand and reductions in coronary blood flow. Greg Brown *et al.* undertook a series of studies in patients with stable coronary artery disease, and performed coronary angiography after hand grip exercise. Although this maneuver produced a 20% increase in heart rate, 24% increase in blood pressure and a 66% increase in blood flow, the lumen area in apparently normal sections of coronary arteries reduced by 15–22%, and in the stenosed segments of coronary arteries by 5–33%[32]. Gage *et al.* have demonstrated a 71% reduction in coronary stenosis area with dynamic exercise which could be prevented by pretreatment with nitroglycerin or by β-blockade[33].

Thus, it is clear that even exercise, which was thought to precipitate myocardial ischemia purely by increasing myocardial oxygen demand, produces vasoconstriction or 'collapse' at the site of atherosclerotic narrowing[32-34]. According to Bernoulli's principle, as velocity increases, the pressure across the lesion falls because part of the pressure is converted into kinetic energy and is dissipated in turbulence. Thus, for example, at a steady flow rate of 65 ml/min, the pressure drop across the 70% coronary stenosis would be 14 mmHg; but doubling the flow would result in a drop of 52 mmHg across the same lesion. This drop in pressure across a compliant lesion with eccentric plaque and preservation of smooth muscle would be at least partly due to passive collapse of the lesion[17].

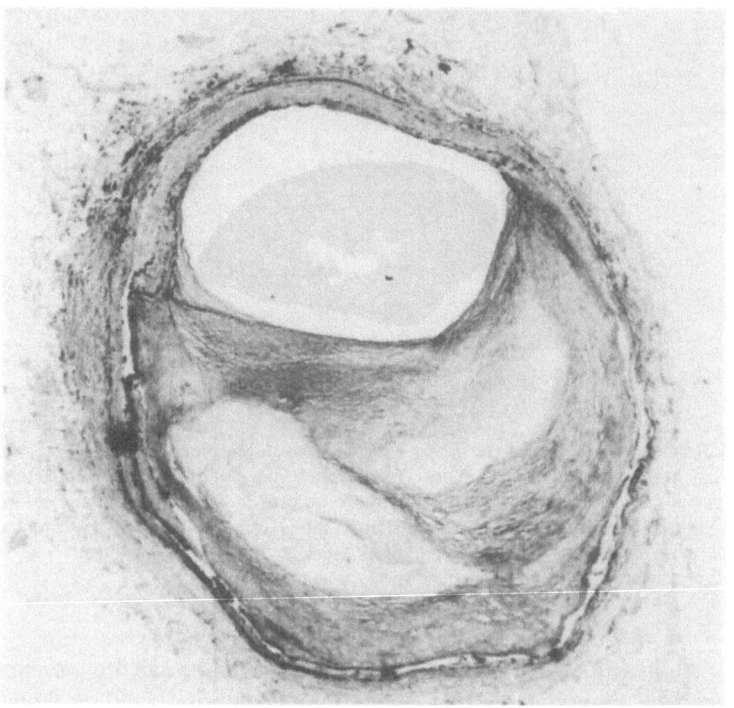

Figure 9.5 Photomicrograph of a section of coronary artery showing eccentric fibroatheromatous intimal thickening without involvement of the remaining intima and with smooth muscle preservations. Reproduced with permission from the *British Heart Journal*

Pathologic sectioning of coronary arteries at 5 mm intervals has demonstrated that approximately three quarters of all sections of epicardial coronary arteries involved in the atherosclerotic process have an eccentric lesion with preservation of smooth muscle in the relatively uninvolved section of the lumen (Figure 9.6)[17,34,35]. It has been hypothesized that vasomotion of medial smooth muscle precipitated by diverse stimuli such as mental stress, cold or norepinephrine could substantially reduce coronary diameter in these sections, and thus dramatically increase resistance, diminish flow and precipitate ischemia[17].

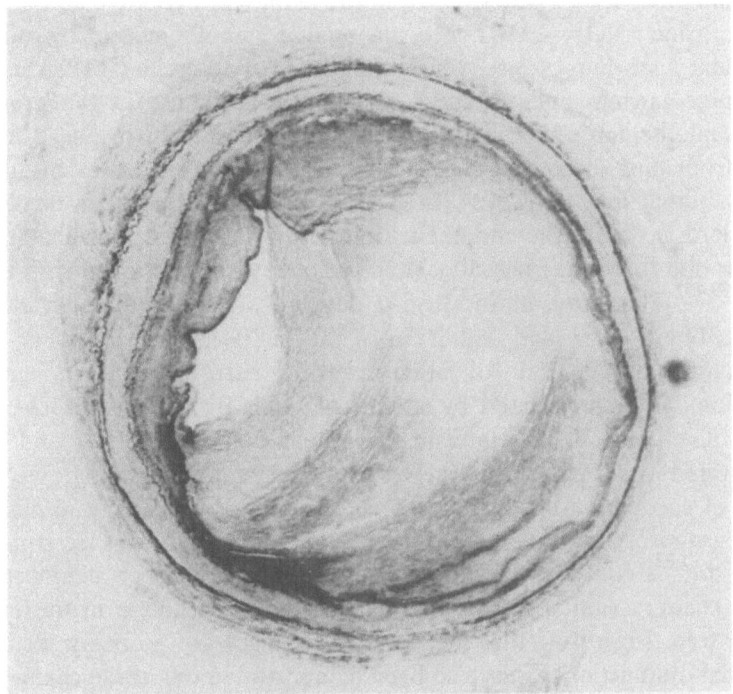

Figure 9.6 Photomicrograph of a section of coronary artery with circumferential fibro-atheromatous intimal thickening where there is no smooth muscle preservation. Reproduced with permission from the *British Heart Journal*

MECHANISMS OF VASOMOTION OF EPICARDIAL CORONARY ARTERIES IN STABLE ANGINA

There is evidence that vasoconstriction at the site of atherosclerotic lesions occurs not only as a result of hydrodynamic changes described above, but also due to factors such as norepinephrine release (causing α-mediated vasoconstriction) or renin–angiotensin system activation. In recent years, the role of two other mechanisms: (a) the endothelium and (b) platelets, in producing epicardial vessel vasomotion has been studied in detail.

IMPORTANCE OF ENDOTHELIUM IN CORONARY VASOMOTION IN STABLE ANGINA

Normal endothelium is capable of releasing a powerful vasodilator, endothelium derived relaxant factor (EDRF) in response to several physiologic and pharmacologic stimuli[36–40]. It is believed that there may be more than one

EDRF and at least one is derived from the amino acid arginine and believed to be nitric oxide (NO). EDRF acts on medial smooth muscle by stimulating intracellular guanylate cyclase, which converts GTP to cyclic GMP. This inhibits intracellular calcium and produces vasodilatation. Thus, in the presence of normal endothelium epicardial vessel dilatation occurs in response to EDRF release from physiologic stimuli such as increasing shear stress by increasing coronary blood flow. However, in sections of coronary arteries involved with atherosclerosis, where the endothelial integrity is disturbed, vasodilatation does not occur and there may be either no change or vasoconstriction with the same stimulus[39,40]. Therefore, an increase in demand would stimulate an increase in coronary blood flow and result in paradoxic vasoconstriction or lack of vasodilatation at the site of atherosclerotic narrowing[41] with endothelial dysfunction, as demonstrated by studies of Greg Brown[17] and Gage et al.[33]. Acetylcholine in low doses stimulates endothelial release of EDRF and has been demonstrated to cause epicardial vessel vasodilatation in apparently normal sections of coronary arteries, but vasoconstriction or no change in diameter in irregular (atherosclerotic) segments of coronary arteries[42]. Diverse stimuli, such as exercise[17,33], cold[42] and increased flow[40,41], have all been demonstrated to produce changes similar to those produced by acetylcholine in the epicardial coronary tree, suggesting that the observed changes are probably secondary to endothelial dysfunction. It has also been demonstrated that these changes can be abolished or reduced by use of nitrates or β-blockers[33,44]. The importance of endothelial integrity and EDRF stimulated vasodilatation of coronary vessels, its role in precipitation and persistence of myocardial ischemia, and its modification with medications, will be clarified further in future studies.

THE ROLE OF PLATELETS IN EPICARDIAL VESSEL VASOMOTION IN STABLE ANGINA

Folts et al. have demonstrated that there are cyclic reductions in coronary blood flow when a fixed stenosis is created in the coronary artery of the dog[45]. These reductions were abolished by aspirin and other platelet inhibitors, and were demonstrated to be caused by intermittent deposition of platelet aggregates. Platelet aggregates may cause reductions in flow either by acute narrowing of the vessel lumen or by vasoconstriction due to local release of platelet extracts such as thromboxane. These studies suggested that platelets may play a role in altering coronary vessel diameter and precipitation of ischemia in patients with obstructive coronary artery disease.

Clinical studies investigating platelet activation in patients with stable coronary artery disease have, however, been confusing mainly because of the inherent difficulties in testing platelet activation and aggregation in vivo. Whereas some studies have shown reduced platelet activity in coronary venous blood due to entrapment of platelet aggregates in the atherosclerotic plaque[47,48], others have shown increased platelet reactivity after exercise and atrial pacing[49]. Hirsch *et al.* did not demonstrate a step-up in thromboxane B2 in coronary venous blood at rest or after induction of ischemia by rapid atrial pacing, isometric exercise or cold[50]. At the present time it appears that platelet activation is not important in precipitating myocardial ischemia in patients with stable coronary artery disease and the observed phenomena are probably a result rather than the cause of ischemia. Furthermore, aspirin therapy has been shown to be ineffective in reducing transient ischemic episodes in patients with stable coronary artery disease[51].

CIRCADIAN RHYTHMS IN TRANSIENT MYOCARDIAL ISCHAEMIA IN STABLE ANGINA

There is no doubt that there is a circadian variation in the occurrence of transient episodes of both silent and symptomatic ischemia in patients with stable coronary artery disease (Figure 9.7)[19,52]. Episodes are more likely to occur in the morning hours, reaching a plateau until noon, with a possible second peak in the late evening, and with the least number of episodes occurring at night. Similar circadian distribution of events has been described with fatal and non-fatal myocardial infarction[53], sudden cardiac death[54] and stroke (Figure 9.7)[55,56]. It also appears that the greatest number of transient ischemic episodes and myocardial infarction occur within the first two hours of awakening[57,58]. Several factors that may be responsible for the observed circadian variation of transient ischemic episodes have been identified. Heart rate[19], blood pressure[59], and probably contractility[60] (measured indirectly as plasma epinephrine levels), all determinants of myocardial oxygen demand, peak in the morning hours between 7 a.m. and noon (Figure 9.8). Factors which may directly or indirectly lead to increases in coronary vasoconstrictor tone also exhibit a circadian variation (Figure 9.9). Plasma norepinephrine level[60] and plasma renin activity[61], both powerful vasoconstrictor influences, are increased in the morning hours. Platelet aggregability is high in the mornings and it has been hypothesized that platelet aggregates over atherosclerotic plaques may result in local release of vasoconstrictor substances such as thromboxane, and cause vasoconstriction[60].

The impact of circadian changes in humoral and neural vasoconstrictor factors on the coronary vasculature in patients with stable coronary artery disease was demonstrated by Quyyumi *et al.*[62]. Patients with stable angina were demonstrated to have a circadian variation in ischemic threshold (heart rate at 1 mm ST segment depression), so that it was easier to precipitate ischemia with treadmill exercise during the morning hours and at night, compared to other times of the day. An inverse and parallel circadian variation in forearm vascular resistance was also demonstrated, suggesting that there is a circadian variation of both coronary and peripheral vascular resistance.

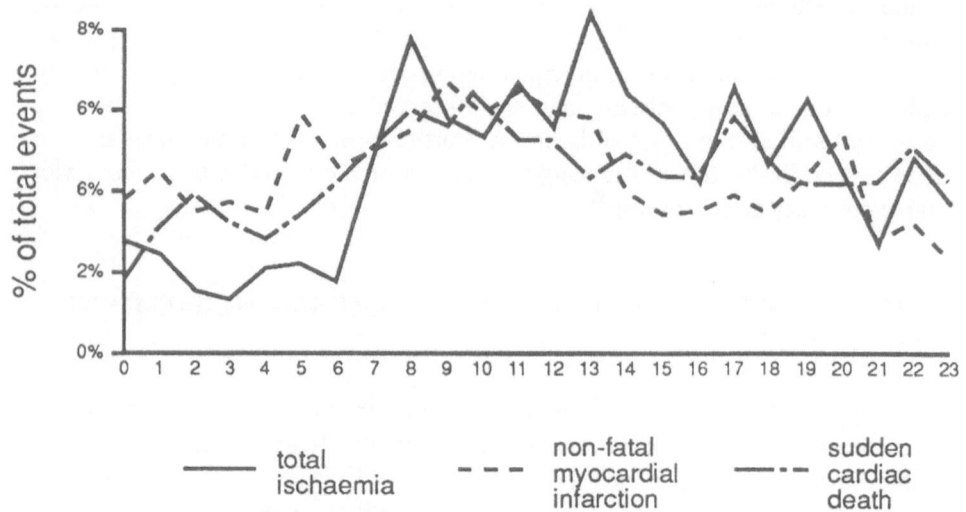

Figure 9.7 Circadian variation in episodes of sudden cardiac death, nonfatal myocardial infarction, and ischemia. (From ref. 52). Adapted from Mulcahy et al.[10]

It is important to emphasize that the variation in physiologic parameters according to the time of day may either have a truly endogenous circadian variation, or be largely determined by awakening and assumption of an upright posture. It is clear that many cardiovascular events occur largely as a result of assumption of the upright posture and awakening. For example, changes in plasma cortisol level appear to have a true endogenous circadian variation[63], whereas increase in platelet aggregability in the morning hours occurs only after assumption of an upright posture[64]. Other factors, such as heart rate, blood pressure, plasma norepinephrine and plasma renin activity have an underlying endogenous circadian variation which is exaggerated by awakening and exercise.

SILENT MYOCARDIAL ISCHEMIA IN STABLE ANGINA PECTORIS

Many patients with coronary artery disease have silent myocardial ischemia during normal daily activities, which can be detected by ambulatory monitoring techniques such as electrocardiography[19,20,52,56] or radionuclide gated blood pool imaging[65]. In a series of 150 unselected patients admitted to hospital with coronary artery disease and a history of chest pain, 48 hour ambulatory ST segment monitoring revealed that 61% had transient episodes of ST segment depression. Of these 91 patients, 30%, had silent ischemia only during 48 hour monitoring, 15% had painful episodes only, and the remaining 55% had both painful and silent episodes. Of the total 598 episodes of ischemia recorded, 75% were silent[20]. Other studies have confirmed these findings[19,56]. Patients with three vessel disease or left main stenosis tend to have more frequent episodes of silent ischemia compared to patients with less extensive disease although there is considerable overlap between these various subsets[19,20]. Patients with resting left ventricular dysfunction and with Q waves on the resting electrocardiogram often do not have electrocardiographic evidence of silent ischemia during daily life but may be more effectively detected by employing radionuclide techniques[19,66,67]. There is also no relation between the frequency of anginal pain and the prevalence and duration of ambulatory ST changes[68]. However, there is a strong relationship between the duration of exercise to ST segment depression during treadmill exercise testing and the presence and frequency of ambulatory silent ischemia[19,20,69].

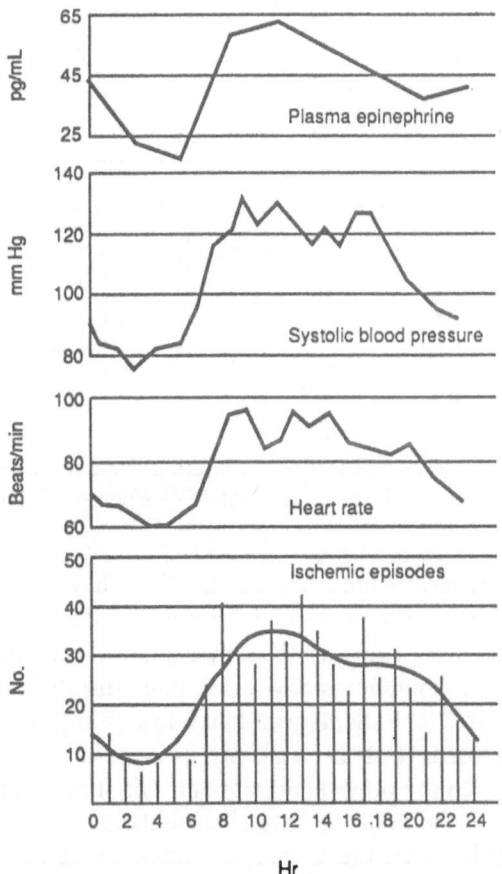

Figure 9.8 Circadian variation in determinants of myocardial oxygen demand. (Adapted from Mulcahy *et al.*[52], Millar-Craig *et al.*[24] and Tofler *et al.*[60]; adapted *Postgraduate Medicine* 1989; 86: 62–75)

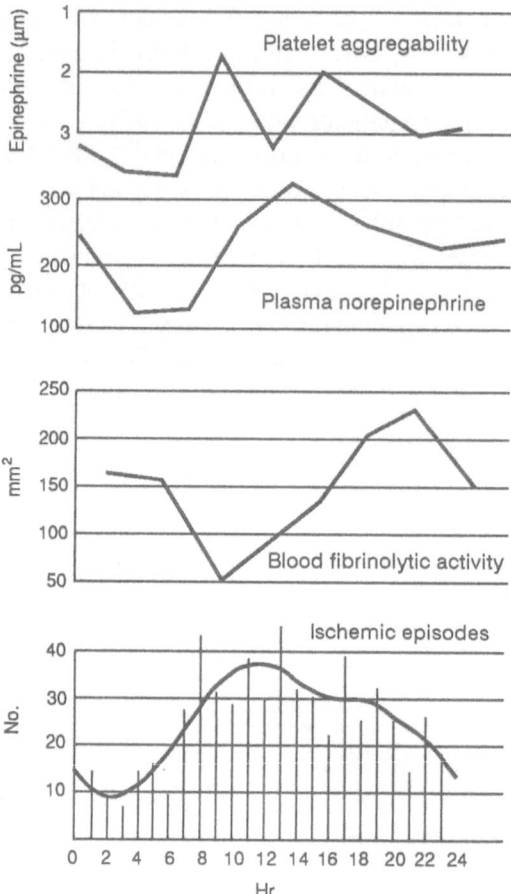

Figure 9.9 Circadian variation in determinants of myocardial blood flow and thrombogenesis. (Adapted from Mulcahy et al.[52] and Tofler et al.[60]; adapted *Postgraduate Medicine* 1989; 86: 62–75)

Why some patients have painful ischemia, others have silent, and yet other patients have a combination of silent and painful ischemia, is not known. There are at least two important factors which may explain these differences. Several studies have examined somatic and visceral pain threshold in patients with coronary artery disease[70,71]. Patients who had a low pain threshold on electrical stimulation, cold pressor test or ischemic pain tests, also had pain with myocardial ischemia. On the other hand, patients who had a high pain threshold with these tests were more likely to have silent ischemia[72]. However, there was considerable overlap between these groups. Patients with neuropathy, such as diabetics, may also be more likely to have silent ischemia. Whether these differences are due to differences in endogenous release of endorphines was also investigated by several groups. Although some have found higher differences in plasma β-endorphine levels in patients who have silent ischemia compared to those who have painful ischemia, other studies have not been able to demonstrate these differences[73,74]. Another factor that may be important in determining whether ischemia is silent or painful is the magnitude of the ischemic insult. When the magnitude of ischemia was measured as the duration and the magnitude of ST segment depression during ambulatory monitoring, it was demonstrated that longer episodes were more likely to be associated with symptoms and the briefer episodes were more likely to be silent[25]. Thus, it is both the patient's pain threshold and the magnitude of the ischemic stimulus which determines whether a given episode is painful or silent. For example, in a patient with a high pain threshold, even a severe episode of ST segment depression may remain silent, and this patient may indeed go on to develop a silent myocardial infarction. On the other hand, a patient with low pain threshold may perceive pain even before the onset of significant ST segment depression during stress testing. There may be other, as yet unknown, factors which may also influence the perception of pain with ischemic episodes.

The pathophysiology of episodes of silent myocardial ischemia in patients with stable coronary artery disease is exactly the same as the mechanisms responsible for precipitation of painful episodes. Silent ischemic episodes can occur in the setting of all other ischemic syndromes, such as variant angina[75] syndrome X[76], unstable angina[77,78] and myocardial infarction[79]. The majority of episodes of variant angina and unstable angina may indeed be silent in some patients, and from the Framingham study it is estimated that up to 30% of myocardial infarcts are unrecognized[79]. Thus, the pathophysiology of silent ischemic events is determined by the clinical presentation of the patient and not whether the episode of ischemia is painful or silent.

VARIANT ANGINA PECTORIS

Even in Heberden's early description of the syndrome of angina pectoris, there were patients whose pain was atypical[1]. He stated 'some have been seized while they are standing still, or sitting, also upon first waking out of sleep'. Wilson and Johnston described electrocardiographic changes similar to those of myocardial infarction in some patients and postulated that ischemia is due to a change in caliber of coronary arteries rather than to increase in work of the heart alone[80]. However, the full description of the syndrome now known as variant angina, or Prinzmetal's angina, was reported by Prinzmetal in 1959, when he described a group of 32 patients with angina pectoris which was different from conventional angina of exertion[81].

Patients with variant angina typically have chest pain at rest rather than with exertion or emotional disturbance. The episodes of pain recur at roughly the same time each day, often in the early hours of the morning between 4 and

6 a.m.[82]. Many episodes are accompanied by ST segment elevation, but others are associated with ST depression or pseudonormalization of the T waves on the electrocardiogram, and are occasionally accompanied by arrhythmias. In general, the pain and the electrocardiographic changes are nitroglycerin responsive. There have been rare reports of patients with normal coronary arteries and a history of exertional angina pectoris who have been demonstrated to develop coronary artery spasm on effort[83,84]. Complete and focal occlusion of an epicardial coronary artery has been angiographically demonstrated during episodes of variant angina by several groups[85-87]. Several arteriographic features have been described[86,87]. The degree of atherosclerotic involvement of the coronary arteries that undergo spasm and total occlusion is variable. This can range from a normal caliber coronary lumen to severely stenosed lumen. Also, the severity of spasm, its duration and electrocardiographic changes accompanying it, vary in the same patient. Thus, with total occlusion, ST segment elevation, peaked T waves or pseudonormalization of inverted T waves occurs. Subtotal occlusion of the lumen by spasm is usually accompanied by ST segment depression.

These angiographic findings have also been confirmed by hemodynamic and cardiac metabolic studies. Maseri et al. monitored left and right ventricular pressures in 22 patients with frequent rest angina[87]. They recorded 153 episodes of ST segment elevation, 92 of which were asymptomatic. No consistent increases in heart rate, blood pressure or left ventricular dp/dt were observed before the onset of ST segment change in any patient. The most typical hemodynamic pattern observed was firstly a reduction of relaxation and contraction peak of the left ventricle (dp/dt). This preceded or accompanied the onset of ST segment or T wave changes. A rise in left ventricular end diastolic pressure followed, and some patients had reduction of systolic arterial pressure. Pulmonary artery wedge pressure rose only after ST segment change had occurred. There was a dramatic decrease in coronary sinus blood flow, coronary sinus oxygen saturation fell often before the onset of ST-T wave changes and lactate production occurred in the coronary sinus. The increase in heart rate and blood pressure was observed some minutes after the onset of ST-T wave changes. The majority of episodes were silent but the sequence of events was similar in painful and silent episodes. Several conclusions were reached by these authors: Firstly, pain was a late phenomenon during ischemia and was often absent; secondly, ST-T wave behavior was often variable in the same patient, and finally, independent of the direction of ST-T wave changes, the episodes were never preceded by increases in indices of myocardial oxygen demand, and were consistent with abrupt reduction of coronary blood flow due to vasospasm. These hemodynamic features are different from the events preceding episodes of ischemia in patients with stable coronary artery disease.

MECHANISMS OF FOCAL SPASM IN EPICARDIAL CORONARY ARTERIES IN VARIANT ANGINA

Medial smooth muscle can constrict and dilate resulting in luminal change by amounts which are determined by geometric constraints of the coronary arteries[89]. The ratio of medial wall thickness to lumen radius is 0.20, which is an average estimate for medium-sized vessels. Normal variations in tone of the coronary artery will cause reductions in outer diameter of coronary arteries by 10%, but may reach up to 25% under certain conditions[70,88,89]. It is clear from geometric calculations made by McAlpin and others, that in the absence of medial or intimal thickening, a 25% reduction in outer diameter will reduce the inner diameter of the lumen by 37%[89]. However, in an artery with intimal thickening, even a smaller increase in vasomotor tone can result in subtotal or total occlusion of the lumen.

Several reports have described total occlusion due to spasm in angiographically normal coronary arteries[85-87]. For this to occur, one has to postulate the existence of localized hyper-reactive and hypercontractile segment of epicardial coronary arteries. With the evidence currently available to us, we have to consider angiographically demonstrated luminal reduction or obliteration as being the result of two probably separate processes. Firstly, as shown above, it may result from a *physiologic* increase in vasomotor tone of the medial smooth muscle, which when superimposed on intimal thickening results in severe luminal narrowing and is probably the mechanism for the variable threshold in patients with stable angina pectoris. Secondly, there may be *pathologic* increase in tone or spasm in a small segment of the epicardial coronary artery, which results in total occlusion and is the likely mechanism responsible for unprovoked episodes of variant angina.

Trigger factors inducing coronary artery spasm have not been identified, although physiologic events such as cold and hyperventilation, or pharmacologic stimuli such as acetylcholine and ergonovine have been demonstrated to precipitate epicardial coronary artery spasm in patients with variant angina. There may be hypersensitivity to α-adrenergic stimulation locally but studies have not demonstrated any increase in receptor density at these sites[17]. There may be local hypersensitivity to and release of vasoconstrictor metabolites, such as thromboxane A2[90]. Other proposed mechanisms include local rise in pH[91], release of histamine, local activation of platelet aggregates[90], or endothelial dysfunction[93].

UNSTABLE ANGINA PECTORIS

Unstable angina, also known as crescendo angina, pre-infarction angina, intermediate coronary syndrome, or coronary insufficiency, is characterized by an increasing frequency, duration and/or magnitude of pain associated with myocardial ischemia. The pain may occur with little or no activity, at rest and sometimes at night, and is less responsive to the usual antianginal medications. Earlier studies had suggested that patients developed unstable angina as a result of progressive severe narrowing of coronary arteries without plaque rupture or thrombus formation[94]. Myocardial ischemia and pain would then occur at rest or with minimal activity due to minor increases in myocardial oxygen demand or vasomotor tone. Recent studies, however, have contradicted this viewpoint. Angiographic studies in patients with unstable angina have suggested the presence of nonocclusive (mural) thrombus in 85 to 100% of patients[94-96] and have been confirmed by angioscopic studies. The beneficial effects of aspirin and thrombolytic therapy in this syndrome are also additional indirect evidence for the role of platelet aggregates and thrombus formation[98,99]. Patients who died after unstable angina have been shown at autopsy to have plaque rupture or fissuring and thrombus formation, as is also invariably seen in myocardial infarction and in most cases of sudden cardiac death[100].

Hemodynamic studies performed by Figueras et al. and Chierchia et al. have demonstrated the importance of coronary vasoconstriction in this syndrome[25,101]. Reduction in coronary sinus oxygen saturation followed by onset of left ventricular dysfunction and ST segment changes and finally chest pain was observed in patients admitted with unstable angina into the Coronary Care Unit. The heart rate–blood pressure product at the onset of electrocardiographic changes remained unchanged in the majority of patients and increased minimally in a few. Maseri et al. have demonstrated coronary artery spasm at sites of previous atherosclerotic narrowing and in normal sections of coronary arteries during both spontaneous and ergonovine-induced episodes of ST segment change in patients presenting with unstable angina[102]. The importance of vasoconstriction in the pathophysiology of unstable angina is further supported by the usefulness of vasodilators in the treatment of chest pain and ischemia in this syndrome[103].

Metabolites of platelet activation are increased in patients with unstable angina pectoris. In separate studies, elevated levels of platelet factor 4 and β-thromboglobulin in peripheral venous blood have been detected in patients with unstable angina, but not in patients with stable angina pectoris[104-106]. Sobel et al. demonstrated a close relation between occurrence of chest pain and platelet activation products in the venous circulation of patients with unstable angina[104]. Hirsch et al. demonstrated that the transcardiac ratio of thromboxane B2 was elevated in patients with unstable angina, but not in those with stable angina pectoris. Although these studies propose a strong association between unstable angina and activation of platelets, the direct causal relation between the two is not proven. Elevated levels of thromboxane B2 and platelet activation products have been detected in the coronary venous circulation only after episodes of spontaneously occurring myocardial ischemia, and therefore may have been secondary to the ischemic injury, rather than the precipitating cause. In a single sample drawn fortuitously a minute before ST segment elevation in one patient, the level of thromboxane B2 was normal. However, the level of thromboxane B2 remained elevated for 6–10 minutes after ST segment elevation resolved, thus providing presumptive evidence that thromboxane A2 alone is not sufficient to cause coronary spasm.

Ambulatory electrocardiographic monitoring for ST segment changes in patients with unstable angina has clearly demonstrated that a number of episodes of myocardial ischemia even in this syndrome are silent[25,27]. However, the pathophysiology and the hemodynamic accompaniments of silent and painful episodes of ischemia are similar. The importance of persistent silent ischemia in determining poor prognosis in unstable angina has also been emphasized by recent studies[77].

MICROVASCULAR ANGINA OR SYNDROME X

Between 10% and 20% of patients undergoing coronary arteriography for angina pectoris have normal epicardial coronary arteries. It is now believed that a number of these patients may in fact have disease affecting the coronary microvasculature. The coronary microvasculature dilates as myocardial work is increased, so that blood flow to the myocardium can be increased proportionately. The arterioles account for the main resistive component of the coronary circulation and would be expected to dilate maximally under ischemic conditions. Microvascular angina or syndrome X is characterized by the failure of maximal dilatation of the coronary resistance bed, resulting in myocardial ischemia and chest pain. Using a variety of stimuli to test maximal vasodilatation, such as atrial pacing, cold pressor test, and dipyridamole, Cannon et al. have demonstrated that, in a group of patients with chest pain and normal coronary arteries, there was evidence of myocardial ischemia with the onset of chest pain after rapid atrial pacing following intravenous ergonovine[105–107]. Patients who had microvascular angina not only developed chest pain, but had inadequate increase in coronary blood flow with pacing after ergonovine compared with control subjects. There was widening of the arterio-venous oxygen content and lactate consumption. No epicardial coronary artery spasm was noted and the authors concluded that the patients with microvascular angina had chest pain despite normal coronary arteries because of an inappropriate coronary vasodilator reserve[107].

Syndrome X is defined as chest pain associated with ST segment depression during treadmill exercise in patients with normal epicardial coronary arteries[76,108]. Opherk et al. demonstrated reduction in maximal coronary blood flow in patients with syndrome X compared with normal individuals in response to intravenous dipyridamole[108]. Ultrastructural examination of myocardial biopsies did not demonstrate physical changes in intramyocardial small vessels, but degenerative changes were noted in the myocardial cells. There has also been demonstrable left ventricular functional impairment on exercise gated blood pool scanning[109]. Many patients with microvascular angina have also been demonstrated to have smooth muscle dysfunction in the esophagus and peripheral vasculature[110,111]. It is likely that syndrome X is pathophysiologically a similar condition to microvascular angina. However, the exact reason for the reduction in vasodilator reserve of the microvasculature is unknown. It has also been hypothesized that it is a metabolic disorder in the myocardial cell or possibly related to endothelial or smooth muscle dysfunction.

RARE SYNDROMES OF ANGINA PECTORIS

Although by far the most common cause of angina pectoris is coronary atherosclerosis, it is not the only pathologic process involving the coronary vasculature that can cause angina. Coronary dissection, vasculitis, and congenital abnormalities have all been described and may cause reduction in coronary blood flow and precipitate angina. Acquired diseases such as syphilis, which may cause osteal stenosis, are now a rare cause of angina pectoris.

Abnormal increase in myocardial oxygen demand due to myocardial hypertrophy may cause ischemia despite the presence of normal epicardial coronary arteries. Thus, it is not unusual for patients with hypertrophic cardiomyopathy, aortic stenosis and severe hypertension to present with angina.

References

1. Heberden W. (1772). Some account of a disorder of the breast. *Med. Trans. Coll. Physicians (London)*, **2**, 59
2. Herrick, J.B. and Nuzum, F.R. (1918). Angina pectoris: Clinical experience with 200 cases. *J. Am. Med. Assoc.*, **70**, 67
3. Zoll, P.M., Wessler, S. and Blumgart, H.L. (1951). Angina pectoris: Clinical and pathological correlation. *Am. J. Med.*, **11**, 331
4. Holland, R.P. and Brooks, H. (1977). TQ-ST segment mapping: critical review and analysis of current concepts. *Am. J. Cardiol.*, **40**, 110
5. Poole-Wilson, P.A. (1983). Angina: pathological mechanisms, clinical expression and treatment. *Postgrad. Med. J.*, **59**, 11
6. Sarnoff, S.J., Braunwald, E., Welch, G.H. *et al.* (1958). Haemodynamic determinants of oxygen consumption of the heart with special reference to the tension time index. *Am. J. Physiol.*, **192**, 148
7. Braunwald, E, Sarnoff, S.J., Case R.B. *et al.* (1958). Hemodynamic determinants of coronary flow. Effect of changes in aortic pressure and cardiac output on the relationship between oxygen consumption and coronary flow. *Am. J. Physiol.*, **192**, 157
8. Hoffman, J.E. and Buckberg, G.D. (1978). The mycardial supply : demand ratio – a critical review. *Am J. Cardiol.*, **41**, 327
9. Krasnow, N., Rolett, E.L., Yurchak, P. *et al.* (1964). Isoproterenol and cardiovascular performance. *Am. J. Med.*, **37**, 514
10. Downey, J.M. and Kirk, E.S. (1975). Inhibition of coronary blood flow by a vascular waterfall mechanism. *Circ. Res.*, **36**, 753
11. Downey, J.M., Downey, H.F. and Kirk, E.S. (1974). Effects of myocardial strains on coronary blood flow. *Circ. Res.*, **34**, 286

12. Downey, J.M. (1900). The extravascular coronary resistance. In Kalsner, S. (ed.). *The Coronary Artery.* pp. 268–91. (London and Canberra: Croom Helm)
13. Weber, K.T. and Janicki, J.S. (1979). The metabolic demand and oxygen supply of the heart. Physiologic and clinical considerations. *Am. J. Cardiol.*, **44**, 722
14. Rubio, R. and Berne, R.M. (1975). Regulation of coronary blood flow. *Prog. Cardiovasc. Dis.*, **18**, 105
15. Wyatt, H.L., Forrester, J.S., Tyber J.V. *et al.* (1975). Effect of graded reductions in regional coronary perfusion on regional and total cardiac function. *Am. J. Cardiol.*, **36**, 185
16. Klocke, F.J. (1983). Measurement of coronary blood flow and degree of stenosis: current clinical implications and continuing uncertainties. *J. Am. Coll. Cardiol.*, **1**, 31
17. Brown, B.G. (1981). Coronary vasospasm: Observations linking the clinical spectrum of ischemic heart disease to the dynamic pathology of coronary atherosclerosis. *Arch. Intern. Med.*, **141**, 716
18. Sabbah, H.N. and Stein, P.D. (1982). Hemodynamics of multiple versus single 50% coronary arterial stenoses. *Am. J. Cardiol.*, **50**, 278
19. Quyyumi, A.A., Mockus, L., Wright, C. and Fox, K.M. (1985). Morphology of ambulatory ST segment changes in patients with varying severity of coronary artery disease. Investigation of the frequency of nocturnal ischaemia and coronary spasm. *Br. Heart J.*, **53**, 186
20. Mulcahy, D., Keege, J., Green, P., Quyyumi, A., Shapiro, L., Wright, C. and Fox, K.M. (1988). Silent myocardial ischaemia in chronic stable angina: a study of its frequency and characteristics in 150 patients. *Br. Heart J.*, **60**, 417
21. Davies, A.B., Bala-Subramanian, V., Cashman, P.M.M. and Raftery, E.T. (1983) Simultaneous recording of continuous arterial pressure, heart rate, and ST segment in ambulant patients with stable angina pectoris. *Br. Heart J.*, **50**, 85
22. Selwyn, A.P., Shea, M., Deanfield, J.E. *et al.* (1986). Character of transient ischemia in angina pectoris. *Am. J. Cardiol.*, **58**(4), 21
23. Cecchi, A.C., Dorvellini, E.V., Marchi, F. *et al.* (1983). Silent myocardial ischemia during ambulatory electrocardiographic monitoring in patients with effort angina. *J. Am. Coll. Cardiol.*, **(3)**, 934
24. Maseri, A., Severi, S., De Nes, M. *et al.* (1978). 'Variant' angina: one aspect of a continuous spectrum of vasospastic myocardial ischaemia. Pathogenetic mechanisms, estimated incidence and clinical and coronary arteriographic findings in 138 patients. *Am. J. Cardiol.*, **42**, 1019
25. Chierchia, S., Brunelli, C., Simonetti, I., Lazzari, M. and Maseri, A. (1980). Sequence of events in angina at rest: primary reduction in coronary flow. *Circulation*, **61**, 759
26. Bertrand, M.E., LeBlanche, J.M., Tilmanc, P.Y. *et al.* (1982). Frequency of provoked coronary arterial spasm in 1089 patients undergoing coronary arteriography. *Circulation*, **65**, 1299
27. Quyyumi, A.A., Wright, C., Mockus, L.J. and Fox, K.M. (1984). Mechanisms of nocturnal angina pectoris: importance of increased myocardial oxygen demand in patients with severe coronary artery disease. *Lancet*, **2**, 1207
28. Quyyumi, A.A., Efthimiou, J., Anees, *et al.* (1984). Mechanisms of rest angina evaluated during sleep. *Br. Heart J.*, **57**, 693
29. Quyyumi, A.A., Crake, T., Wright, C.M., Mockus, L.J. and Fox. K.M. (1987). Medical treatment of patients with severe and rest angina: double blind comparison of beta blocker, calcium antagonist and nitrate. *Br. Heart J.*, **57**, 505
30. Deanfield, J.E., Maseri, A., Selwyn, A.P. *et al.* (1983). Myocardial ischemia during daily life in patients with stable angina: its relation to symptoms and heart rate changes. *Lancet*, **2**, 753
31. Rozanski, A., Bairey, C.N., Krantz, D.S., Friedman, J., Resser, K.J., Morell, M., Hilton-Chalfen, S., Hestrim, L., Bietendorf, J. and Berman, D.S. (1988). Mental stress and the induction of silent myocardial ischemia in patients with coronary artery disease. *N. Engl. J. Med.*, **318**, 1005
32. Brown, B.G., Lee, A.B., Bolson, E.L. and Dodge, H.T. (1984). Reflex constriction of significant coronary stenosis as a mechanism contributing to ischemic left ventricular dysfunction during isometric exercise. *Circulation*, **70**, 18
33. Gage, J.E., Hess, O.M., Murakami, T., Ritter, M., Gramm, J. and Krayenbuehl, H.P. (1986). Vasoconstriction of stenotic coronary arteries during dynamic exercise in patients with classic angina pectoris: Reversibility by nitroglycerin. *Circulation*, **73**, 865
34. Quyyumi, A.A., Rufaie, H.K., Olsen, E.G.J. and Fox, K.M. (1985). Coronary anatomy in patients with various manifestations of three vessel coronary artery disease. *Br. Heart J.*, **54**, 362

35. Roberts, W.C. and Jones, A.A. (1980), Quantification of coronary arterial narrowing at necropsy in sudden coronary death. Analysis of 31 patients and comparison with 25 control subjects. *Am. J. Cardiol.*, **44**, 39
36. Furchgott, R.F. and Zawadski, J.V. (1980). The obligatory role of endothelial cells in the relaxation of arterial smooth muscle by acetylcholine. *Nature*, **288**, 373
37. Griffith, T.M., Lewis, M.J., Newby, A.C. and Henderson, A.H. (1988). Endothelium-derived relaxing factor. *J. Am. Coll. Cardiol.*, **12**, 797
38. Vanhoutte, P.M. and Shimokawa, H. (1989). Endothelium-derived relaxing factor and coronary vasospasm. *Circulation*, **80**, 1
39. Holtz, J., Forstermann, U., Pohl, U., Giesler, M. and Bassenge, E. (1984). Flow-dependent, endothelium-mediated dilatation of epicardial coronary arteries in conscious dogs: effects of cycloxygenase inhibition. *J. Cardiovasc. Pharmacol.*, **6**, 1161
40. Rubanyi, G.M., Romero, J.C. and Vanhoutte, P.M. (1986). Flow-induced release of endothelium-derived relaxing factor. *Am. J. Physiol.*, **250**, H1145
41. Cox, D.A., Vita, J.A., Treasure, C.B., Fish, R.D., Alexandra, R.W., Ganz, O.P. and Selwyn, A.P. (1989). Atherosclerosis impairs flow-mediated dilatation of coronary arteries in humans. *Circulation*, **80**, 458
42. Ludmer, P.L., Selwyn, A.P., Shook, T.L., Wayne, R.R., Mudge, G.H., Alexander, R.W. and Ganz, P. (1986). Paradoxical vasoconstriction induced by acetylcholine in atherosclerotic coronary arteries. *N. Engl. J. Med.*, **315**, 1046
43. Nabel, E.G., Ganz, P., Gordon, J.R., Alexander, R.W. and Selwyn, A.P. (1988). Dilation of normal and constriction of atherosclerotic coronary arteries caused by the cold pressor test. *Circulation*, **77**, 43
44. Griffith, T.M., Edwards, D.H., Davies, R.U., Harrison, T.J. and Evans, K.T. (1988). Endothelium-derived relaxing factor (EDRF) and resistance vessels in an intact vascular bed: a micro-angiographic study of the rabbit isolated ear. *Br. J. Pharmacol.*, **93**, 654
45. Folts, J.D., Crowell, E.B. Jr and Rowe, G.G. (1976). Platelet aggregation in partially obstructed vessels and its elimination with aspirin. *Circulation*, **54**, 365
46. Folts, J.D., Gallagher, K. and Rowe, G.G. (1982). Blood flow reductions in stenosed canine coronary arteries: vasospasm or platelet aggregation? *Circulation*, **65**, 245
47. Moschos, C.B., Lahiri, K., Manskopf, G. *et al.* (1973). Effect of experimental coronary thrombosis upon platelet kinetics. *Thromb. Diath. Haem.*, **30**, 339
48. Davis, H.H., Siegel, B.A., Joist, J.H. *et al.* (1978). Scintigraphic detection of atherosclerotic lesions and venous thrombi in man by indium-111 labelled autologous platelets. *Lancet*, **1**, 1185
49. Mehta, J., Mehta, P., Pepine, C.J. *et al.* (1980). Platelet function studies in coronary artery disease. VII. Effect of aspirin and tachycardia stress on aortic and coronary venous blood. *Am. J. Cardiol.*, **45**, 945
50. Hirsch, P.D., Hillis, L.D., Campbell, W.B. *et al.* (1981). Release of prostaglandins and thromboxane into the coronary circulation in patients with ischemic heart disease. *N. Engl. J. Med.*, **304**, 685
51. Frishman, W.H., Christodoulou, J., Weksler, B. *et al.* (1976). Aspirin therapy in angina pectoris. Effects on platelet aggregation, exercise tolerance, and electrocardiographic manifestations of ischaemia. *Am. Heart J.*, **92**, 3
52. Mulcahy, D., Keegan, J., Cunningham, D., Quyyumi, A., Crean, P., Park, A., Wright, C. and Fox, K. (1988). Circadian variation of total ischemic burden and its alteration with anti-anginal agents. *Lancet*, **2**, 755
53. Muller, J.E., Stone, P.H., Turi, Z.G., Rutherford, J.D., Czeisler, C.A., Parker, C., Poole, W.K., Passamani, E., Roberts, R., Robertson, T., Sobel, B.E., Willerson, J.T., Braunwald, E., and the MILIS Study Group (1985). Circadian variation in the frequency of onset of acute myocardial infarction. *N. Engl. J. Med.*, **313**, 1215
54. Muller, J.E., Ludmer, P.L., Willich, S.N., Tobes, G.H., Aytmer, G., Ksangos, I. and Stone, P.H. (1987). Circadian variation in the frequency of sudden cardiac death. *Circulation*, **75**, 131
55. Marler J.R., Price, T.R., Clark, G.L., Muller J.E., Robertson, T., Mohr, J.P., Hier, D.B., Wolf, P.A., Caplan, L.R. and Foulkes, M.A. (1989). Morning increase in onset of ischemic stroke. *Stroke*, **20**, 473
56. Tsementzis, S.A., Gill, J.S., Hitchcock, E.R., Gil, S.K. and Beevers, D.G. (1985). Diurnal variation of and activity during the onset of stroke. *Neurosurgery*, **17**, 901

57. Rocco, M.B., Barry, J., Campbell, S., Nabel, E., Cook, E.F., Goldman, L. and Selwyn, A.P. (1987). Circadian variation of transient myocardial ischemia in patients with coronary artery disease. *Circulation*, **76**, 395
58. Goldberg, R., Brady, P., Chen, Z., Grore, J., Flessas, A., Greenberg, J., Thedosiou, G., Dalen, J. and Muller, J.E. (1989). Time of onset of acute myocardial infarction after awakening (abstract). *J. Am. Coll. Cardiol.*, **13**, 133A
59. Millar-Craig, M.W., Bishop, C.N. and Raftery, E.B. (1978). Circadian variation of blood pressure. *Lancet*, **1**, 795
60. Tofler, G.H., Brenzinski, D.A., Schafer, A., Czeisler, C.A., Rutherford, J.D., Willich, S.N., Gleason, R.E., Williams, G.H. and Muller, J.E. (1987). Concurrent morning increase in platelet aggregability and the risk of myocardial infarction and sudden cardiac death. *N. Engl. J. Med.*, **316**, 1514
61. Gordon, R.D., Wolfe, L.K., Island, D.P. and Liddle, G.W. (1966). A diurnal rhythm in plasma renin activity in man. *J. Clin. Invest.*, **45**, 1587
62. Quyyumi, A.A., Panza, J.A., Lakatos, E. and Epstein, S.E. (1988). Circadian variation in ischemic events: Causal role of variation in ischemic threshold due to changes in vascular resistance (abstract). *Circulation*, **78** (Suppl II), 11
63. Weitzman, E.D., Fukushima, D., Nogeire, C., Roffwarg, H., Gallagher, T.F. and Hellman, L. (1971). Twenty-four hour pattern of the episodic secretion of cortisol in normal subjects. *J. Clin. Endocrinol. Metab.*, **33**, 14
64. Brezinski, D.A., Tofler, G.H., Muller J.E., Pohjola-Sintonen, S., Willich, S.N., Schafer, A.L., Czeisler, C.A. and Williams, G.H. (1988). Morning increase in platelet aggregability: Association with assumption of the upright posture. *Circulation*, **78**, 35
65. Kayden, D.S., Wackers, F.J., Francis, C.K. and Zaret, B.L. (1988). Silent left ventricular dysfunction during ambulatory radionuclide monitoring following thrombolysis: a potential predictor of subsequent cardiac morbidity. *J. Am. Coll. Cardiol.*, **11**, 25A
66. Quyyumi, A.A., Panza, J.A., McCarthy, K.E., Callahan, T.S., Bonow, R.O. and Epstein, S.E. (1989). Left ventricular function at rest and the prevalence of ambulatory silent ischemia in coronary artery disease. *J. Am. Coll. Cardiol.*, **13**, 203A
67. Quyyumi, A.A., Dilsizian, V., Panza, J.A., Callahan, T.S., Scheffnecht, B.H.B. and Bonow, R.O. (1989). Lack of relation between thallium scintigraphy and ambulatory silent ischemia in coronary artery disease. *Circulation*, **80** (Suppl II), 208
68. Quyyumi, A.A., Wright, C., Mockus, L. and Fox, K. M. (1985). How important is the history of pain in determining the degree of ischaemia in patients with angina pectoris? *Br. Heart J.*, **54**, 22
69. Panza, J.A., Quyyumi, A.A., Callahan, T.S. and Epstein, S.E. (1988). Silent ischemia on Holter monitoring in asymptomatic and mildy symptomatic patients with coronary artery disease: relation to exercise ischemic threshold. *Circulation*, **78** (Suppl II), 42
70. Droste, C. and Roskamm, H. (1983). Experimental pain measurement in patients with asymptomatic myocardial ischemia. *J. Am. Coll. Cardiol.*, **1**(3), 940
71. Glazier, J.J., Chierchia, S., Brown, M.J. *et al.* (1986). Importance of generalized defective perception of painful stimuli as a cause of silent myocardial ischemia in chronic stable angina pectoris. *Am. J. Cardiol.*, **58**(9), 667
72. Chiariello, M., Indolfi, C., Cotecchia, M.R.T. *et al.* (1985). Asymptomatic transient ST changes during ambulatory ECG monitoring in diabetic patients. *Am. Heart J.*, **110**(3), 529
73. Droste, C., Meier-Blankenberg, H., Greenlee, M.W. and Roskamm, H. (1988). Measurement of experimental pain and serum B-endorphin in patients with symptomatic (SMI) and asymptomatic myocardial ischemia (AMI) – modification by naloxone. *Am. J. Coll. Cardiol.*, **11**, 47A
74. Ellestad, M.H. and Kuan, P. (1984). Naloxone and asymptomatic ischemia: failure to induce angina during exercise testing. *Am. J. Cardiol.* **54**, 982
75. Arak, H., Koiwaya, Y., Nakagaki, D. and Nakamura, M. (1983). Duirnal distribution of ST-segment elevation and related arrhythmias in patients with variant angina: a study by ambulatory ECG monitoring. *Circulation*, **67**, 995
76. Kaski, J.C., Crea, F., Nihoyannopoulos, P., Hackett, D. and Maseri, A. (1986). Transient myocardial ischemia during daily life in patients with syndrome X. *Am. J. Cardiol.*, **58**, 1242
77. Gottlieb, S.O., Weisfeldt, M.L., Ouyang, P., Mellits, E.D. and Gerstenblith G. (1986). Silent ischemia as a marker for early unfavorable outcomes in patients with unstable angina. *N. Engl. J. Med.*, **314**, 1214

78. Nademanee, K., Intarachot, V., Josephson, M.A., Rieders, D., Mody, F.V. and Singh, B.N. (1987). Prognostic significance of silent myocardial ischemia in patients with unstable angina. *J. Am. Coll. Cardiol.*, **10**, 1

79. Kannel, W.B. and Abbott, R.D. (1984). Incidence and prognosis of unrecognized myocardial infarction: an update on the Framingham Study. *N. Engl. J. Med.*, **311**, 1144

80. Wilson, F. and Johnston, F. (1941), The occurrence in angina pectoris of electrocardiographic changes similar in magnitude and in kind to those produced by myocardial infarction. *Am. Heart J.*, **22**, 64

81. Prinzmetal, M., Kemnamer, R., Merliss, R. *et al.* (1959). The variant form of angina pectoris. *Am. J. Med.*, **27**, 375

82. Nademanee, K., Intrachot, V., Josephson, M.A. and Singh, B.N. (1987). Circadian variation in occurrence of transient overt and silent myocardial ischemia in chronic stable angina and compansion with Prinzmetal angina in men. *Am. J. Cardiol.*, **60**, 494

83. Specchia, G., De Servi S., Falcone, C. *et al.* (1979). Coronary arterial spasm as a cause of exercise induced ST segment elevation in patients with variant angina. *Circulation*, **59**, 948

84. Freedman, B., Dunn, R.F., Richmond, D. *et al.* (1981). Coronary artery spasm during exercise treatment with verapamil. *Circulation*, **64**, 68

85. Gensini, G.C., Di Giorgi, S., Murad-Netto, D. *et al.* (1963). The coronary circulation: An experimental and clinical study. In: *Memorias del IV Congres. Mondial de Cardiologie IA Mexico*, 325

86. Oliva, R.B., Potts, D.E. and Pluss, R.G. (1973). Coronary arterial spasm in Prinzmetal angina: documentation by coronary arteriography. *N. Engl. J. Med.*, **788**, 745

87. Maseri, A., Severi, S., DeNes, M. *et al.* (1978). 'Variant angina': One aspect of a continuous spectrum of vasospastic myocardial ischaemia. *Am. J. Cardiol.*, **42**, 1019

88. Freedman, M.B., Richmond, D.R. and Kelly, D.T. (1982). Pathophysiology of coronary artery spasm. *Circulation*, **66**, 705

89. Brown, B.G. (1985). Response of normal and diseased epicardial coronary arteries to vasoactive drugs: quantitative arteriographic studies. *Am. J. Cardiol.*, **56**, 23

90. Levy, R.I., Smith, J.B., Silver, M.J. *et al.* (1979). Detection of thromboxane B_2 in the peripheral blood of patients with Prinztmetal's angina. *Prostaglandins Med.*, **2**, 243

91. Weber, S., Pasquier, G., Guiomard, A. *et al.* (1981). Clinical applications of alkalosis stress testing for coronary artery spasm. *Arch. Mal. Coeur*, **74**, 1389

92. Ginsburg, R., Bristow, M.R., Kantrowitz, N. *et al.* (1981). Histamine provocation of clinical coronary artery spasm: implications concerning pathogenesis of variant angina pectoris. *Am. Heart J.*, **102**, 809

93. Demura, K., Yasue, H., Matzuyama, K. *et al.* (1988). Sensitivity and specificity of intracoronary injection of acetylcholine for the induction of coronary artery spasm. *J. Am. Coll. Cardiol.*, **12**, 883

94. Roberts, W.C. and Virmani, R. (1979). Quantification of coronary arterial narrowing in clinically isolated unstable angina pectoris. An analysis of 22 necropsy patients. *Am. J. Med.*, **67**, 792

95. Vetrovec, G.W., Cowley, M.J., Overton, H. and Richardson, D.W. (1981). Intracoronary thrombus in syndromes of unstable myocardial ischemia. *Am. Heart J.*, **102**, 1202

96. Homes, D.R. Jr, Hartzler, G.O., Smith, H.C. and Fuster, V. (1981). Coronary artery thrombosis in patients with unstable angina. *Br. Heart J.*, **45**, 411

97. Sherman, C.T., Litvack, F., Grundfest, W., *et al.* (1986). Coronary angioscopy in patients with unstable angina pectoris. *N. Engl. J. Med.*, **315**, 913

98. Brunelli, C., Spallarosse, P., Ghighliotti, G., Iannetti, M. and Capounetto, S. (1988). Thrombolysis in patients with unstable angina refractory to maximal medical therapy. *J. Am. Coll. Cardiol.*, **11**, 233A

99. Cairns, J.A., Gent, M., Singer, J. *et al.* (1984). A study of aspirin and sulphinpyrazone in unstable angina pectoris. *Circulation*, **70**, 415

100. Davies, M.J. and Thomas, A.C. (1985). Plaque fissuring – the cause of acute myocardial infarction, sudden ischaemic death, and crescendo angina. *Br. Heart J.*, **53**, 363

101. Figueras, J., Singh, B.N., Ganz, W. *et al.* (1979). Mechanism of rest and nocturnal angina: Observations during continuous hemodynamic and electrocardiographic monitoring. *Circulation*, **59**, 995

102. Maseri, A., Pesola, A., Marzilli, M. *et al.* (1977). Coronary vasospasm in angina pectoris. *Lancet*, **1**, 713

103. Theroux, P., Taeymans, Y., Morissette, D., Bosch, Z., Pelletier, G. and Waters, D. (1985). A randomized study comparing propranolol and diltiazem in the treatment of unstable angina. *J. Am. Coll. Cardiol.*, **5**, 717

104. Sobel, M., Salzman, E.W., Davies, G.C. *et al.* (1981). Circulating platelet products in unstable angina pectoris. *Circulation*, **63**, 300

105. Ellis, J.B., Krentz, L.S. and Levine, S.P. (1978), Increased plasma platelet factor 4(PF4) in patients with coronary artery disease. *Circulation*, **58**, 116

106. Smitherman, T.C., Milatn, M., Wood, J. *et al.* (1981). Elevated beta-thromboglobulin in peripheral venous blood of patients with acute myocardial ischaemia: Direct evidence for enhanced platelet reactivity in vivo. *Am. J. Cardiol.*, **48**, 395

107. Cannon, R.O. and Epstein, S.E. (1988). 'Microvascular angina' as a cause of chest pain with angiographically normal coronary arteries. *Am. J. Cardiol.*, **61**, 1338

108. Opherk, D., Zebe, H., Weihe, E. *et al.* (1981). Reduced coronary dilatory capacity and ultra-structural changes of the myocardium in patients with angina pectoris but normal coronary arteriograms. *Circulation*, **63**, 817

109. Cannon, R.O., Bonow, R.O., Bacharach, S.L., Green, M.V., Rosing, D.R., Leon, M.B., Watson, R.M. and Epstein, S.E. (1985). Left ventricualr dysfunction in patients with angina pectoris, normal epicardial coronary arteries and abnormal vasodilator reserve. *Circulation*, **71**, 218

110. Cannon, R.O., Hirszel, R., Cattau, E.L. and Epstein, S.E. (1987). Abnormalities of coronary flow reserve and esophageal motility in syndrome X: a systemic disorder of smooth muscle reactivity? (abstr) *J.A.C.C.*, **9**, 249A

111. Sax, F.L., Cannon, R.O. and Epstein, S.E. (1987). Forearm flow in patients with microvascular angina: evidence of a generalized disorder of vascular tone? *N. Engl. J. Med.* **317**, 1366

10
Investigation and management of acute myocardial infarction

A. CHENG and C.D.J. ILSLEY

INTRODUCTION

The management of acute myocardial infarction has changed radically in the past decade. The interruption of blood supply which leads to infarction usually relates to acute coronary thrombosis upon a pre-existing coronary athero-sclerotic plaque but recent studies involving coronary angiography in the early stages of infarction have also demonstrated the dynamic nature of coronary thrombosis. Although sudden occlusion of a major epicardial coronary artery can be catastrophic, the effects may be mitigated by collateral flow from other arteries or a stuttering thrombotic process. Myocardial infarction can occur in the presence of ostensibly normal vessels, with coronary embolism, spasm or trauma or indeed with rarer specific coronary arterial disease. However, the current approach to management targets the removal or amelioration of thrombotic occlusion as the prime therapeutic objective.

In the initial hours following a 'heart attack', as many as 50% of subjects die from ventricular fibrillation or acute left ventricular failure. For the survivors who reach hospital, or who are treated at home, left ventricular function, reflecting the amount of viable myocardium that remains, is the single most important determinant of both short and long term morbidity and mortality. Patients with a large infarction will demonstrate poor left ventricular function and a high percentage will develop cardiogenic shock, late ventricular tachy-arrhythmias, or subsequent (often unheralded) ventricular fibrillation. Though coronary care units, introduced in the early 1960s, have decreased the in-hospital mortality from arrhythmias, in the 1970s there was only a slight reduction in mortality from the other principal causes of death, such as cardiogenic shock, heart failure or further myocardial infarction. The introduction of an aggressive early interventional approach to the management of acute myocardial infarction will improve prognosis but at what cost and with what degree of risk? Large multicentre trials have answered many of the questions set by clinical investigators at the beginning of the 1980s but in doing so have raised others that will need ongoing research in the coming years.

Considerable effort in current research relating to myocardial infarction is aimed towards the recognition of high risk groups, particularly those at the high risk of early sudden death. The coronary care unit does not merely fulfil the function of an arrhythmia detection centre, but is necessarily a starting point for ongoing research and the development of a more rational approach to the management of patients with acute myocardial infarction and indeed other cardiac diseases. Patients who have unequivocal evidence of acute myocardial infarction, or those in whom a strong suspicion that a myocardial infarction is an evolution, should be admitted to a coronary care unit for the first 48 hours of their illness.

It is nearly 20 years since it was suggested that the quantity of myocardium that becomes necrotic following coronary artery occlusion might be limited by specific interventions[1]. Since then, evidence has become available from studies in experimental animals indicating that an infarct was not a sudden catastrophic event but rather one that evolved and was therefore subject to modification. Experimental studies suggest that substantial quantities of myocardium can be salvaged by treatment with β-adrenergic blockers, nitrates, hyaluronidase and other agents[2]. More recently, direct revascularization with thrombolysis, percutaneous transluminal coronary angioplasty (PTCA) and aorto-coronary bypass surgery have been advocated with the former becoming pre-eminent by the end of the 1980s. Despite apparently unequivocal laboratory findings in experimental animals, there have been no clear guidelines for the use of any modality designed to protect ischaemic myocardium in patients with acute myocardial infarction. Perhaps the single most important factor hampering such research is the inability to predict the infarct size in patients with evolving myocardial infarction and perhaps more importantly the inability to assess the amount of ischaemic myocardium salvaged by intervention. Such predictions may be difficult, or indeed impossible, at the present time; but it is likely that there are several interventions which are clinically useful.

CLINICAL FEATURES Of ACUTE MYOCARDIAL INFARCTION[3]

Chest pain, evolving electrocardiographic changes and elevated serum enzymes remain the necessary building blocks to establish a diagnosis of acute myocardial infarction. The chest pain is variable in intensity but in most patients is severe, typically lasting for more than 30 minutes and resembling classic angina pectoris. A prodromal history can be elicited in up to 60% of patients with myocardial infarction and though the onset is often at rest (in over 50%), severe exertion, emotional stress, trauma or surgical procedures are well-known precipitating factors. Up to one quarter of non-fatal myocardial infarctions may be unrecognized by the patient and discovered only on routine electrocardiography. Unrecognized or silent infarction occurs but rarely in patients with angina pectoris and is more common in patients with diabetes and hypertension.

Patients with myocardial infarction are usually classified into two groups on the basis of well-known electrocardiographic criteria: 'transmural', 'Q-wave infarction'; and 'non-transmural', 'non-Q-wave' infarction occurring without the development of Q waves with associated isolated ST or T wave changes. The term Q-wave infarction has replaced transmural infarction because morphological studies have shown a lack of specificity of Q waves as a marker for infarction involving all layers of the myocardium. Similarly with non-Q-wave infarction. Myocardial infarction may occur in the absence of significant electrocardiographic changes. Irreversibly injured myocardial cells release enzymes causing the serum creatinine phosphokinase (CPK) activity to exceed the normal range within about 6 hours of infarction, elevating the aspartate transaminase (AST) levels within 12 to 14 hours and elevating the serum hydroxybutyric dehydrogenase (HBD) activity beyond the normal within 24 hours. Peak activity in these enzymes occurs at approximately 24 hours, 48 hours and 4–5 days respectively (Figure 10.1).

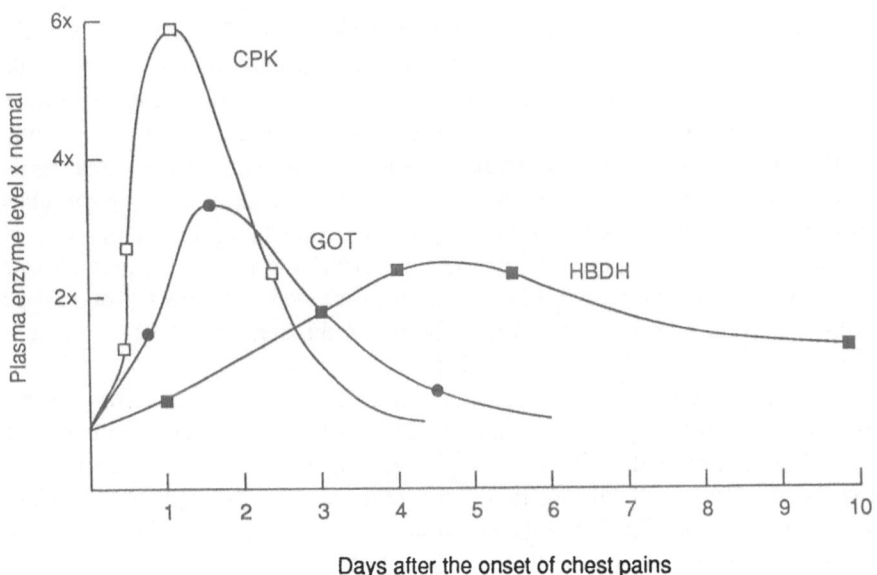

Figure 10.1 Plasma profiles for creatine kinase (CPK), glutamine–oxaloacetic transaminase (GOT) and hydroxybutyrate dehydrogenase (HBDH, LDH) activities following the onset of acute myocardial infarction

Patients with acute myocardial infarction are usually anxious and in considerable pain. The heart rate may vary from a marked bradycardia – either naturally occurring or induced by therapy, such as β-adrenergic blockade or morphine – or may be rapid and regular or irregular depending on the underlying rhythm and the degree of left ventricular failure. The blood pressure is usually normal or low, but a minority of patients may show a hypertensive response with the arterial pressure exceeding 160/90 mmHg. Patients with a tachycardia and elevated blood pressure are at greater risk, presumably as a consequence of adrenergic discharge secondary to pain and agitation. Arrhythmias are common and some abnormality of cardiac rhythm is noted in 75% of patients. Moreover, many arrhythmias occur prior to hospitalization and thus the overall incidence of rhythm disturbance in acute myocardial infarction may be as high as 100%. Sinus bradycardia is the commonest arrhythmia, but 1 in 3 patients will have a sinus tachycardia at some stage in the early period following infarction and atrial premature extrasystoles, supraventricular tachycardia, atrial flutter, ventricular extrasystoles and ventricular tachy-arrhythmias are all common.

Ventricular extrasystoles are so frequent as to be almost universal. 'Warning arrhythmias' have been defined as frequent ventricular extrasystoles (more than 5 min^{-1}), multiform configuration, early coupling (the R on T phenomenon) and repetitive extrasystoles in the form of couplets or salvos. However, primary ventricular fibrillation (ventricular fibrillation in the absence of congestive failure, pulmonary oedema and cardiogenic shock) occurs without warning arrhythmias in as many as 80% of cases and frequent and complex extrasystoles are commonly observed in patients with acute myocardial infarction, who never develop ventricular fibrillation. Although the suppression of ventricular premature beats is traditional, most physicians treat simple unifocal extrasystoles (whatever the frequency) conservatively. Conduction disturbances, particularly atrioventricular block, carry varying prognostic importance depending on site and haemodynamic consequences of the myocardial infarction. It is well known that complete atrio-ventricular block in association with an anterior myocardial infarction carries a grave prognosis; whereas mild degrees of heart block in inferior infarction carry little additional risk.

The major haemodynamic derangement in acute myocardial infarction is consequent on left ventricular dysfunction. However, catastrophic events such as the development of acute ventricular septal defect, papillary muscle rupture, and left ventricular free wall rupture in a small proportion of patients are associated with a very high mortality. Patients with non-Q-wave infarction appear to behave as if they have had partial reperfusion. Though there is a reduced early mortality compared to those with Q-wave infarction they are at higher risk of early re-infarction, and are more likely to demonstrate a patent but severely stenosed infarct-related coronary artery. This in turn increases the likelihood of residual coronary ischaemia.

The investigation of a patient presenting with chest pain consistent with acute myocardial infarction is designed to confirm the diagnosis and provide an indirect estimate of infarct size. The management is directed at limiting infarct size as much as possible and in treating the haemodynamic disturbance, whatever the mechanism, with appropriate therapy. Myocardial infarction is usually the result of acute coronary thrombosis and early full reperfusion offers a logical and most likely the best method of reducing infarct size. However, it appears that mortality related to large infarcts can be reduced by a host of different agents and since these agents act through independent mechanisms, combinations of all or some of them are likely to be more beneficial than any single treatment modality. As such, modern treatment may make a considerable impact upon the risk of death due to left ventricular failure associated with acute myocardial infarction.

Estimation of infarct size[2]

Myocardial infarct size can be estimated indirectly by the use of electro-cardiographic changes, enzyme release, myocardial scintigraphy and two-dimensional echocardiography. Although these techniques have been validated experimentally, each method has its limitations.

ST segment elevation obtained from multiple precordial ECG leads is a useful indicator of the extent of myocardial ischaemia in patients with anterior infarction who have no conduction defect. A normal or near normal ECG on admission with suspected myocardial infarction carries a good prognosis[4]. Although ST segment mapping may be criticized for its lack of reproducibility or lack of correlation with other markers of necrosis, if very early peak ST segment elevation is compared with enzyme release or the development of subsequent Q waves, good correlations can be demonstrated. Loss of R wave amplitude and the development of Q waves have been shown to correlate well with pathological measurements in experimental infarction and total enzyme release.

Persistent ST segment depression or elevation (especially if the latter occurs without objective evidence of pericarditis), persistent T wave inversion and abnormal Q waves in multiple leads correlates with a poor prognosis following infarction. In addition, patients demonstrating persistent repetitive ventricular extrasystolic activity, atrioventricular and intraventricular conduction defects, atrial fibrillation and left ventricular hypertrophy have an increased mortality.

A relationship exists between prognosis and high serum enzyme levels and several studies have demonstrated that infarct size estimated from serial CPK measurements correlates with pathological infarct size. In this regard, the measurement of the MB isoenzyme of CPK appears to be the most useful test for myocardial necrosis. However, highly elevated cardiac enzymes may be found in patients undergoing spontaneous or therapeutic thrombolysis and such patients may go on to have a good clinical result. Patients with cardiogenic shock, who may have poor blood flow through the infarct, demonstrate greater enzyme release than those without cardiogenic shock and thus it is possible that the size of the infarct has actually little effect on the kinetics of enzyme release.

Myocardial scintigraphy can be performed with a variety of techniques and it appears that infarct estimates using technetium-99 correlate well with infarct size in dogs and a good correlation has also been reported between thallium scanning and post mortem estimation of infarct size in man. Good correlations have been obtained between quantitative QRS scoring systems and ventricular function assessed by radionuclide studies.

With the advent of two-dimensional echocardiography, repeated non-invasive measurements of left ventricular wall motion may be performed at the bedside. Though actual infarct size is overestimated by this technique, its very ready application to the coronary care setting makes it a more attractive clinical option than radionuclear methods.

Survival following myocardial infarction depends on a number of factors, the most important of these being the state of left ventricular function. Overall, there appears to be an in-hospital mortality of 15% in patients admitted with acute myocardial infarction, though in the absence of clinically apparent cardiac failure on admission mortality is 8% or less. In the smaller number of patients admitted with established left ventricular failure or shock, mortality is 45% and 75–100% respectively.

The Norris coronary prognostic index (CPI) is a useful and clinically relevant index derived from the patient's age, the admission ECG, blood pressure, heart size and pulmonary vasculature[5]. The major value of the Norris index, however, lies in the stratification of groups of patients rather than the ability to define any individual course. Such factors as male sex, increasing age, history of diabetes mellitus, hypertension, prior angina pectoris or previous myocardial infarction have been considered related to a worse prognosis, but are not predictive (apart from increasing age) of in-hospital mortality according to Norris's data.

MANAGEMENT OF ACUTE MYOCARDIAL INFARCTION[6]

Bed rest, the establishment of electrocardiographic monitoring, analgesia for the relief of chest pain and the provision of oxygen (when necessary) may be regarded as routine measures in all patients admitted with chest pain in whom myocardial infarction is suspected. In addition, all patients should be anticoagulated with systemic administration of full dose heparin therapy, most frequently at a dose of 1000 units hourly. The initial management of chest pain is to administer morphine, supplemented by intravenous nitroglycerine infusion and β-adrenergic blockade. Therapy with calcium antagonists is usually reserved for the treatment of ongoing angina in patients in whom β-adrenergic blockade is contraindicated, or where antianginal therapy is required in addition to established β-blockade. Oxygen is only administered when clear arterial hypoxaemia has been demonstrated. An ECG is taken on admission and subsequently every 12 hours, or more frequently if the patient's progress is complicated. Blood is taken for haemoglobin, white count, urea, electrolytes, glucose and serially for cardiac enzymes estimation.

Anticoagulation in the early stages of acute myocardial infarction has three main benefits. Since acute coronary thrombosis is usually responsible for infarction, herapin may enhance natural thrombolytic mechanisms. Anticoagulants also diminish the formation of intracardiac thrombi and therefore the risk of systemic embolization – especially in acute anterior myocardial infarction. Anticoagulant therapy certainly exerts a favourable effect on survival in patients with a high risk of embolism – i.e. those with ventricular aneurysm and/or demonstrable intraventricular thrombus, patients with marked obesity, low output state, or a past history of deep vein thrombosis or pulmonary embolism. However, the long term benefit of anticoagulants remains controversial.

It is pertinent that this 'routine' management has been available for two decades with little demonstrable improvement in patient survival. For example, an analysis of results of all the coronary care units in Boston, Massachusetts, failed to show any demonstrable improvement in hospital mortality calculated for the years 1973/74 and compared to 1978/79 – a period in which the United States mortality for ischaemic heart disease was consistently falling. Overall admission rates, with approximately 8500 patients admitted in both years, were accompanied by similar mortalities of 22% and 23% respectively[7]. Most attention during this period related to the consequences of myocardial infarction rather than its cause.

Interventions that may be expected to limit infarct size revolve around the basic principles of supply and demand. It is obviously attractive to remove the initiating thrombus and re-establish coronary arterial perfusion in the infarct-related vessel; but an equally favourable result might be obtained by improving collateral flow from non-obstructed arterial beds. Alternatively, the provision of metabolites – such as glucose, insulin and potassium – may limit the effects of hypoxaemia, if sufficient perfusion exists to deliver them to the site of infarction. Indirectly, oxygen demand may be reduced by β-adrenergic blockade or decreasing the 'load' on the heart by systemic arteriolar or venous vasodilation. All of these approaches have been evaluated and demonstrated as effective in the experimental laboratory but perhaps only a few have been properly evaluated in man[2].

Acute myocardial infarction usually occurs as thrombosis on an established coronary atherosclerotic plaque. Thrombosis leading to infarction may also occur in apparently normal epicardial vessels. Equally, although spontaneous thrombolysis is recognized, it may not occur until irreversible damage has been sustained. Activation and augmentation of the thrombolytic system offers the prospect of effective reperfusion within a sufficiently short time frame to allow for some or complete myocardial salvage. If instigated very early in the evolution of a myocardial infarction, complete recovery is possible. After several small studies supported this hypothesis publications of the GISSI Study[8], and the ISIS-2[9], ASSET[10] and APSAC-AIMS[11] studies amongst others have firmly established thrombolytic therapy in addition to 'routine' therapy for myocardial infarction. The further implication is that the greatest benefit will come from the earliest interventions. Nevertheless however far we progress with in-hospital treatment of myocardial infarction a major effect on national mortality will not occur until active thrombolytic therapy is delivered to patients in the community. The parallel with out-of-hospital cardiopulmonary resuscitation for ventricular fibrillation is obvious.

EARLY IN-HOSPITAL INTERVENTION IN ACUTE MYOCARDIAL INFARCTION

The specific management in any individual with suspected myocardial infarction depends upon the clinical presentation. Figure 8.2 outlines a basic scheme of management undertaken for patients admitted to the coronary care unit (CCU). Such units should be supported by an intermediate care unit and telemetry for post-infarction monitoring in the general cardiology ward. In addition to routine tests we would place an emphasis on the non-invasive assessment of infarct size by use of two-dimensional echocardiography (2D–echo). Access to a cardiac catheter laboratory is extremely attractive but not mandatory for successful management of acute myocardial ischaemia and infarction.

Traditionally, the diagnosis of acute myocardial infarction relies on history, serial ECG changes and a characteristic enzyme pattern. Once all these criteria are satisfied that infarction has occurred, the time for active intervention has long passed. In some cases a questionable history or ECG changes on admission can be supported by the use of 2D-echo demonstrating regional wall motion abnormalities. Once a diagnosis of acute myocardial infarction has been made, it is possible to consider the various therapeutic options.

The role of thrombolytic therapy in acute myocardial infarction

We would use streptokinase in all patients presenting within six hours of the onset of pain (1) in which the electrocardiogram demonstrates typical ST segment elevation, (2) in some individuals with relatively normal ECGs (those with a convincing history within one to two hours of the onset of pain), and (3) occasional patients with myocardial infarction complicated by hypotension or ongoing chest pain (Figure 10.2). In patients selected for streptokinase therapy, a dose of corticosteroids (either 200 mg of hydrocortisone or 2 g of methyl-prednisolone, depending on physician preference) is given followed by 1.5 million units of streptokinase administered by intravenous infusion over 20 minutes. Streptokinase may also be administered either directly, or during cardiac catheterization into the infarct-related vessel where a much lower dose may be given – an initial 40 000 units and then 10 000 units each minute (up to a maximum of 250 000 units) until restoration of blood flow in the infarct vessel has been demonstrated. However, many studies are available to suggest that the rate of coronary thrombolysis (either recanalization or reperfusion, depending

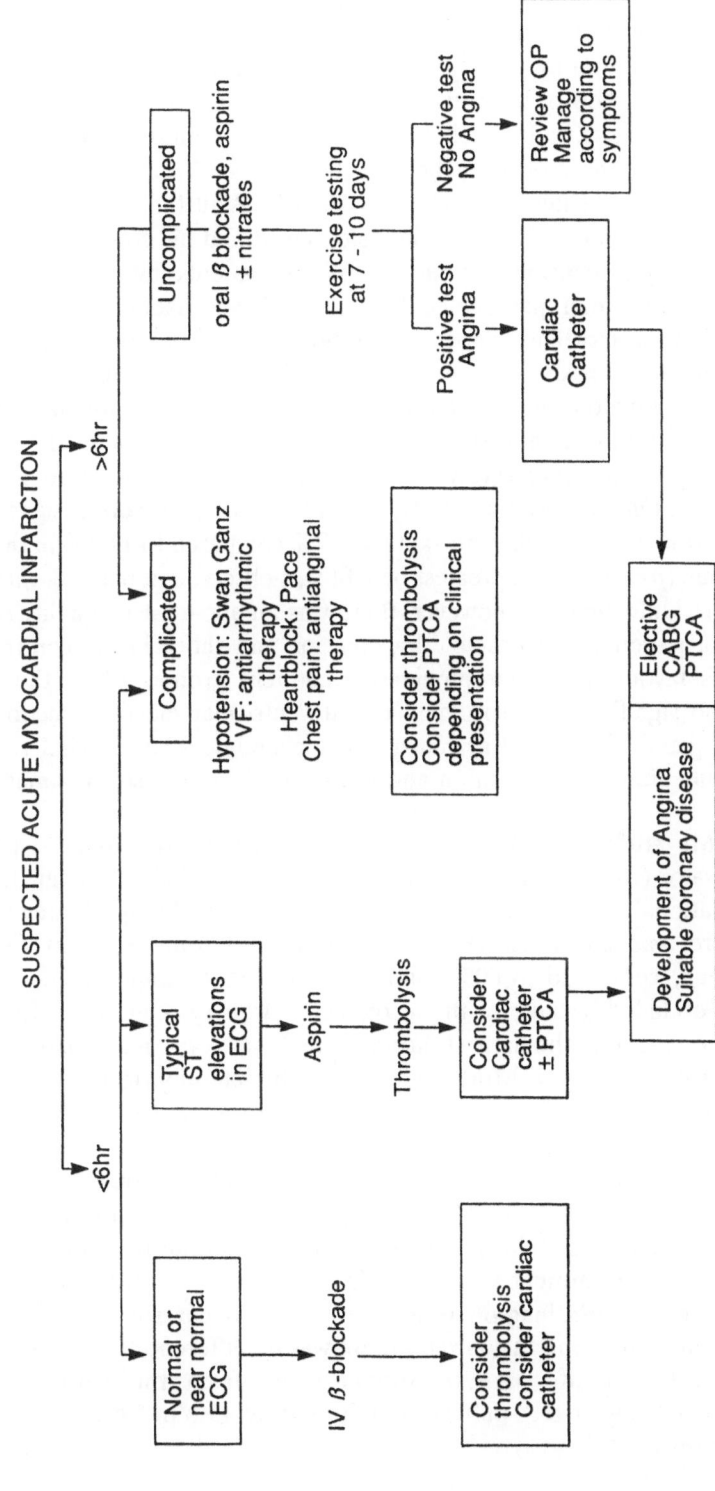

SUSPECTED ACUTE MYOCARDIAL INFARCTION

<6hr

>6hr

Normal or near normal ECG

IV β-blockade

Consider thrombolysis
Consider cardiac catheter

Typical ST elevations in ECG

Aspirin

Thrombolysis

Consider Cardiac catheter ± PTCA

Complicated

Hypotension: Swan Ganz
VF: antiarrhythmic therapy
Heartblock: Pace
Chest pain: antianginal therapy

Consider thrombolysis
Consider PTCA depending on clinical presentation

Uncomplicated

oral β blockade, aspirin ± nitrates

Exercise testing at 7 - 10 days

Positive test Angina

Negative test No Angina

Cardiac Catheter

Review OP Manage according to symptoms

Development of Angina
Suitable coronary disease

Elective CABG PTCA

CABG = coronary atery bypass grafting, OP = outpatient, VF = ventricular fibrillation
PTCA = percutaneous transluminal coronary angioplasty

Figure 10.2 Outline of the management of acute myocardial infarction

on coronary dye flow) is similar. As peripheral administration is logistically easier, this has a more widespread appeal.

Despite the vast literature produced in recent years many questions remained[12,13]. In their review of intravenous and intracoronary fibrolytic therapy in myocardial infarction, Yusuf and his colleagues have summarized all the available information on the mortality, the infarction rate and side effects from 33 randomized controlled trials from 1959 to 1985[14]. Whilst the wisdom of pooling results from several trials is questionable, Yusuf and his colleagues did draw some interesting conclusions. Whilst 0–15% of patients suffered minor bleeding, only a very small percentage had a significant haemorrhage. A moderate reduction in mortality appeared to be gained from thrombolytic therapy (streptokinase or urokinase) and the rate of reinfarction was also lower.

The Western Washington randomized trial of intracoronary streptokinase in acute myocardial infarction demonstrated a three fold improvement in the 30 day mortality in those patients receiving streptokinase as compared to the control population[15]. One hundred and thirty-four of 250 patients were assigned to the treatment group with a 30 day mortality of 3.7% compared to 11.2% in the 116 control patients ($p = 0.02$). The greatest benefit was observed in patients with anterior infarction. Unfortunately, however, there was an apparent inequality in the distribution of patients with baseline hypotension and shock in the control patients, perhaps favouring the streptokinase treatment group. Also, there appeared to be no significant improvement in left ventricular ejection fraction (as measured by gated blood pool scanning and technetium-99m labelled red cells) in all patients after catheterization and at two weeks in the streptokinase treated patients.

The first TIMI study randomized intravenous recombinant tissue type plasminogen activator (rt-PA) vs intravenous streptokinase carried out under the auspices of the National Heart, Lung and Blood Institute in the United States of America[16]. There was an observed reperfusion rate of only 35% in the streptokinase group, compared to 60% following rt-PA at 90 minutes. Of 290 patients, 76 were excluded because of the incomplete coronary occlusion before drug infusion, demonstrating the natural thrombolytic tendency in many patients with acute myocardial infarction. Mortality, analysed by intention to treat, was 5% (7/143) and 8% (12/147) of those originally assigned to rt-PA and streptokinase therapy respectively. Despite the theoretical advantages of rt-PA over streptokinase, it was important to note that haemorrhagic problems were not demonstrably eliminated with r-tPA. Once again, methodological criticisms are easy to assemble and it should be noted that the mean time from onset of pain to the initiation of treatment was nearly five hours in the TIMI trial. In contrast to the Western Washington trial, there was no control group and despite the apparent better reperfusion rates there was no difference in mortality between the two treatments. An additional study from the European Cooperative study group for r-tPA published in the *Lancet*, also in 1985, showed essentially similar results[17].

In the GISSI trial, 11 806 patients in 176 units were enrolled over 17 months[8]. Patients admitted within 12 hours after the onset of pain were randomized with respect to streptokinase but otherwise had additional 'usual treatment'. At 21 days there was an 18% reduction in overall mortality ($p = 0.0002$) with reported mortality of 10.7% (628/5860) in the streptokinase treated patients compared with 13% (758/5852) in the control group.

In contrast to our own practice, and that advocated by others, it should be remembered that the GISSI study enrolled patients within 12 hours of the onset of symptoms and the authors conclude that:

> In view of the high consistency of our findings with those obtained in small, more rigidly controlled studies, intravenous infusion of 1.5 million units of streptokinase can be recommended as a safe treatment for all patients with no positive contraindication, who can be treated within six hours from the onset of pain.

But within the trial, subgroup analysis clearly demonstrated greatest mortality reduction in patients treated within one hour (50%) and no reduction in those treated after six hours. Further data from the GISSI group showed that streptokinase was of little benefit in small infarcts (assessed by 12-lead electrocardiographic changes) where the overall mortality risk was only about 6%. In contrast a significant decrease was noted in modest (8% vs 11%), large (13% vs 17%) and extensive (20% vs 24%) infarction leading the authors to conclude that the extent of infarction was more relevant than the site in determining the in-hospital mortality and efficacy of thrombolytic therapy.

Following on from the GISSI trial, ISIS-2 confirmed and established the role of thrombolytic therapy and also examined the contribution of aspirin in the treatment of myocardial infarction[9]. 17 187 patients were enrolled and randomized to receive 1.5 mega units streptokinase i.v. over one hour and also randomized to additional 160 mg enteric coated aspirin for a month. Both streptokinase and aspirin were placebo controlled in the study, and study design ensured a quarter of the patients received both. Placebo mortality was 12–13% with the greatest advantage observed when aspirin and streptokinase were given together (mortality 8% (343/4292) vs 13.2% (568/4300)). Both streptokinase and aspirin individually provided a highly significant improvement in five week mortality. Of interest was the fact that treatment was initiated within 24 hours of the onset of pain and over 400 patients aged 80 years and over were enrolled in this study with no reported intracerebral haemorrhage.

The Anglo Scandinavian Study of early thrombolysis (ASSET)[10] enrolled over 5000 patients in a double blind randomized trial of intravenous r-tPA and heparin versus placebo and heparin. A 26% reduction in nine month mortality was observed in the treatment group (7% versus 10%).

An alternative agent is anisoylated plasminogen streptokinase activator complex (APSAC), now called anistreplase. This is concentrated at the site of recent thrombus and has the singular advantage in being administered as a single bolus injection of 20 units. It results in reperfusion in about 65% and the British APSAC AIMS double blind placebo controlled trial showed a near 50% reduction in 30 day mortality (6.4% versus 12.2%)[11]. There was a similar reduction at one year (10.8% versus 19.4%).

Thrombolytic therapy *per se* has great benefit in the management of patients with acute myocardial infarction and the choice of agent is dependent on physician preference. Anistreplase may well be the best of the agents because it can be administered as a single intravenous injection rather than an infusion over 30 to 60 minutes as in the case of streptokinase and r-tPA. Within the next couple of years, however, the results of the ISIS-3 study will become available. Once again ISIS will enroll a formidable number of patients comparing the three major thrombolytic agents. Currently, in the UK, streptokinase is favoured because it is significantly cheaper and more readily available than the other agents. No comparable studies exist for urokinase, and other hybrid thrombolytic agents are being developed and will undergo trial in the forthcoming decade.

Aspirin also has a firmly established role in the treatment of acute myocardial ischaemia and infarction. Enthusiasm for thrombolysis should not lead us to forget the value of β-blockade and though the early acute administration of an intravenous agent such as metoprolol may not provide any additional benefit as regards mortality, it certainly reduces cardiac pain, and the incidence of serious ventricular arrhythmias in the peri- and post-infarction period in patients who can tolerate such agents.

When presented with a patient one to two hours after the onset of chest pain, it can often be difficult to differentiate infarction from unstable or severe angina unless there is typical ST segment elevation. Patients with a normal or near normal ECG in this setting are known to have a good prognosis and it is not necessary to administer to all such individuals thrombolytic therapy unless they are clinically ill. Some authorities have recommended thrombolysis when the ECG shows only ST segment depression (and thus more likely unstable angina) but this is not yet routine practice. Trials of thrombolytic therapy in patients with ST segment depression or T wave infarction are under way.

THE ROLE OF PERCUTANEOUS TRANSLUMINAL CORONARY ANGIOPLASTY IN ACUTE MYOCARDIAL INFARCTION

Thrombolysis will only be successful in reopening up to 75% of occluded arteries, and the majority of such patients will be left with a high grade stenosis in the infarct-related vessel. PTCA is now firmly established in the treatment of ischaemic heart disease with a large number of cardiologists having sufficient expertise to perform this procedure. Successful coronary thrombolysis might be expected to limit infarction but leave a region of ischaemia, and some studies suggest a higher rate of reinfarction or post-infarction angina in patients after thrombolysis. It was logical to assume that additional PTCA might add to the prognostic benefit of thrombolysis.

The first account of immediate PTCA after successful intracoronary thrombolysis was reported by Meyer and colleagues in 1982[18]. In their study 17 of 21 patients (81%) underwent successful PTCA within 24 hours of successful thrombolysis and the results compared favourably to a retrospective control group of 18 patients with similar clinical characteristics that had been treated with intracoronary streptokinase alone. Similar results have been described from other centres, though usually with relatively small numbers of patients and accepting the fact that it is exceedingly difficult to provide a scientifically satisfactory control group in such studies. In this regard it may be seen that the open study from Simoons and colleagues, who reported the Dutch experience, provides a reasonable clinical framework for the use of PTCA in acute infarction[17]. They performed an open study comparing a highly invasive approach with both thrombolysis and PTCA in some patients and compared the results to patients treated with more conventional management without acute catheterization or the use of thrombolytic drugs. Of 44 patients who underwent PTCA immediately after thrombolysis, three had non-fatal reinfarctions and one died. Overall, the long term survival was much improved by their invasive approach compared to 'conservative management'.

In 1983, Hartzler and colleagues provided the first study in which PTCA was used without associated thrombolytic therapy for myocardial infarction[19]. PTCA alone was performed in 37 patients and was successful in 78%. Streptokinase was applied as the primary intervention in 39 patients (50%) and in the 80% for whom streptokinase produced coronary recanalization, PTCA was performed with a high grade residual stenosis with an 81% success. The incidence of early ischaemic events was only 6% after acute PTCA with a late re-occlusion rate of 17% at a mean follow-up of six months.

However, larger, randomized studies have tested the strategy of electively performing PTCA in the early post-infarction period. Both TIMI[20,21] and the TAMI[22] trials have shown that thrombolysis combined with early PTCA offers no clear advantage. Indeed, mortality and morbidity are slightly higher in the PTCA treated patients in the first week. In the TAMI study, r-tPA was given within four hours of onset of symptoms, and coronary angiography performed 90 minutes later. 288 (75%) patients had a patent infarct-related artery and 197 were randomized to immediate PTCA (99 patients) or elective PTCA (97 patients) seven days post-infarction[22]. There was no difference in overall left ventricular function in the two groups. In the TIMI-IIA study, the aim was to investigate whether immediate cardiac catheterization with PTCA within two hours of treatment confers any advantage over the same procedure performed at 24 hours[21]. PTCA was attempted in 72% of the 195 patients randomized to PTCA and 55% of the 194 randomized to a slightly more delayed attempt. Mortality and reinfarction were numerically more significant (13% vs 9%) in the two hour group, though with relatively small numbers this was not statistically significant. There was no difference in left ventricular function but the risk of complications, especially those leading to coronary bypass grafting, was significantly higher in the two hour PTCA treated group.

In the full TIMI-II trial[20], 3262 patients were randomized to invasive (coronary angiography and PTCA treatment where possible to residual stenosis) or conservative (angiography and PTCA only in individuals with spontaneous or exercise induced ischaemia) strategies. 57% underwent PTCA in the former group compared to only 13% in the latter with no difference in the mortality or reinfarction rate in the six week period of follow-up (11% vs 10% respectively). The one year follow-up results also show no difference between the groups.

Given the logistic difficulties of considering early PTCA in all patients with myocardial infarction in this country, these results are very reassuring. Elective PTCA is not indicated though individuals with suitable anatomy showing signs of ongoing ischaemia may need PTCA, and in such patients it can be life saving. The APSAC-SWIFT study comparing conservative therapy with an intervention policy involving either PTCA or coronary bypass showed broadly comparable results to the TIMI-II trial, but this study has not yet been reported in full.

On the other hand, another chapter in this story is about to be written. Some patients with known coronary anatomy who develop acute infarction after diagnostic coronary angiography can undergo PTCA without thrombolysis with excellent clinical results. No trial has yet been performed comparing immediate

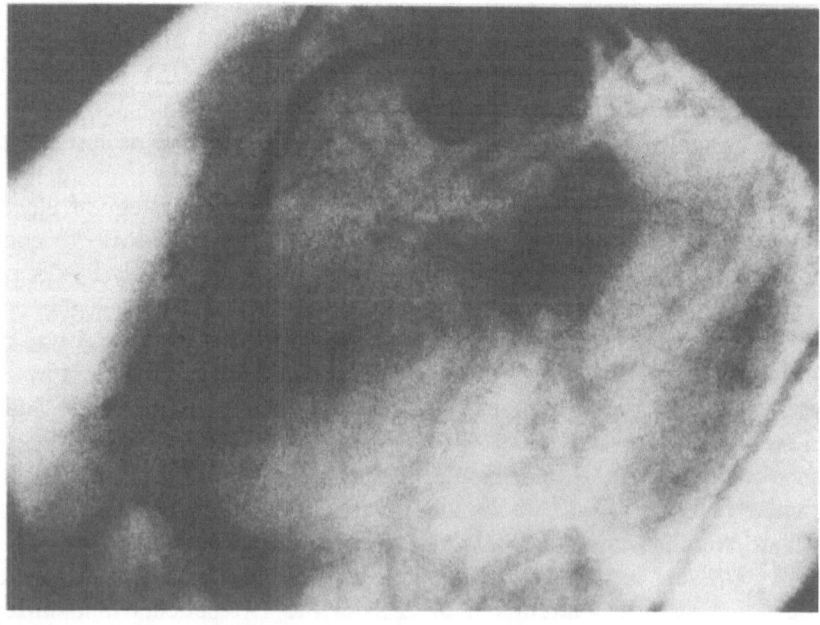

(a)

Figure 10.3
(a) Acute inferior infarction: Right coronary angiogram taken in a 48-year-old man. He presented with chest pain and the ECG demonstrated hyperacute ST segment elevation in leads II, III, aVF. The artery is completely occluded. Taken 1.5 hours after the onset of pain

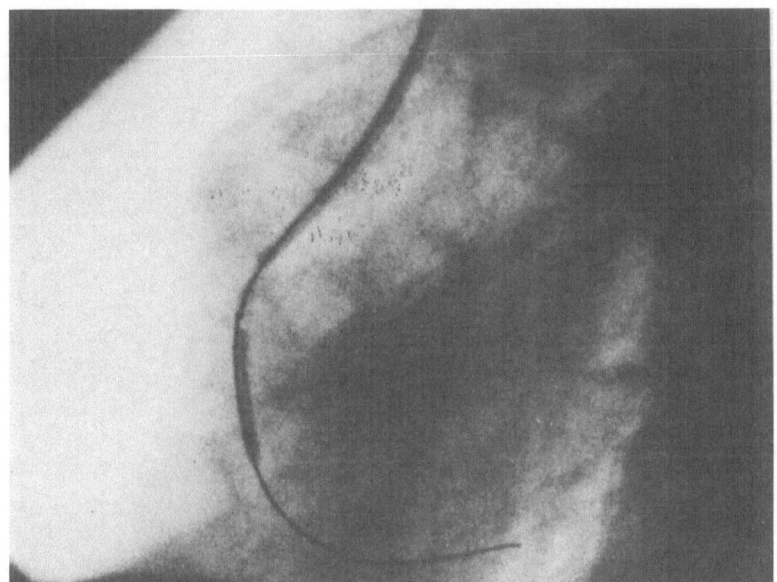

(b)

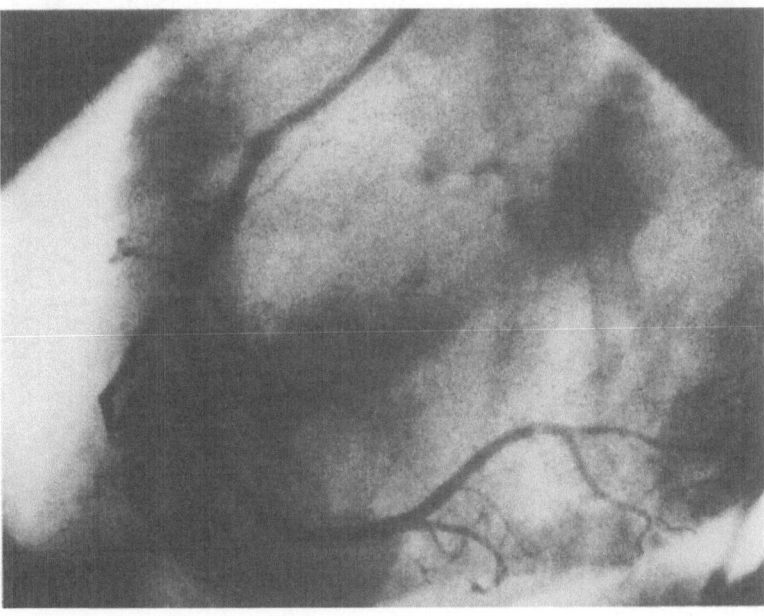

(c)

(b) The occlusion was probed and crossed with a guide wire, which allowed the balloon dilation catheter to be positioned and inflated

(c) After PTCA, showing complete restoration of right coronary flow. In this patient there were no other stenoses in the coronary arterial system, the ECG and left ventricular function returned to normal. Peak enzyme 'rises' were within the normal range

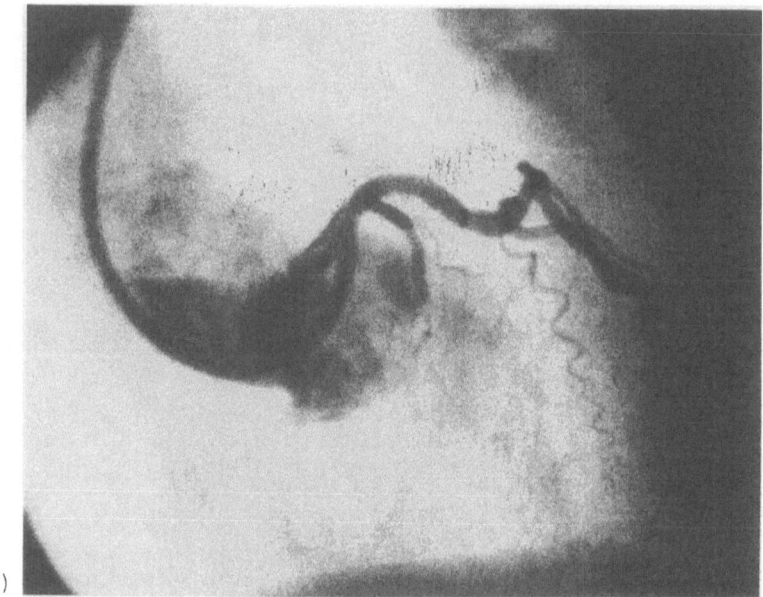

(a)

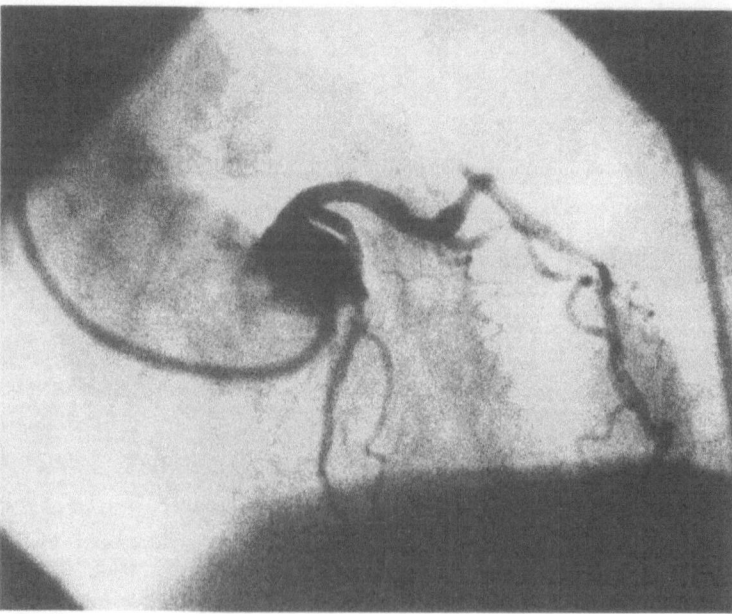

(b)

Figure 10.4
(a) Acute anterior infarction. Left coronary angiogram (left anterior oblique view) in a 63-year-old woman who presented with chest pain two hours prior to angiography. The anterior descending artery shows a moderate proximal stenosis with subsequent total occlusion

(b) After streptokinase (40 000 units intracoronary, followed by 10 000 units per minute for 10 minutes) the acute thrombus has disappeared to reveal a ragged, moderately severe stenosis just proximal to the diagonal artery. PTCA was then performed [See Figure 10.3(c)]

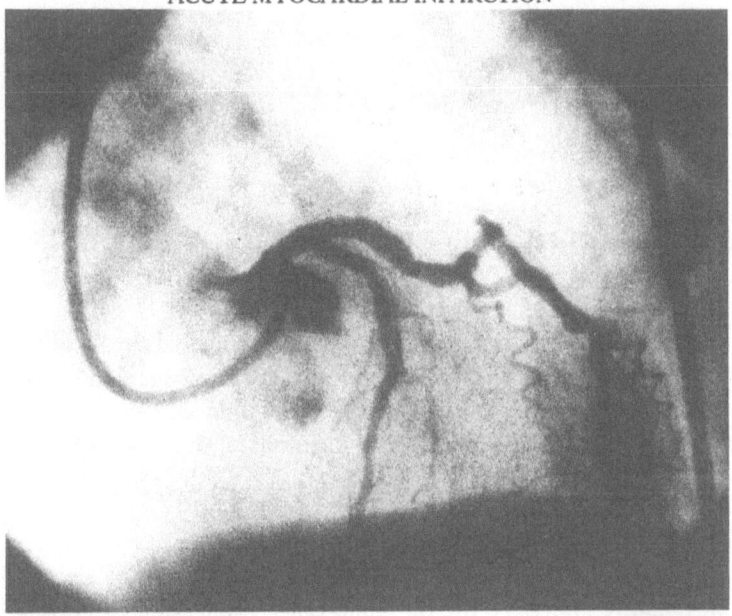

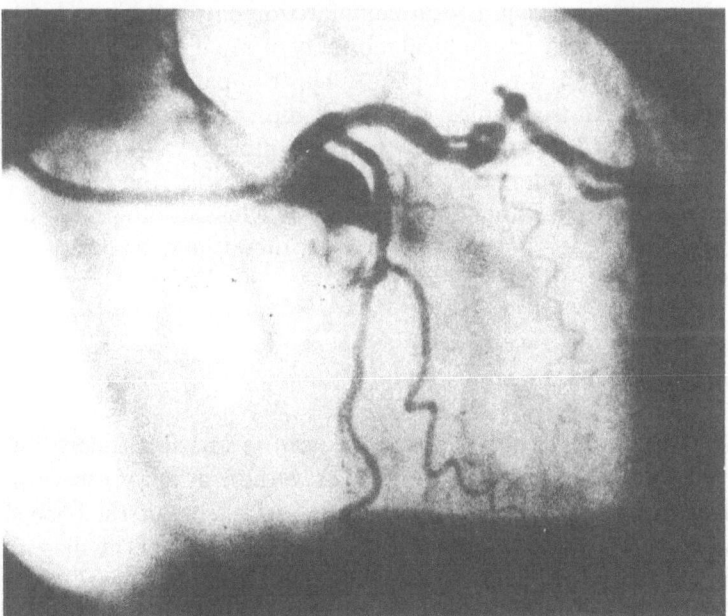

(c) After PTCA – dilation of anterior descending artery with a 2.5 mm balloon catheter. Note good perfusion in anterior descending artery, but relatively poor flow in the diagonal. There is an easily visible intimal tear

(d) Same patient – elective restudy at six months following the acute intervention. The anterior descending artery remains widely patent, the intimal tear has healed and diagonal flow is excellent. The ECG showed Q waves in VI-3 left ventricular function remained well preserved with an ejection fraction of 63%

PTCA without thrombolysis against thrombolysis alone. Hartzler and his colleagues have excellent uncontrolled data advocating this approach, and a direct comparison of PTCA versus thrombolysis within four hours of the onset of pain will be started in the United States in 1990.

THE ROLE OF CARDIAC SURGERY IN ACUTE MYOCARDIAL INFARCTION

Despite the relatively high risk in patients with established myocardial infarction undergoing cardiac surgery, a small number of such patients will inevitably require cardiac surgery for the treatment of ongoing unstable angina, residual stable angina pectoris or mechanical complications of the infarction.

Revascularization of acute myocardial infarction

Whilst the benefits and risks for the aggressive application of coronary bypass surgery in an acute evolving myocardial infarction have not been clearly defined, some centres report an early surgical mortality of 2% if surgery is performed less than six hours after onset of chest pain[23]. This compares to a mortality of about 11.5% with conventional medical therapy at the same institutions. One surgical group also reported an extremely low first year mortality of only 1.4%. Although these results appear superficially to be very favourable, the absence of proper control groups makes it difficult to draw any conclusions other than if surgery is necessary, for example, for persistent angina, then it may be performed with an acceptable risk.

Threatened extension of myocardial infarction

The clinical presentation of this syndrome may be varied. Broadly, but perhaps oversimply, it could be represented as either a non-Q-wave infarction threatening to extend to a full thickness infarction or an established Q-wave infarction that threatens to extend laterally. The essence of diagnosis is the presence of continued pain with additional ECG changes. Early cardiac catheterization is important and many such patients demonstrate left main coronary artery disease or extensive disease involving all three of the major epicardial coronary arteries, which may not be suitable for PTCA. If aggressive medical therapy, comprising continuous nitroglycerin infusion with or without intra-aortic balloon pumping, fails to control the pain, then surgery is indicated. The risks of surgery in this setting are relatively high, possibly as much as 20% depending on the age and state of left ventricular function[24]. This must be compared to studies that have demonstrated that the 'natural history' of post-infarction angina is very gloomy with as much as a 70% mortality at six months in patients treated conservatively[25].

Mechanical complications of acute myocardial infarction[26]

Mitral regurgitation in association with myocardial infarction may be caused by dilatation of the left ventricle and papillary muscle dysfunction. Less frequently, infarction may produce rupture of some or all of the papillary muscle, resulting in torrential acute mitral regurgitation and severe pulmonary oedema. Rupture of the papillary muscle is usually fatal, with death in a few hours occurring in a third and within 24 hours in 50% of these patients without surgical intervention. Mitral valve replacement in this group itself carries a 20–25% risk but surgery is inevitable in the face of the otherwise gloomy prognosis – assuming that sufficient ventricular function is demonstrated to allow postoperative recovery.

Rupture of the ventricular septum is a complication occurring in about 1% of acute myocardial infarctions and most usually occurs between 7 and 10 days. The sudden appearance of a loud murmur with clinical deterioration may make it difficult to distinguish acute ventricular septal rupture from acute mitral regurgitation, but in cases of doubt the diagnosis of septal rupture can be confirmed by right heart catheterization with associated two-dimensional echocardiography. Clinically, it is useful to note that patients with acute mitral regurgitation demonstrate extremely severe pulmonary oedema, whereas the majority of those with ventricular septal defects can lie at least semi-prone with less marked pulmonary oedema. Defects in the distal ventricular septum are usually amenable to surgical repair; defects which develop high in the ventricular septum, usually in the context of extensive infarction, tend to have a high mortality irrespective of surgical intervention. In those patients in whom the haemodynamic consequences of septal rupture can be controlled, surgery should be delayed for about four weeks.

Ventricular free wall rupture

This occurs in about 8% of acute Q-wave infarction and is perhaps responsible for about 10% of post-infarction deaths in hospital. It usually occurs in older patients and appears to be more common in women. Death is the most common sequel but surgical successful repair has followed 'subacute heart rupture' and the prognosis for such patients appears to be surprisingly good if they survive the surgery.

Left ventricular aneurysm

This may develop after acute infarction, classically acute Q-wave anterior infarction. It presents usually several weeks or possibly months later with either tachyarrhythmias, left ventricular thrombus and embolism or the signs and symptoms of left ventricular failure. Excision of left ventricular aneurysm will remove the thrombus, improve ventricular function where sufficient viable muscle exists to provide for an adequate left ventricular cavity post-surgery, and many patients (but by no means all) may lose their recurrent ventricular tachyarrhythmia. In this latter situation, tachycardia control might be provided by alternative surgical techniques, such as endocardial resection or the encircling ventriculotomy approach.

Cardiac transplantation

Occasionally it is possible to perform cardiac transplantation in selected individuals with irreversible left ventricular failure, and we have treated a number of such individuals at Harefield. However, this approach will not be widely applicable even though the number of centres capable of cardiac transplantation will increase. In young patients, with continuing normal renal, liver and cerebral function it is sometimes logistically possible to insert an intra-aortic balloon pump to temporarily support the circulation whilst awaiting a donor. If an artificial heart can be successfully developed and applied the possibility of providing cardiac transplantation to individuals with irreversible left ventricular failure will increase.

β-ADRENERGIC BLOCKING DRUGS IN ACUTE MYOCARDIAL INFARCTION

Following the initial observations from Snow in 1966, there is a wealth of literature pertaining to the use of nearly all of the currently available β-blockers in the context of myocardial infarction[27]. Studies with various intravenous β-blockers given within 4 to 12 hours of the onset of pain have reliably demonstrated an average reduction in enzyme release by about a third and there is also greater preservation of the R wave in treated compared to control groups. These apparently beneficial effects, linked and attributed to reduction in infarct size, have been accompanied by reduction in chest pain, ventricular tachy-arrhythmias and in particular ventricular fibrillation, and present a persuasive case that early intravenous β-blockade is likely to be beneficial in the absence of any contraindications. However, randomized placebo controlled trials in acute myocardial infarction are notoriously difficult to set up and the results of the available data are open to the criticism that a majority of apparently 'high risk' patients (i.e. those with significant left ventricular failure or cardiogenic shock) are consistently excluded from such trials. Reduced infarct size by the early administration of intravenous metoprolol and timolol published recently show a 10% reduction in mortality.

The recent MIAMI (metoprolol in acute myocardial infarction) trial provides a representative example of such studies[28]. Between December 1982 and March 1984, 5778 patients with suspected acute infarction were randomized for treatment with intravenous followed by oral metoprolol ($n = 2877$) or placebo ($n = 2901$). The trial was double blind and conducted at 104 centres in 17 countries. Mortality rates for the 15 day study period were 4.9% (142 deaths) in the control group and 4.3% (123 deaths) in those treated with metoprolol; representing a 13% mortality reduction in the treated group, which did not achieve statistical significance. In one of those 104 centres a local analysis of results underlined the fact that those people actually eligible for inclusion in the MIAMI trial ($n = 56$) had a low risk Norris coronary prognostic index (4.7 ± 0.2) with no deaths in the 15 day follow-up period. During the same period, 137 patients who fulfilled the basic entry criteria (age under 75 years, chest pain of at least 15 minutes duration) were excluded for one reason or another with a total of 16 deaths (12%, CPI 6.9 ± 0.3, $p < 0.01$). Subgroup analysis showed that only one of five patients (2%) who had pretreatment with β-blockers prior to the onset of suspected infarction, died. We interpret these results as confirming β-blockade as a useful therapy in the context of acute myocardial infarction.

It must be acknowledged that definitive proof that substantial quantities of myocardium can be salvaged and prognosis thereby improved is not yet available. However, those that advocate that 'even a 10% mortality reduction' in patients with acute myocardial infarction treated world-wide, present an impressive (if somewhat emotive) message.

It appears certain that patients treated with the oral administration of a β-blocker after an acute infarction carry a significantly lower mortality[29]. After initially impressive short term improvements in mortality with timolol (Norwegian study), metopropol (Swedish studies), propranolol (BHAT, β-blocker heart attack trial) and atenolol (ISIS-1) it would appear that long term benefits are maintained and continue with prolonged therapy. Only the sotolol trial failed to show any statistical demonstrable improvement, though mortality was 18% less in the treated group.

Our recommendation is that all patients who are eligible for treatment with β-blockers should receive them in the early stages of acute myocardial infarction.

Other therapeutic interventions

Although intravenous β-blockers have been the most common therapeutic modality to be investigated, various agents have been shown to have an effect on different indices of infarct size. Many of these studies involve only small numbers of patients but are supported by good experimental evidence. Glucose-insulin-potassium therapy, the vasodilator drugs (nitroprusside and nitroglycerin), and hyaluronidase have all been demonstrated to have efficacy. Several excellent detailed reviews of the results of all these trials are available but the question of reduced mortality in association with apparent reduction in infarct size is less clearly established[2,29]. On the other hand, the published early intervention studies with either verapamil[30] or nifedipine[31] have been disappointing. The results with diltiazem are more complex and quite interesting[32]. Though there was no major difference overall, subgroup analysis did show improved prognosis in patients with good ventricular function but increased mortality in those with reduced left ventricular function. More studies are under-way to explore this important clinical difference.

THE ROLE OF TWO-DIMENSIONAL ECHOCARDIOGRAPHY IN ACUTE MYOCARDIAL INFARCTION

Two-dimensional echocardiography (2D-echo) has an important role to play in the management of patients presenting with acute chest pain[33]. The indications and expectations of 2D-echo in this context may be summarized as:

(1)   The provision of diagnostic information as to the extent and site of regional areas of left ventricular dysfunction confirming the diagnosis of myocardial infarction. Whilst this will not necessarily distinguish between old and current infarction, increasing experience suggests that even subtle abnormalities of myocardial systolic performance can be appreciated and provide a clue that ischaemic heart disease underlies the symptoms rather than one of the many other causes of chest pain.

(2)   Ejection fraction may be accurately assessed and in patients in whom multiple views are possible (about 85% in our experience) the estimated ejection fraction correlates closely with both angiography and radio-nuclide methods. An assessment of ejection fraction will necessarily provide an index of risk, especially when it is correlated to either clinical or haemodynamic information available from the same patient.

(3)   Major complications, such as acute mitral regurgitation, right ventricular infarction and ventricular septal defects may be quickly and readily identified. In addition, the presence of intra-ventricular thrombus may be appreciated and managed with extended anticoagulant therapy.

(4)   The effect of interventions on left ventricular function may be established serially. In this regard, major regional hypokinetic segments recover to normal after successful PTCA and thrombolysis.

(5)   In those patients requiring cardiac catheterization, knowledge of left ventricular function derived from 2D-echo data can simplify the procedure to involve only coronary angiography and thus remove the potential hazards involved in emergency left ventricular angiography.

The major limitation of 2D-echo is the fact that not all patients are suitable echocardiographic subjects and thus not all patients have entirely accurate evaluation of, for example, their ventricular function. On the other hand, the ease with which studies may be repeated as frequently as necessary, provides a major advantage over other methods of assessing the left ventricle.

In our experience, the patient at high risk can be identified from the admission 2D-echo. Multiple views allow for analysis of the left ventricular wall in 14 segments, each of which is ascribed a score (normal = 1, hypokinetic = 2, akinetic = 3). A wall motion score index (WMSI) is derived by dividing the sum of wall motion by the number of segments visualized. High risk patients are predicted as those with a WMSI > 2. In our first 50 consecutive patients undergoing echocardiographic assessment within 48 hours of acute infarction, 20% (4/20) of the high risk group died compared to none of the remaining 30 patients ($p < 0.02$). Thirteen of 18 anterior infarcts fell into the high risk group compared with only 7 of 31 with inferior infarction ($p < 0.01$).

Future developments with computer-assisted methods, such as edge detection and image processing, will increase objectivity and perhaps allow differentiation of ischaemic from infarcted myocardium. Doppler echocardiography will also help in detecting and quantifying intracardiac lesions (such as mitral regurgitation) and providing an estimation of cardiac output.

ROLE OF CARDIAC CATHETERIZATION IN HOSPITAL IN-PATIENTS AFTER MYOCARDIAL INFARCTION

The indications for cardiac catheterization in patients with acute and recent myocardial infarction remain controversial. As the prognosis in these patients depends on left ventricular function and the extent of coronary artery disease, however, we currently advocate and practise an aggressive approach to early coronary angiography in acute infarction. The indications for coronary angiography in the setting of acute myocardial infarction include[34]:

(1)   Selected individuals with hyperacute ST segment elevation presenting within two to four hours of the onset of pain.

(2)   Ongoing angina after either Q-wave infarction or non-Q-wave infarction.

(3)   'High risk' patients (e.g. patients with occasional angina yet significantly reduced left ventricular function, those threatening to extend a previous

infarction, those with recurrent ventricular tachyarrhythmias or survivors of the 'sudden death' syndrome).

(4)   Patients requiring emergency surgery for other than ongoing angina.

(5)   Elective study at 7–10 days in those following a non-Q-wave infarction in order to plan a future strategy.

(6)   'Young' (defined in our institution as patients under 50 years) patients after Q-wave infarction in order to plan a future strategy.

Although patients can often be separated into high risk and low risk subsets by a non-invasive assessment during and after myocardial infarction, several other factors are also considered when making the decision to proceed – including the availability of accurate non-invasive tests at each individual institution (Figures 10.5 and 10.6).

Persistent angina pectoris following myocardial infarction is a bad prognostic sign. However, cardiac catheterization is not necessary for all patients if the left ventricular function is severely depressed, even though the prognosis is bad in this group, unless surgical therapy is contemplated. Patients with persistent ventricular arrhythmias, which are either symptomatic, producing cardiac arrest or detected on post-infarction monitoring, should be considered for further investigation since preliminary evidence suggests that even in the absence of angina pectoris, patients with severe coronary artery disease and associated ventricular tachyarrhythmias may have a better prognosis following surgery.

Though the acute hospital mortality for non-Q wave myocardial infarction is less than that of Q wave infarction, it has been shown repeatedly that patients with such 'minor infarctions' have a high instance of early complications[35]. This is particularly true in those with left main disease, proximal anterior descending artery lesions and patients with triple vessel involvement. With PTCA, it is now possible to treat a majority of patients with advanced coronary artery disease underlying the apparently minor infarction, but proof that this results in an objective improvement in prognosis remains to be demonstrated. As the risk in such patients is within the first two months of the infarction, we see little merit in delaying cardiac catheterization beyond 7–10 days in such patients where the facilities are available. We recently completed a study of early in-hospital angiography on a consecutive series of 103 patients following acute myocardial infarction: 39 had non-Q-wave infarctions and 14 were demonstrated to have triple vessel disease, 8 double and 17 single vessel disease. Of these 39 patients only 13 were asymptomatic and had negative exercise tests, 10 underwent elective coronary bypass grafting, 8 PTCA and two declined the offer of intervention. Only one of these 39 patients died in over 12 months follow up and this patient had two vessel coronary artery disease with no residual angina and a negative exercise electrocardiogram.

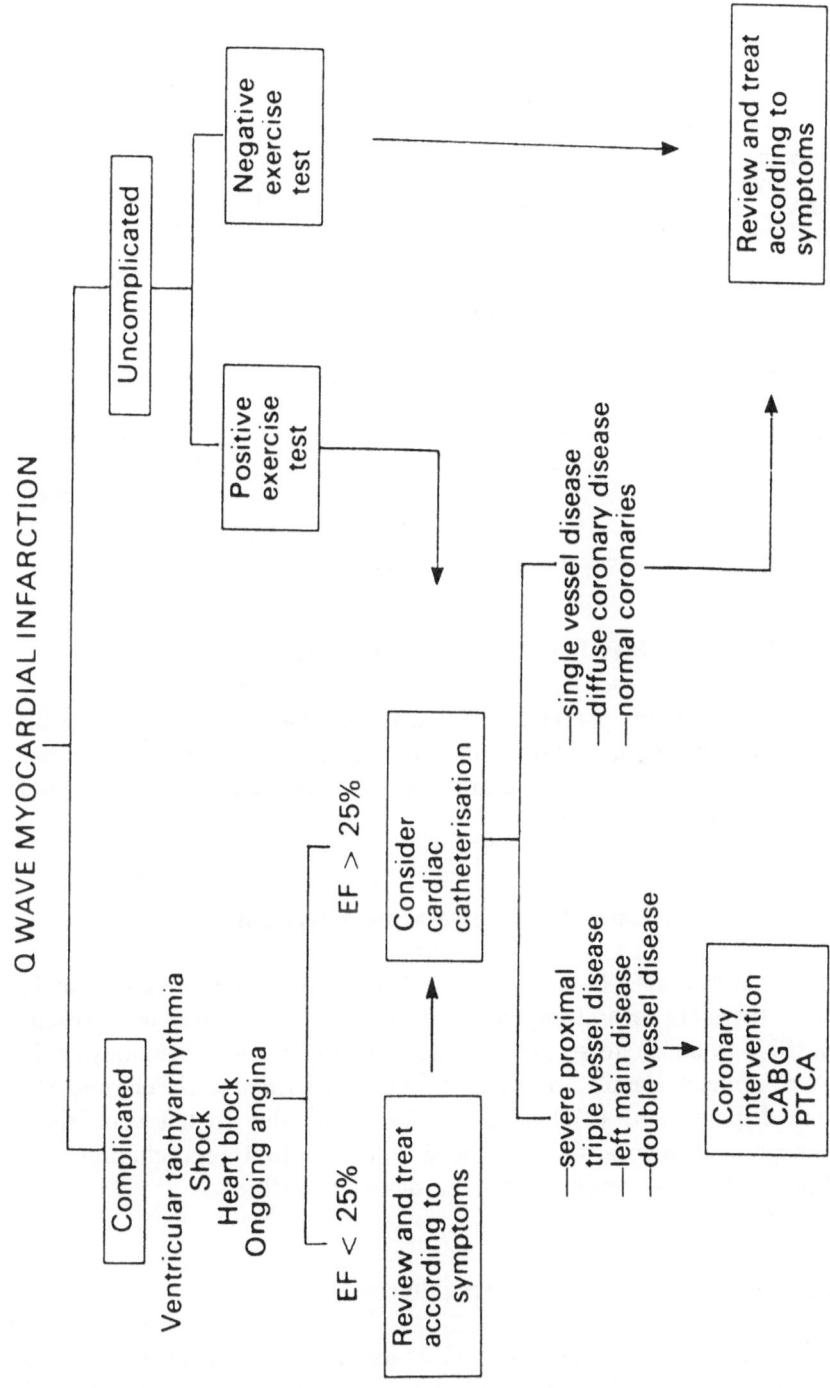

Figure 10.5 Strategy for the management of Q-wave infarction

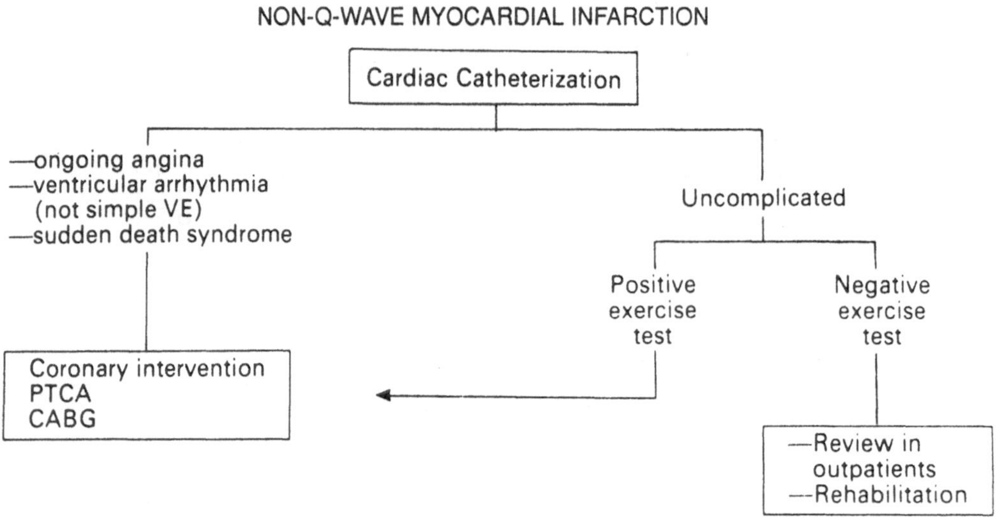

NON-Q-WAVE MYOCARDIAL INFARCTION

```
                    ┌──────────────────────────┐
                    │  Cardiac Catheterization │
                    └──────────────────────────┘

—ongoing angina
—ventricular arrhythmia
  (not simple VE)                      Uncomplicated
—sudden death syndrome

                                    Positive        Negative
                                    exercise        exercise
                                      test            test

┌──────────────────────┐
│ Coronary intervention│  ◄─────────────────
│ PTCA                 │                          ┌──────────────────┐
│ CABG                 │                          │ —Review in       │
└──────────────────────┘                          │   outpatients    │
                                                  │ —-Rehabilitation │
                                                  └──────────────────┘
```

Figure 10.6 Strategy for the management of non-Q-wave infarction

MANAGEMENT OF COMPLICATED MYOCARDIAL INFARCTION

There are a number of potential complications that beset patients with established acute myocardial infarction[3,6]. In the main, however, the more common and clinically relevant ones are those that cause cardiac failure and rhythm disturbances.

Haemodynamic complications of acute myocardial infarction

Haemodynamic disturbance in association with acute infarction is usual; but in general terms, there are several ways in which abnormal haemodynamics present and it is possible to delineate several subsets with characteristic haemodynamic profiles. A convenient classification may be (1) hyperdynamic circulation, (2) hypovolaemic hypotension, (3) left ventricular failure due to left ventricular muscle damage and myocardial ischaemia, acute mitral regurgitation and rupture of the ventricular septum, and (4) cardiogenic shock.

Indications for invasive haemodynamic monitoring

Invasive monitoring is generally not necessary in the truly uncomplicated infarction or in patients with a hyperdynamic state, but it should be instituted early in patients in whom it is apparent that complications are developing or in patients in whom complications are very likely. Invasive monitoring consists of inserting an arterial line for continuous measurement of arterial pressure (most usually in a radial artery) and inserting a balloon flotation catheter (Swan Ganz) for measurement of pulmonary artery, pulmonary capillary wedge and right atrial pressures and cardiac output by thermodilution. In patients with severe haemodynamic impairment, a urinary catheter to provide accurate and continuous measurement of urinary output is also recommended.

We would suggest the following to be indications for invasive haemodynamic monitoring in patients with acute infarction:

(1)   Hypotension where the cause is not obvious (such as excessive morphine administration or heart block).
(2)   Evidence of left ventricular failure and hypoxaemia which does not respond immediately to simple diuretic and oxygen therapy.
(3)   Unexplained or frequent tachyarrhythmias requiring high dose anti-arrhythmic therapy or cardiac pacing in which Swan Ganz catheters can be inserted at the same time as a pacing catheter without additional risk.
(4)   Unexplained or severe cyanosis, hypoxia or acidosis.
(5)   Acute mitral regurgitation.
(6)   Ventricular septal defect.

The importance of invasive haemodynamic monitoring is related to the difficulty of interpreting clinical and radiographic findings, especially in patients with left ventricular failure and hypotension in whom the usual cardiac therapies may be either beneficial or detrimental. Hypovolaemia and right ventricular infarction will be treated differently, as it is not usual to give a fluid load to patients following myocardial infarction. Haemodynamic monitoring of cardiac output and wedge pressure make therapeutic intervention with such agents as nitroprusside, dopamine and other vasoactive drugs a much more controlled intervention. It can be difficult to assess the severity and sometimes even the presence of acute mitral valve insufficiency and ventricular septal defect, especially when cardiac output and systemic pressure are reduced.

Hyperdynamic circulation

In patients with a high sinus rate, elevated arterial pressure and a high cardiac output occurring either singly or together, treatment with β-adrenergic blockade is indicated. If hypertension is the prime problem, virtually irrespective of cardiac output, the treatment of choice is intravenous nitroprusside therapy monitored by continuous haemodynamic measurement using a Swan Ganz catheter.

Hypovolaemic hypotension

Exclusion of hypovolaemia as the cause of hypotension requires documentation of reduced cardiac output despite an adequate left ventricular filling pressure (pulmonary capillary wedge pressure or pulmonary diastolic pressure in excess of 12–15 mmHg). In this situation, two-dimensional echocardiography is an extremely useful adjunct to therapy, since not only does it give a direct indication of the extent of left ventricular damage but it also provides data on right ventricular function. Significant right ventricular infarction[36] may be confused with hypovolaemia because both are characteristically associated with a low left ventricular filling pressure. The characteristic triad of hypotension in association with elevated right atrial or jugular venous pressure and a low left ventricular filling pressure often responds to the vigorous administration of fluid. Some patients may need additional support in this situation by means of dopamine (or dobutamine) infusion.

Left ventricular failure

All patients with established myocardial infarction have a degree of left ventricular failure as evidenced by mild sinus tachycardia, the presence of a gallop rhythm or clinical evidence of pulmonary congestion. Once failure has developed to the extent that the patient is hypoxaemic, invasive haemodynamic monitoring is particularly helpful. The intravenous administration of a diuretic reduces pulmonary vascular congestion and pulmonary venous pressure both by direct vasodilation and subsequent diuresis. Active vasodilator therapy, however, is very important and the judicious use of nitroprusside, with frequent monitoring of cardiac output and intracardiac pressures, is usually the treatment of choice. Depending on the haemodynamic profile and severity, intravenous nitroglycerin may be an equally acceptable and 'easier' alternative in CCUs not used to dealing with nitroprusside. In addition to vasodilator therapy, with either nitroprusside or nitroglycerin, inotropic support may be indicated to improve cardiac output. Dopamine is the drug most favoured in this situation and usually doses of 2–5 μg kg^{-1} min^{-1} are all that is necessary. Dopamine is particularly useful where the haemodynamics situation has been reasonably controlled and yet renal function, as evidenced by urinary output, is depressed. In such patients, the addition of dopamine usually provides immediate improvement in diuresis, especially if administered early in the course of left ventricular failure. Once the acute episode is under control the institution of oral vasodilator therapy is achieved early and we currently favour angiotensin converting enzyme inhibitors, such as captopril or enalapril, as drugs of choice in this situation. Digitalis is not administered routinely but in patients already taking digoxin it is continued. Other newer agents such as enoxamone and milrinone may find a place in the future.

It is well known that β-adrenergic blockade may cause or precipitate left ventricular failure in patients with extensive infarction, but in clinical practice this association is relatively uncommon. Occasional patients, especially those with inappropriate tachycardia in relation to reduced cardiac output, may actually improve with judicious use of small doses of a β-blocker.

Cardiogenic shock

Massive myocardial infarction, or a further myocardial infarction in patients with previous ventricular damage may produce global impairment of ventricular function, which is so profound that cardiogenic shock develops. Such shock is characterized by marked hypotension (systolic arterial pressure <80 mmHg) and a marked reduction of cardiac output (cardiac index <1.7 l min^{-1} m^{-2}) in the face of elevated left ventricular filling pressure (pulmonary capillary wedge pressure in excess of 20 mmHg). Clinically, such patients in addition to pulmonary congestion will also demonstrate the signs of low output failure with cold, pale extremities, sweating and either poor or absent urinary output. In patients with hypotension, two-dimensional echocardiography is particularly useful as this technique can either confirm the profound depression of left ventricular function or identify particularly reversible situations – such as hypovolaemia, right ventricular infarction (dilated right ventricle with reasonably good left ventricular function), acute mitral valve rupture (papillary muscle rupture) or evidence of ventricular septal defect. In patients presenting with profound hypotension, once left ventricular impairment has been demonstrated as the cause, invasive haemodynamic monitoring is set up with a radial arterial line, Swan Ganz catheterization and the insertion of a urinary catheter.

Inotropic agents are employed extensively in the treatment of cardiogenic shock, but provide only a short term improvement and have not been demonstrated to affect overall mortality. Similarly, vasodilator therapy, particularly nitroprusside, may provide a satisfactory improvement in haemodynamics early after administration, but such improvement is usually short lived in the absence of left ventricular recovery. In uncommon instances, the systemic vascular resistance may, instead of being elevated, actually be either normal or in some cases low. In these cases, noradrenaline or adrenaline are better inotropic agents compared to dopamine or dobutamine.

Intra-aortic balloon counter pulsation (IABCP) is rarely used but on occasion, can be lifesaving – particularly if used in the preoperative resuscitation of surgically correctable, mechanical left ventricular failure. Although IABCP used to be advocated for the treatment of persistent and ongoing cardiac pain (augmenting coronary flow), since the introduction of nitroglycerin it is rarely needed. IABCP may be required for control of the patient undergoing emergency coronary angiography as a prelude to cardiac surgery.

Surgical intervention is most successful in patients where the circulatory collapse is due to such mechanical complications as ventricular septal defect, acute mitral regurgitation and (more rarely) left ventricular aneurysm. Emergency surgery in such acutely ill patients carries a high mortality.

Treatment or prophylaxis of arrhythmia

Any cardiac arrhythmia may be seen to complicate the early phase of acute myocardial infarction. Those of special significance comprise (1) sinus bradycardia, (2) atrioventricular block, (3) atrial fibrillation, (4) ventricular extrasystoles, (5) ventricular tachycardia, and (6) ventricular fibrillation.

Sinus bradycardia

Sinus bradycardia in the early few hours of the myocardial infarction occurs more commonly in patients with inferior and posterior infarctions, which are more likely to be associated with marked vagotonia. Atropine in small dosage, repeated as necessary, is indicated where the sinus bradycardia is associated with symptoms. Sinus bradycardia is also commonly caused by analgesic therapy with morphine and of course β-blockade. Temporary cardiac pacing is not indicated for simple sinus bradycardia. Whereas atropine may be useful in the presence of sinus node dysfunction, temporary cardiac pacing (particularly atrioventricular sequential pacing) may be indicated if there is haemodynamic disturbance.

Atrioventricular block

First degree and Mobitz Type I, second degree AV block (Wenckebach) are seen but usually do not require specific therapy. Mobitz Type II, second degree AV block is relatively uncommon in acute myocardial infarction and it should be treated with a temporary cardiac pacemaker. Traditionally, these lower grades of heart block tended to be treated conservatively in patients with inferior myocardial infarction as they are often transient and related to relatively short lived ischaemia of the AV node, being consequent on its anatomic supply from the posterior descending artery. In patients with anterior myocardial infarction, however, even low grade atrioventricular block may indicate relatively extensive infarction and thus be associated with poorer prognosis. Although there is no evidence that temporary cardiac pacing affects mortality, in practice, temporary pacing is often used in second degree heart block in patients with anterior myocardial infarction. Ventricular or atrioventricular sequential pacing is indicated in patients with complete AV block in the early stages of an infarction. Atropine is of little use in such patients. The prognosis of patients with complete AV block associated with anterior infarction is very poor regardless of therapy.

Complete bundle branch block (either left or right) or the combination of right bundle branch block and axis deviation ('bifascicular' block) are more often associated with anterior than inferior or posterior infarction. Temporary cardiac pacing is not automatic in such patients, but one must review these with specific regard to progressive development of high grade AV block. The prognosis in these patients is worse, but again, temporary cardiac pacing has not been demonstrated to improve mortality.

The question of permanent cardiac pacing in survivors of myocardial infarction with associated conduction defects remains controversial. Clearly, patients with ongoing symptomatic sick sinus syndrome or high grade AV block will require permanent cardiac pacing. Although the survivors of infarction complicated by AV block or bundle branch block have a poorer prognosis, this is not necessarily due to subsequent recurrent complete heart block. These patients have a high instance of late in-hospital ventricular fibrillation and clearly, a cardiac pacemaker will have no effect on this situation. On the other hand, a retrospective multicentre study has demonstrated a reduced incidence of sudden death in patients treated by insertion of a permanent pacemaker having experienced transient high grade block during infarction. It is our practice not to insert a permanent cardiac pacemaker in the absence of symptomatic bradycardia.

Atrial fibrillation

Both atrial fibrillation and atrial flutter are relatively more common in the first 24 hours following myocardial infarction than subsequently and are associated with increased mortality, particularly in patients with anterior myocardial infarction. This association is probably not an independent risk factor, however, as atrial fibrillation is more common where there is clinical and haemodynamic evidence of extensive damage. β-Adrenergic blockade is to be preferred to digitalis for heart rate control, but if there is acute haemodynamic deterioration related to the onset of atrial fibrillation, then DC cardioversion remains the treatment of choice. In view of the Danish multicentre study showing an increased mortality in patients given verapamil in the early stages of myocardial infarction, we currently do not favour this particular drug. On the other hand, flecainide, a new Class Ic anti-arrhythmic agent, is extremely potent and usually controls the heart rate, often reverting the rhythm to sinus without electrical intervention. In patients with extensive infarction, however, flecainide may have major adverse haemodynamic consequences.

Ventricular extrasystoles

The suppression of ventricular extrasystoles in the early stages of myocardial infarction was based on the premise that ventricular extrasystoles trigger ventricular fibrillation. This is far from proven and indeed there are several studies to suggest that the ventricular fibrillation occurs as an unheralded event with no premonitory ventricular extrasystoles. The concept that ventricular extrasystoles are 'warning arrhythmias' for ventricular tachycardia, however, has much more merit and intravenous lignocaine (2 mg kg^{-1} as a bolus followed by continuous infusion of 1–4 mg min^{-1}) is the standard treatment for either frequent (in excess of 10 min^{-1}) unifocal extrasystoles or high grade extrasystoles. Hypokalaemia should be corrected. Large numbers of randomized trials have compared the routine administration of several Vaughan Williams Class I agents (lignocaine, quinidine, procainamide, disopyramide and mexilitine) against placebo. All of these agents reduced the frequency of ventricular extrasystoles and occasional studies show reduced incidence of ventricular fibrillation. However, none of these agents administered in this fashion demonstrate reduced in-hospital mortality. Arguably, the routine use of β-blockade has reduced the frequency of ventricular extrasystoles seen in the coronary care unit and many studies have now been shown to demonstrate reduced mortality though the overall effect is small[37,38].

Class 1c agents have now been discredited as elective treatment of ventricular extrasystoles occurring in the post-infarction period. Although CAPS (cardiac arrhythmia pilot study)[39] suggested that drugs such as flecainide and encainide might improve the longer term mortality risk when they came to be tested in the larger CAST (cardiac arrhythmia suppression trial) study this hope was not realized[40]. 2309 patients with symptomatic or mildly symptomatic ventricular arrhythmias (65 or more PVCs per hour) were randomly assigned to a variety of drugs or placebo. Both encainide and flecainide treated patients showed an excess mortality compared with the placebo treated group. Admittedly the placebo mortality was surprisingly low and over-reaction was the order of the day. Class 1c drugs such as flecainide and encainide should not be used to electively treat ventricular extrasystoles in patients with a recent history of myocardial infarction.

Lignocaine, or related drugs, are indicated if there are any extrasystoles following a previously documented ventricular arrhythmia – occasionally a clinically important negative inotropic effect occurs, especially with higher doses. In such circumstances, intravenous amiodarone with continued oral therapy may be used in selected cases.

Ventricular tachycardia

Accelerated idioventricular tachycardia (sequential ventricular complexes with a rate of between 60 and 100 beats per minute) do not require active drug therapy. However, since they are often seen in the presence of relative bradycardia and may degenerate to ventricular tachycardia or ventricular fibrillation, we use temporary pacing to 'overdrive' the rhythm if necessary. There is no evidence of increased mortality in association with an accelerated idioventricular arrhythmia.

Definite ventricular tachycardia (usually with a rate of between 120 and 160 beats per minute) requires immediate therapy. In instances of non-sustained ventricular tachycardia (less than 15 consecutive beats) lignocaine and associated β-blockade are usually adequate to suppress the rhythm. Following intravenous suppression, a short term therapy with oral anti-arrhythmias, usually Class I agents, is recommended. In cases of sustained ventricular tachycardia, DC cardioversion is the treatment of choice, with subsequent oral anti-arrhythmia therapy to suppress the rhythm. If ventricular tachycardia occurs in a coronary care unit, immediate treatment usually prevents severe hypoxia, hypotension, acidosis or electrolyte disturbance, but if these supervene they must be treated appropriately. Hypokalaemia (serum potassium < 4.2 mmol l^{-1}) is a frequent clinical association with ventricular tachycardia in acute myocardial infarction and simple potassium replacement may be all that is necessary to control the acute episodes. Digoxin at toxic levels is an important iatrogenic cause of ventricular tachycardia in the early stages of myocardial infarction.

Ventricular fibrillation

Since the advent of well-appointed coronary care units, ventricular fibrillation as a primary cause of death is a rare phenomenon in ECG monitored patients. However, late in-hospital ventricular fibrillation (usually occurring after the third or fourth day) is much more common in patients with intraventricular conduction defects, extensive anterior infarction, persistent sinus tachycardia, atrial flutter or fibrillation during the first 24 hours, or those who have demonstrated ventricular tachyarrhythmias in the period 12–36 hours following infarction[41].

The treatment of ventricular fibrillation is immediate DC cardioversion. The likelihood of success declines rapidly with time and with the development of acidosis and electrolyte imbalance consequent on severe hypoxia. Ventricular fibrillation often recurs rapidly and repeatedly when patients are metabolically unstable or simply severely hypokalaemic. In patients with resistant ventricular fibrillation, assuming lignocaine has been tried, the administration of amiodarone intravenously (5 mg kg^{-1} to a maximum of 350 mg over 20 min) or bretylium tosylate (5 mg kg^{-1} intravenously) may ultimately be successful but require prolonged cardiopulmonary resuscitation to allow time for these drugs to work (at least 20 min). Amiodarone has a rather strange pharmaco- dynamic profile and may be better in the prevention rather than the treatment of ventricular fibrillation, but nevertheless is worth trying especially in patients where echocardiography has demonstrated that cardiac function is preserved. In such individuals, even prolonged cardiopulmonary resuscitation, if administered adequately, can result in excellent patient salvage.

Bretylium tosylate is not available in oral form; therefore, there are three longer term therapeutic alternatives in patients who have suffered serious ventricular arrhythmias or ventricular fibrillation. Vaughan Williams Class I agents have not been demonstrated to be effective, but β-blockers do reduce the incidence of late death following myocardial infarction. Patients who have ventricular fibrillation after the first four to six hours ('secondary' ventricular fibrillation) and have heart failure or cardiogenic shock have a poor prognosis irrespective of therapy. In those who have late in-hospital ventricular fibrillation with good left ventricular function, the prognosis may be excellent and this group of patients should have on-going cardiac therapy with either β-blockade or amiodarone.

Role of electrophysiological testing after acute myocardial infarction

Although programmed ventricular stimulation of the heart has proved useful in the treatment of patients with recurrent sustained ventricular tachycardia in general, its role in the hospital phase immediately after an acute infarction is unclear. The Westmeade Group provide the only prospective analysis of routine detailed electrophysiological assessment in patients 7–28 days after an uncomplicated myocardial infarction[42]. All 228 clinically well survivors of acute myocardial infarction underwent both exercise electrocardiography and programmed stimulation. In the 62% of their patients in whom both tests were negative, only 1% died in the first year of follow-up; but those patients in whom it was possible to induce ventricular arrhythmias during electrophysiological testing, had a poor prognosis. However, the specific role of electrophysiological testing remains in doubt. Despite the Westmeade experience, most physicians question the validity and logistic demands of routine electrophysiological testing.

THE ROLE OF EXERCISE TESTING IN THE EARLY PERIOD AFTER MYOCARDIAL INFARCTION

Exercise testing is a safe and non-invasive method that can provide information not only on residual ischaemia as evidenced by ST segment change, but also on prognostically important changes, such as an abnormal blood pressure response, exercise capacity and the presence of exercise induced ventricular arrhythmias. There are several excellent reviews of the status of exercise testing after myocardial infarction[43,44].

Exercise electrocardiography

Most reports on early exercise tests after myocardial infarction have analysed only data collected during exercise and have failed to take into account other prognostic variables such as patient age, history of previous infarction and left ventricular function. It would appear from several studies that the annual mortality of patients who develop ST segment depression during exercise testing approaches 20% compared to only about 2–3% in those who do not. A poor exercise tolerance, indicating poor residual left ventricular function, is a relatively non-specific variable, but in multivariate analysis it becomes a very significant prognostic indicator. For example in a study from Weld and colleagues in a series of 250 patients undergoing a nine minute treadmill test before hospital discharge, an exercise duration of less than six minutes was a powerful independent prognostic index – indeed, more so than the presence of ST segment depression[45]. Ventricular arrhythmias occurring during exercise have also been considered by many to indicate a poor prognosis but others have reported that they are not relevant.

Nuclear stress testing

Exercise thallium-201 scintigraphy may be regarded as more sensitive and specific than the exercise electrocardiogram *per se*, but few studies provide a comparison between the two. Radionuclide angiography at rest and particularly during exercise offer excellent information about left ventricular function.

Summary

A negative exercise test (normal electrocardiographic response or good left ventricular function on exercise determined by radionuclide angiography) is a better indicator of good prognosis than an abnormal exercise test is an individual prognostic index for a bad prognosis in a specific patient. We, therefore, limit the use of exercise tests after myocardial infarction to specific sub-groups. In patients who have had an uncomplicated myocardial infarction, 12-lead bicycle or treadmill exercise testing is performed at 7–10 days; and if it is positive by ST segment criteria, or if exercise-induced angina develops, then the patients may be considered for early cardiac catheterization possibly to proceed to PTCA or elective coronary bypass grafting depending on the coronary anatomy and the exercise test response. Patients in whom the early exercise test is negative are reviewed after discharge and managed according to the presence or absence of symptoms.

CONCLUSIONS

In the United Kingdom approximately 160 000 deaths occur each year as a direct result of coronary artery disease. A large variety of potential interventions, therapies and investigations are currently available for the investigation and management of patients presenting with acute myocardial infarction. There is no definite agreement, and probably never will be, on the exact treatment for all patients. However, physicians must continue to emphasize the importance of reducing primary risk factors, in particular – cessation of cigarette smoking, improved levels of exercise and modified diet. After a myocardial infarction, investigations should be aimed at identifying the high risk patient for coronary intervention and the low risk patient for lifestyle modification and long term β-adrenergic blockade therapy where possible.

What one used to regard as the 'natural history' of a myocardial infarction has been radically altered by the modern interventional approach. Indeed, in some tertiary referral institutions, iatrogenic myocardial infarction (occurring after coronary angioplasty or bypass surgery) may be the predominant occurrence. Does an abnormal exercise test mean the same after an 'uncomplicated' event as after infarction treated with thrombolysis or coronary angioplasty? Which thrombolytic agent, administered to which patients at what time in association with which drugs will yield the best results? Can we prevent coronary disease occurring in the first place? What physical and dietary recommendations should be made? Does hyperlipidaemia require treatment and which drug and at what level of abnormality should be introduced? The list of questions seems endless but we must continue to provide carefully controlled studies to test these and other issues.

The incidence of ischaemic heart disease and myocardial infarction appears to be falling in many countries. However, we cannot be complacent – data from the Framingham study show that 1 in 5 men and 1 in 17 women under the age of 60 will suffer acute myocardial infarction and 1 in 3 of the population will die from ischaemic heart disease. Further investigation and research into the causes and treatment of myocardial infarction remains of paramount importance.

REFERENCES

1. Braunwald, E. (1967). Pathogenesis and treatment of shock in myocardial infraction. *Johns Hopkins Med. J.*, **121**, 421–9
2. Rude, R.E., Muller, J.E. and Braunwald, E. (1981). Efforts to limit the size of myocardial infarcts. *Ann. Intern. Med.*, **95**, 736–61
3. Pasternak, R.C., Braunwald, E. and Sobel, B.E. (1988). Acute myocardial infarction: pathological, pathophysiological and clinical manifestations, In Braunwald, E. (ed.) *Heart Disease*. pp. 1223–1244 (Saunders)
4. Brush, J.E., Brand, D.A., Acampora D., Chalmer B. and Wackers, F.J. (1985). Use of initial electrocardiogram to predict in-hospital complications of acute myocardial infarction. *N. Engl. J. Med.*, **312**, 1137–41

5. Norris, R.M., Brandt, P.W.T., Caughey, D.E., Lee, A.J. and Scott, P.J. (1969). A new coronary prognostic index. *Lancet*, **1**, 274–8
6. Sobel, B.E. and Braunwald, E. (1984). The management of acute myocardial infarction. In Braunwald, E. (ed.) *Heart Disease*. pp. 1301–33 (Eastbourne: Saunders)
7. Goldman, L., Cook, F., Hashimoto, B., Stone, P., Muller, J. and Loscalzo, A. (1982). Evidence that hospital care for acute myocardial infarction has not contributed to the decline in coronary mortality between 1973–74 and 1978–79. *Circulation*, **65**, 936–42
8. Gruppo Italiano per lo studio della streptochinasi nell'infarcto miocardico (GISSI). (1986). Effectiveness of intravenous thrombolytic treatment in acute myocardial infarction. *Lancet*, **1**, 397–401
9. ISIS-2 (second international study of infarct survival) collaborative group (1988). Randomized trial of intravenous streptokinase, oral aspirin, both, or neither among 17,187 cases of suspected acute myocardial infarction: ISIS-2. *Lancet*, **2**, 349–60
10. Wilcox, R.G., Olsson, C.G., Skene, A.M., von der Lippe, C., Jensen, G. and Hampton, J.R. for the Asset Study Group (1988). Trial of tissue plasminogen activator for mortality reduction in acute myocardial infarction. Anglo-Scandinavian Study of Early Thrombolysis (ASSET). *Lancet*, **2**, 525–30
11. AIMS Trial Study Group (1988). Effect of intravenous APSAC on mortality after acute myocardial infarction: preliminary report of a placebo-controlled clinical trial. *Lancet*, **1**, 545–49
12. Rentrop, K.P. (1985). Thrombolytic therapy in patients with acute myocardial infarction. *Circulation*, **71**, 627–31
13. Laffel, G.L. and Braunwald, E. (1984). Thrombolytic therapy. A new strategy for the treatment of acute myocardial infarction (2 parts). *N. Engl. J. Med.*, **311**, 710–17 and 770–6
14. Yusuf, S., Collins, R., Peto, R., Furberg, C., Stampfer, M.J., Goldhaber, S.Z. and Hennekens, C.H. (1985). Intravenous and intracoronary fibrinolytic therapy in acute myocardial infarction: Overview of the results on mortality, reinfarction and side effects from 33 randomised controlled trials. *Eur. Heart J.*, **6**, 556–85
15. Kennedy, J.W., Richie, J.L., Davis, K.B. and Fritz, J.K. (1983). Western Washington randomised trial of intracoronary streptokinase in acute myocardial infarction. *N. Engl. J. Med.*, **309**, 1477–8113
16. Thrombolysis in Myocardial Infarction Study Group. (1985). The thrombolysis in acute myocardial infarction (TIMI) trial. Phase 1 findings. *N. Engl. J. Med.*, **312**, 932–6
17. Simoons, M.L., Serruys, P.W., Brand, M.V., Bar, F., DeZwaan, C., *et al.* (1985). Improved survival after thrombolysis in acute myocardial infarction. *Lancet*, **2**, 578–81
18. Meyer, J., Merx, W., Schmitz, H., Erbel, R., Kiesslich, T., Dorr, R., Lanbedz, H. *et al.* (1982). Percutaneous transluminal coronary angioplasty immediately after intra-coronary streptolysis of transmural myocardial infarction. *Circulation*, **66**, 905–13
19. Hartzler, G.O., Rutherford, B.D., McConahay, D.R., Johnson, W.L. Jr, McCallister, B.D., Gura, G.M., Conn, R.C. and Crockett, J.E. (1983). Percutaneous transluminal coronary angioplasty with and without thrombolytic therapy for treatment of acute myocardial infarction. *Am. Heart. J.*, **106**, 965–73
20. The TIMI Study Group (1989). Comparison of invasive and conservative strategies after treatment with intravenous tissue plasminogen activator in acute myocardial infarction. Results of the Thrombolysis in Myocardial Infarction (TIMI) Phase II Trial. *N. Engl. J. Med.*, **320**, 618–27
21. The TIMI Research Group (1988). Immediate vs delayed catheterization and angioplasty following thrombolytic therapy for acute myocardial infacrtion. *J. Am. Med. Assoc.*, **260**, 2849–58
22. Califf, R.M., Topol, E.J., George, B.S., Boswick, J.M., Lee, K.L., Stump, D., Dillon, J. Abbottsmith, C., Candela, R.J., Kereiakes, D.J., O'Neill, W.W. and Stack, R.S. and the TAMI Study Group (1988). Characteristics and outcome of patients in whom reperfusion with intravenous tissue-type plasminogen activator fails: results of the Thrombolysis and Angioplasty in Myocardial Infarction (TAMI) I trial. *Circulation*, **77**(5), 1090–99
23. DeWood, M.A. and Berg, R. Jr (1984). The role of surgical reperfusion in myocardial infarction. In Robeds, R. (ed.). *Prognosis after Myocardial Infarction. Cardiology Clinics*, **2** (1), pp. 113–22. (Philadelphia: W. B. Saunders Co)

24. Gray, R.J., Sethna, D. and Matloff, J.M. (1983). The role of cardiac surgery in acute myocardial infarction. II. Without mechanical complications. *Am. Heart J.*, **106**, 728–35
25. Schuster, E.H. and Bulkley, B.H. (1981). Early post infarction angina. *N. Engl. J. Med.*, **305**, 1101–5
26. Gray, R.J., Sethna, D. and Matloff, J.M. (1983). The role of cardiac surgery in acute myocardial infarction. I. With mechanical complications. *Am. Heart J.*, **106**, 723–8
27. Yusuf, S., Peto, R., Lewis, J., Collins, R. and Sleight, P. (1985). β blockade during and after myocardial infarction: An overview of the randomised trials. *Prog. Cardiovasc. Dis.*, **27**, 335–71
28. The MIAMI trial research group (1985). Metoprolol in acute myocardial infarction (MIAMI). A randomised placebo-controlled international trial. *Eur. Heart J.*, 1985, **6**, 199–226
29. Muller, J.E. and Braunwald, E. (1983). Can infarct size be limited in patients with acute myocardial infarction? *Cardiovasc. Clin.*, **13**(1), 147–61
30. The Danish Study Group on verapamil in acute myocardial infarction (1984). Verapamil in acute myocardial infarction. *Eur. Heart J.*, **5**, 516–28
31. Muller, J.E., Morrison, J., Stone, P.H., Rude, R.E., Rosner, B. *et al.* (1984). Nifedepine therapy for patients with threatened and acute myocardial infarction: a randomised, double blind, placebo controlled comparison. *Circulation*, **69**, 740–7
32. Boden, W.E., Kleiger, R.E., Miller, J.M., Greenberg, H., Krone, R.J., Hager, W.D., Abrams, J. and Moss, A.J. MDPIT Research Group (1989). Favourable effect of diltiazem on late mortality and reinfarction after non-Q-wave myocardial infarction: Multicenter diltiazem post-infarction trial (MDPIT). *J. Am. Coll. Cardiol.*, **13**, 6A
33. Quinones, M.A. (1984). Echocardiography in acute myocardial infarction. *Cardiol. Clin.*, **2**(1), 123–34
34. Epstein, S.E., Palmeri, S.T. and Patterson, R.D. (1982). Evaluation of patients after acute myocardial infarction. Indications for cardiac catheterisation and surgical intervention. *N. Engl. J. Med.*, **307**, 1487–92
35. Maisel, A.S., A hvre, S., Gilpin, E., Henning, H., Goldberger, A.L., Collins, D., LeWinter, M. and Ross, J. Jr (1985). Prognosis after extension of myocardial infarct: the role of Q wave or non-Q wave infarction. *Circulation*, **71**, 211–17
36. Roberts, R. and Marmor, A.T. (1983). Right ventricular infarction. *Ann. Rev. Med.*, **34**, 377–90
37. May, G.S., Furberg, C.D., Eberlain, K.A. and Geraci, B.J. (1983). Secondary prevention after acute myocardial infarction: a review of the short term acute phase trials. *Prog. Cardiovasc. Dis.*, **25**, 335–59
38. May, G.S., Eberlein, K.A., Furberg, C.D., Passamani, E.R. and DeMets, D.L. (1982). Secondary prevention after myocardial infarction. A review of long-term trials. *Prog. Cardiovasc. Dis.*, **24**, 331–52
39. The Cardiac Arrhythmia Pilot Study (CAPS) Investigators (1988). Effect of encainide, flecainide, imipramine and moricizine on ventricular arrhythmias during the year after acute myocardial infarction: The CAPS. *Am. J. Cardiol.*, **61**, 501–9
40. The Cardiac Arrhythmia Suppression Trial (CAST) Investigators (1989). Preliminary report: effect of encainide and flecainide on mortality in a randomized trial of arrhythmia suppression after myocardial infarction. *N. Engl. J. Med.*, **321**, 406–12
41. Graboys, D.B. (1975). In hospital sudden death after coronary care unit discharge: A high risk profile. *Arch. Intern. Med.*, **135**, 512–14
42. Denniss, A.R., Baaijens, H., Cody, D.V., Richards, D.A., Russell, P.A., Young, A.A., Ross, D.L. and Uther, J.B. (1985). Value of programmed stimulation and exercise testing in predicting one year mortality after acute myocardial infarction. *Am. J. Cardiol.*, **56**, 213–20
43. Baron, D.B., Light, J.R. and Ellestad, M.H. (1984). Status of exercise stress testing after myocardial infarction. *Arch. Intern. Med.*, **144**, 595–601
44. Cohn, P.F. (1983). The role of non-invasive cardiac testing after an uncomplicated myocardial infarction. *N. Engl. J. Med.*, **308**, 90–3
45. Weld, F.M., Chu, K.L. and Bigger, J.T. (1981). Risk stratification with low level exercise testing two weeks after acute myocardial infarction. *Circulation*, **64**, 306–14

11

The use of gene probes to investigate the aetiology of arterial diseases

A. TYBJÆRG-HANSEN and S.E. HUMPHRIES

INTRODUCTION

There are a number of advantages in using molecular biology techniques to study human pathology. With a few minor exceptions, the DNA is the same in all the cells of the body. This means that by analysing the DNA from a tissue that is easy to obtain, such as peripheral blood lymphocytes, it is possible to obtain information about genes that are expressed in tissues that are hard to biopsy, such as the heart, aorta or liver. It is also possible to detect mutations in genes that will be expressed only at a later stage in the development of the individual. The best example of this is the use of DNA tests for antenatal diagnosis of thalassaemia, which is caused by a defect in the gene for either the α- or β-globin protein. Diagnosis of the defect can be carried out using a sample from a non-haemopoietic tissue such as the chorionic villi of the fetal placenta. At this early developmental stage only the fetal, and not the adult, globin proteins are being made.

In order to study the role of genetic variation in the development of a disease, we need to be able to distinguish variants of the gene or genes involved. At the protein level this can be carried out using biochemical or physical techniques, for example using a functional assay for the protein, or by detecting alterations in the size or charge of the protein. DNA techniques take advantage of the considerably greater amount of variation that is occurring at the level of the gene, compared to the level of the protein. The application of this powerful approach to genetic studies has already resulted in major breakthroughs in the study of diseases caused by single gene defects, such as cystic fibrosis and Huntington's chorea. It should also be possible to use these same techniques to study diseases where the products of several genes interact to cause the development of the pathology.

It is widely accepted that there are many factors involved in the development of coronary artery disease (CAD). Some of the risk factors are environmental, such as cigarette smoking and diet. However, the susceptibility to arterial disease varies among individuals, even when they are exposed to a similar environment. This variation in response must be under genetic control, and these genetic processes can be studied using recombinant DNA technology.

In the last few years a great deal of progress has been made in the application of DNA techniques to the study of the genes involved in lipid metabolism (reviewed in refs 1 and 2). Many genes must be involved in the development of hyperlipidaemia and atherosclerosis, with different defects (or combinations of defects) occurring in different patients. All genes that are involved in lipid metabolism are good 'candidate genes' for the study of atherosclerosis. Subtle or minor defects in one or more of these genes, when inherited together, may predispose an individual to develop hyperlipidaemia and atherosclerosis. If individuals carrying such defective genes could be identified before they have developed the symptoms of arterial disease, they could be monitored closely, and given specific preventive advice to reduce their subsequent risk.

Ultimately it should be possible to determine, at the DNA level, the 'mutations' that are contributing to the increased risk of arterial disease. The problem is which of the candidate genes to study first, and how to tell whether genetic variation in any particular gene does indeed contribute to the development of hyperlipidaemia. There are three different ways to approach this problem which will be examined in turn: family studies, studies in groups of patients, and studies within the normal population.

FAMILY STUDIES – FAMILIAL HYPERCHOLESTEROLAEMIA AS AN EXAMPLE

The cholesterol-rich low density lipoprotein (LDL), is removed from the blood by a specific receptor. This receptor is found on nearly all cells, but most importantly in the liver, which has the capacity for cholesterol catabolism and excretion. In familial hypercholesterolaemia (FH), a defect has occurred in this receptor[3-5]. Individuals with one normal and one defective receptor gene have only one half the normal number of receptors on each cell, and have roughly twice the normal levels of serum LDL. These individuals have an increased rate of atherosclerosis and an increased frequency of heart attacks in mid-life. On average, 50% of the first degree relatives of an individual with FH will inherit the defective allele of the gene, and therefore will themselves develop FH. The LDL-receptor gene is therefore a clear candidate for study.

A DNA probe for the human LDL-receptor gene was isolated by Brown and Goldstein and their co-workers in 1984[6]. They have made this probe available for research purposes, and it has been used by them and others to study the defects occurring in FH[7,8] and to develop methods of diagnosis[9]. The techniques required to identify the LDL-receptor gene in a sample of DNA from an individual are straightforward, and are carried out in the research laboratory in about 7 days[10-12]. The technique used was developed by Dr Ed Southern in Edinburgh, and is named after him as the 'Southern blot'[10]. DNA from a patient can be isolated from the leukocytes in a small peripheral venous blood sample. A 10 ml blood sample yields enough DNA for up to 100 different analyses; 5 μg of this DNA is incubated with a restriction enzyme[13]. These enzymes are purified from different species of bacteria, and recognize and cleave DNA at particular sequences of 4, 5 or 6 bases. The DNA will be cut into many millions of specific fragments, one or more of which will contain the LDL-receptor gene. These fragments are separated according to size by electrophoresis in an agarose gel. The normally double-stranded DNA is made single-stranded by soaking the gel in alkali, and the DNA transferred to a sheet of nitrocellulose filter or nylon membrane by the blotting procedure (Figure 11.1). The gel is placed onto a 'wick' of filter paper, immersed in a trough containing concentrated salt solution. The sheet of nitrocellulose is then placed on top of the gel, and a layer of dry absorbent paper towels laid on top of this. The salt solution is drawn up by the absorbent paper towels, passes through the gel and the nitrocellulose, and carries the single-stranded DNA out of the gel onto the membrane filter. The final result is a single-strand DNA replica of the pattern of fragments on the original agarose gel, that are now bound to the membrane.

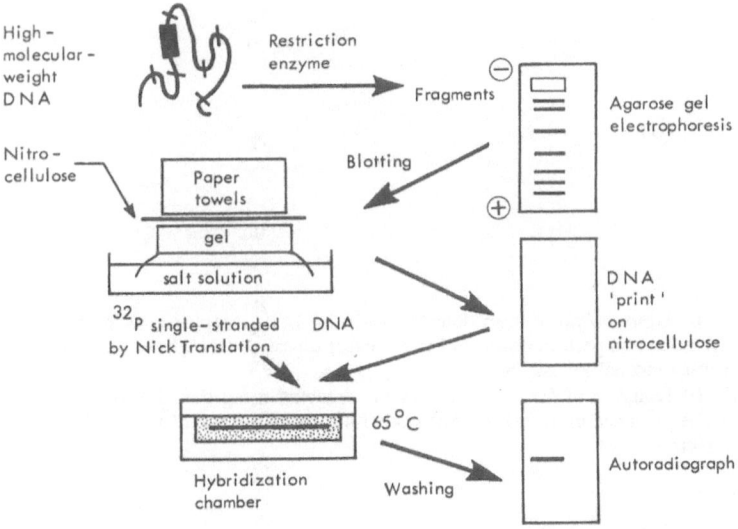

Figure 11.1 The Southern blot procedure to detect the LDL-receptor gene in a DNA sample from an individual

The next step is to make the DNA probe for the LDL-receptor highly radioactive. This is done in the test-tube, using a commercially available kit and radioactive phosphorus-labelled nucleotides. The probe can then be used to detect the normal or defective LDL-receptor genes present on the membrane. The membrane is incubated with the probe, which finds the matching single-stranded LDL-receptor gene fragments bound to the membrane and 'hybridizes' with them by reforming the DNA double helix. This process is highly specific, and the probe does not hybridize to any of the other millions of gene fragments on the membrane. Radioactive probe that has not hybridized is washed off and an X-ray film is exposed to the membrane. On the resulting autoradiogram, only the DNA fragments from the two LDL-receptor genes are detected as black bands because the radioactive probe has bound to them specifically (Figure 11.2).

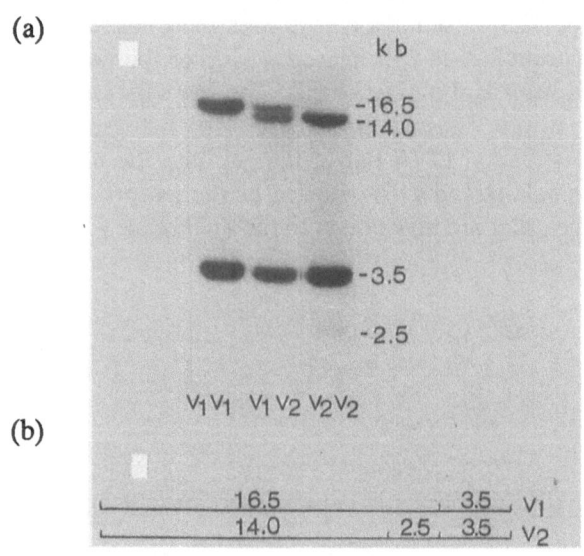

(a)

(b)

Figure 11.2 (a) DNA polymorphism detected with the LDL-receptor gene probe. Southern blot analysis of hybridization pattern obtained from a PvuII digest of DNA from three individuals (sizes of the fragments detected are shown)
Figure 11.2 (b) Diagram of how DNA fragments detected using the LDL-receptor probe can be produced by the presence of an extra PvuII site within the sequence of the gene. Cutting sites for PvuII are indicated

The aim of the research is to use these techniques to study genetic variation in the population, and in individuals. We are able to detect the variation because of the specificity of the restriction enzymes. The DNA sequences around a particular gene have been slowly changing through evolutionary time. Most of these changes are neutral and have no pathological significance, although a few will alter the function or level of expression of the gene of interest. However, by chance, these changes may have created or destroyed the DNA sequence that is the recognition and cutting site for a particular restriction enzyme. The consequence of this will be that when we digest different DNA samples with this particular enzyme, we will be able to distinguish two different sizes of gene fragments. In an individual who, by chance, has one chromosome with this site, and one chromosome lacking the site, we will be able to distinguish the two alleles of the gene of interest (Figure 11.2 (a and b)). This change will be inherited and this restriction fragment length polymorphism (RFLP) allows us to follow the inheritance of the alleles of a gene in a family, by taking advantage of the existence of a polymorphism at the DNA level. By analogy, the ABO blood group system is an example of a polymorphism at the protein level.

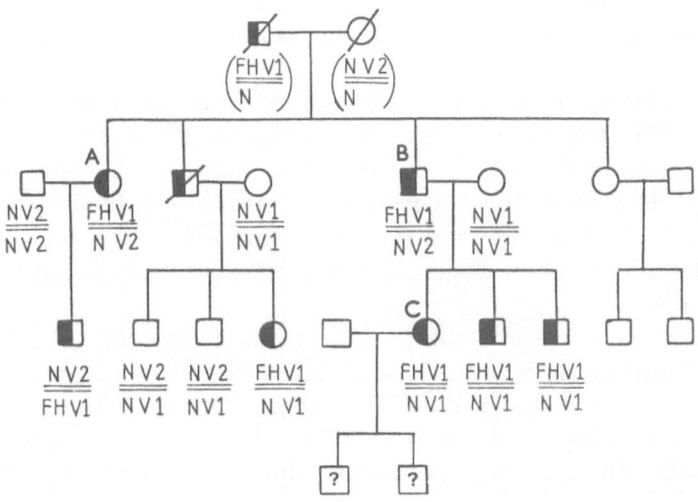

Figure 11.3 Segregation of familial hypercholesterolaemia and the LDL-receptor gene polymorphism in a model family. The deduced combinations of alleles on the chromosomes of the various individuals are shown. N, normal LDL gene; FH, familial hypercholesterolaemia gene. The sons of individual (C) are under 10 years old, and have serum LDL-concentrations in the 75th–80th centile for their age. It is not possible on these grounds alone to determine if they will develop FH

For the LDL-receptor there is a DNA polymorphism detected with the enzyme PvuII, with the common allele designated *V1* and the rare allele designated *V2* (Figure 11.2 (b)). The use of this polymorphism to study a family with FH is shown in Figure 11.3. For any individual with FH, we have no way of knowing, *a priori*, whether the defective LDL-receptor gene is on the chromosome with the cutting site for PvuII (*V2* allele) or without the cutting site (*V1*). This has to be deduced by inspection of the pedigree, and determining which chromosome is inherited by the affected and unaffected family members. In this family, the eldest sister (A) has FH and the genotype *V1V2*. Her husband is normal and has the genotype *V2V2*, and her affected son has the genotype *V1V2*. The son must have inherited the normal allele of the LDL-receptor gene from his father on a chromosome carrying the cutting site (*V2*), and the defective gene from his mother on a chromosome without the site (*V1*). We can, therefore, predict that in this family the defective LDL-receptor gene will co-segregate with the *V1* allele of the DNA polymorphism. As can be seen, this is indeed the case, and we can carry out diagnosis for the children of the propositus of this family (B), before they develop high serum lipid levels. However, we cannot carry out diagnosis in the next generation, since we cannot distinguish the normal and defective alleles of the LDL-receptor gene in the mother (C). In order to be able to do this, other RFLPs of the gene will need to be detected, and for the LDL receptor there are now over a dozen such RFLPs reported[14] and using only four of these roughly 80% of individuals are heterozygous for at least one[15] and thus potentially informative for family studies.

It should be noted that neither allele of the PvuII polymorphism is itself a marker for FH. The DNA change that creates the RFLP occurs outside the coding sequence of the gene[16] and, therefore, does not alter the amino acid sequence of the protein. The frequency of the rare allele of the RFLP is 27% in both the general population and in patients with FH[15]. This means that the polymorphism is useful for diagnosis only in situations where family studies can be carried out.

However when several DNA polymorphisms around the gene have been detected, it may be possible to carry out direct diagnosis in some populations, using these RFLPs in conjunction. For example, for five RFLPs, there are 32 possible combinations of the pairs of alleles that can occur together on one chromosome. This genetic information defines the 'haplotypes' of the two chromosomes in an individual. When a base change occurs, creating a mutation in the LDL-receptor gene, it will occur on one particular haplotype in an individual in the population. From then on, all the individuals who inherit this defective LDL-receptor gene will also have inherited the haplotype, which will be diagnostic for that mutation. This approach has been very fruitful in the analysis of the haemoglobinopathies[17], and is also applicable to FH. For example in South Africa there is a high frequency of FH in the Afrikaaner population[18]. Most of these individuals have probably inherited the defect from a common ancestor. In this population, therefore, there may be only a few defects causing FH, and these will be found on a particular chromosomal haplotype defined by several RFLPs[19]. Using these RFLPs, it may be possible to distinguish these chromosomes from all others in the population. This would then give a population-specific diagnostic test for FH, since all individuals in the population carrying this unique chromosome will also have inherited the defective LDL-receptor gene. This will probably only be applicable in isolated communities or regions where there has not been migration, immigration or the occurrence of many different mutations.

In the future it may be possible in some individuals with FH, to carry out direct diagnosis using DNA techniques. For example, in the UK in about 5% of affected individuals have deletions of a large part of the LDL-receptor gene, which give rise to correspondingly reduced restriction enzyme fragments of the gene. These can be detected easily by the blotting technique[20]. In FH patients in Canada of French origin over 60% have an identical 10,000 base pair deletion of the 5' part of the gene[21]. This deletion renders the gene non-functional, and must have been passed on from one of the founding immigrants to all the affected descendants. A second rarer deletion (about 4% of patients) has also been recently reported in French Canadians[22]. In the rest of the patients there are many different defects in the LDL-receptor gene that cause FH. These defects are deletions of a few DNA bases from the gene, or single base changes that critically alter the function of the protein. There are a number of techniques that are available, or that are being developed, that will enable these single base changes to be detected and, although time-consuming, these may be applicable for diagnosis of FH. For example, two common single base change mutations have recently been detected in Afrikaaner FH patients that create or destroy a site for a specific restriction enzyme. These can be detected easily by DNA techniques, and taken together allow a direct unambiguous diagnosis in approximately 95% of patients in this region[23]. In geographical areas of genetic heterogeneity such as the UK such a high frequency for any single defect causing FH is unlikely. However, if it were available, information about specific mutations might be useful in developing therapeutic strategies, if for example patients with a particular defect respond best to a certain drug. Research in the area continues.

FH is a common disease, occurring in roughly 1 in 500 members of the population[1]. In some families, early diagnosis using a DNA test[24], may allow the affected children to start an appropriate lipid-lowering lifestyle before hyperlipidaemia and atherosclerosis have developed. FH thus provides an excellent model for the use of DNA techniques to develop diagnostic methods, and to study disorders where hyperlipidaemia is caused by a defect in a single gene. However, in the majority of individuals with hyperlipidaemia, there is no single gene defect causing the elevated serum lipid levels. Other techniques, therefore, have to be applied to analyse the problem.

POPULATION ASSOCIATION IN PATIENTS. THE APO AI GENE COMPLEX AS AN EXAMPLE

The second example of the use of RFLPs in the study of genetic hyperlipidaemia, is the search for population associations between the neutral genetic variation detected by the RFLP, and functionally significant genetic variation of a nearby gene. There are a number of reports of such associations for the polymorphisms of the apo AI gene complex (Table 1)[25-34].

It is now known that there are three apolipoprotein genes on human chromosome 11[35]. They are the genes for apo AI, apo CIII and apo AIV. They are in a cluster, with only 12 kb of DNA (1 kb (kilobase) = 1000 base pairs) separating the 5' end of the apo AI gene (amino terminal end of the protein) and the 3' end of the apo AIV gene (carboxy terminal end of the protein). Many common RFLPs have been detected within this gene cluster (see refs 1 and 2) and the locations of the variable sites detected with some of these enzymes are shown in Figure 11.4. Most of these polymorphisms are caused by sequence changes outside the coding regions of the genes, and therefore do not, in themselves, alter the amino acid sequence of any of the proteins. The variant SstI site is within the 3' untranslated region of the gene for apo CIII but, as far as is known, this does not alter the function of the protein or mRNA[36].

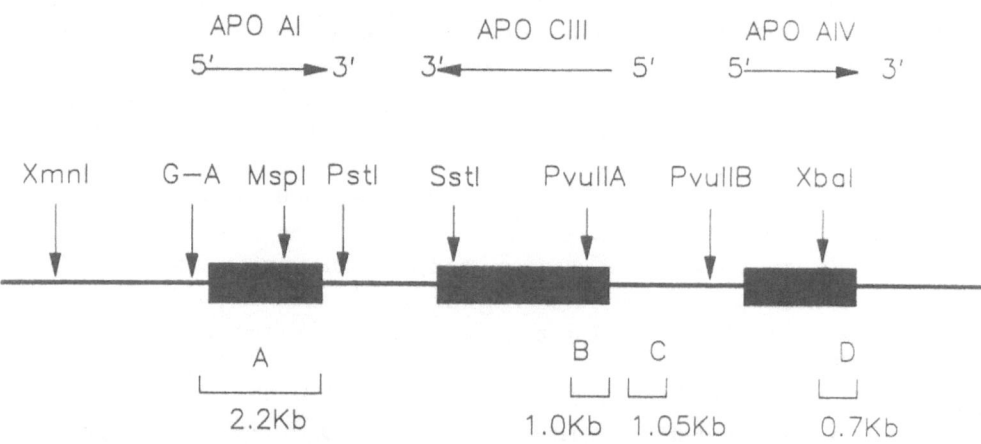

Figure 11.4 Map of the apo AI-CIII-AIV RFLPs showing the varying sites, the direction of transcription of the genes and the probes used to identify the fragments[25,34]

In the first reports describing the SstI RFLP it was found that the rare allele (designated *S2*) was present in a higher frequency in a group of patients with hypertriglyceridaemia than in the normal population[30,31]. The *S2* allele frequency was higher only in a group of patients with Type IV and V hyperlipidaemia, and not significantly different in patients with Type IIb, or Type III[37]. Similar results have been obtained by others[33], though some studies have detected a significant difference in allele frequency only in groups of patients with Type V hyperlipidaemia[32]. This discrepancy may be explained by chance variations due to the small sample sizes involved, or real differences due to the samples being drawn from different populations.

It is also possible to analyse the data by ranking all the patients and normolipidaemic individuals by triglyceride levels, and comparing the allele frequency of the RFLPs in the lowest and highest group, or the frequency below and above the 95th centile of the normal population[39]. This will give information about genetic variation involved in the determination of triglyceride levels in general, and not specifically in the development of a particular lipoprotein pattern, such as Type V hyperlipidaemia.

Table 11.1 Some reported associations between apolipoprotein gene RFLPs and clinically important phenotypes

Gene	RFLP	Trait	Ref
AI-CIII-AIV	XmnI	AI	25
	PstI	AI, HDL, CAD	25–29
	SstI	TRIG, CAD	30–33
	PvuII	HDL	34
B	EcoRI	CAD/TRIG	49–51
	XbaI	CHOL/TRIG Apo B/LDL	52–54
	MspI	OBESITY	56

A model to explain these findings, based on evolutionary history, is shown in Figure 11.5. In the original normolipidaemic population, there were individuals who had chromosomes both with and without the SstI cutting site. In one individual, a mutation occurred in this gene cluster and predisposed the individual to develop hypertriglyceridaemia (HTG). By chance, the mutation occurred on a chromosome containing the cutting site – the S2 allele. In the population there were now three types of chromosomes, S1-normal, S2-normal and S2-HTG. This would mean that when the population was analysed many generations later, as a result of its historical association, many people with hypertriglyceridaemia would have the genotype S1S2 or S2S2, but the S2 allele would also be found in normolipidaemic individuals. We may also find hypertriglyceridaemic individuals with the genotype S1S1. This may be the result of independent events causing the same or a different mutation, or by a loss of association between the mutation and the S2 allele of the SstI RFLP, because of recombination occurring in the region of DNA between them.

Recombination occurs during meiosis, and is an important mechanism in the creation of new genetic diversity. It is the result of crossing over and exchange of DNA between two chromosomes, in this case the paternal and maternal chromosome 11s. In general, the rate of recombination between two gene loci is dependent on the distance between them. For the apoAI/CIII/AIV gene cluster, the small physical distance separating the genes means that it will take many hundreds of generations for recombination to lead to the loss of association between the allele of an RFLP and a mutation causing hypertriglyceridaemia.

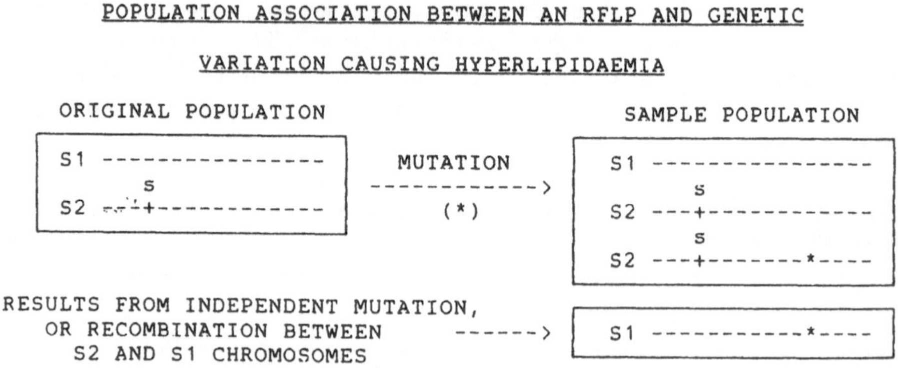

POPULATION ASSOCIATION BETWEEN AN RFLP AND GENETIC

VARIATION CAUSING HYPERLIPIDAEMIA

ORIGINAL POPULATION   SAMPLE POPULATION

```
 _____          MUTATION        _____
| S1 ----------------    |      ------------>     | S1 ----------------    |
|         s              |          (*)           |         s              |
| S2 --.-+-----------    |                        | S2 ---+------------    |
|_____|                        |         s              |
                                                  | S2 ---+-------*----    |
                                                  |_____|
```

RESULTS FROM INDEPENDENT MUTATION,
   OR RECOMBINATION BETWEEN   ------>
   S2 AND S1 CHROMOSOMES

```
 _____
| S1 -----------*----    |
|_____|
```

Figure 11.5 Model to explain the observed population association between the Apo AI, SstI, RFLP and mutation causing hypertriglyceridaemia. *S1, S2,* chromosomes respectively without, and with the cutting site for SstI (shown as S). *, the mutation in the gene cluster causing the development of hypertriglyceridaemia

One of the consequences of evolutionary history is that the allele frequency of protein and DNA polymorphisms may alter in populations with different ethnic backgrounds. For example, the frequency of the ABO blood group, or the HLA surface antigens varies among the different races, and even among different groups in Europe. The frequency of the apo E protein isoforms, E3, E2 and E4, varies significantly between the German and the Finnish populations[38], and there are larger differences when more distantly related groups, such as the Asian population, are compared. These frequency differences may be the result of selection pressure, or due to the fact that the DNA changes causing the variation may have arisen independently, in the different populations. They may also arise by chance differences in the frequency of the polymorphism in the group of individuals who originally founded the population.

It is, therefore, not surprising that the allele frequency of many of the RFLPs so far examined has been shown to vary in different populations (Table 2). There are clear differences in the allele frequency of the SstI RfLP between the UK, Norwegian, Italian, and Japanese populations. These observations mean that caution must be exercised in extrapolating results of RFLP frequency obtained in one population to another. It is possible that in a second, distantly related population, genetic variation predisposing to hypertriglyceridaemia may be associated with a different allele of an RFLP (i.e. the 'mutation' occurred on a chromosome bearing a different RFLP allele). This appears to be the case in the Japanese population, where there is evidence that individuals with hyper-triglyceridaemia have a higher frequency of the SstI *S1* allele as compared with Japanese normolipidaemic individuals[41].

It is unlikely that selection pressures, either positive or negative, have produced any of the variants of the apolipoprotein genes. Even individuals with FH have passed reproductive age before the deleterious effects of mutation in the LDL-receptor gene become manifest. In the sense of reproductive fitness (the frequency of passing on genes to the next generation), both FH and genetic variation predisposing to any of the hyperlipidaemias appears to have no selective disadvantage, at least acting through the development of athero-sclerosis.

Table 11.2 Frequency of SstI RFLP in different ethnic groups

Group	Frequency of S2 allele	Reference
London	0.05–0.08	30, 25
Norway	0.17	39
African	0.15	31
Asian	0.18	31
Amerindian	0.25	40
Italy	0.35	29
Japan	0.48	31, 41

In 1986 there was a report of a population association in patients with coronary artery disease, between low levels of HDL and the PstI RPLP of the apo AI gene[26]. The frequency of the rare allele, P2, was significantly higher in patients with low levels of HDL. This observation has been confirmed in a UK study[27] but not in a study in Austria[28]. However, in one study in normo-lipidaemic clinically well individuals, those with low levels of HDL do not have a higher frequency of the P2 allele[25]. This suggests a polygenic model, where genetic variation associated with the P2 allele predisposes an individual to develop low levels of HDL, but another factor, possibly genetic, is required to develop low levels of HDL. Such a model has been proposed for the development of Type III hyperlipidaemia[38], with individuals who are homozygous for the E2 isoform of apo E having low levels of serum cholesterol, but being predisposed (when they co-inherit a second, as yet unidentified, gene variant) to develop hyperlipidaemia.

As with FH, it should be possible to refine the diagnostic power of the RFLPs by using several of them in conjunction. The haplotypes that can be identified may be more specific for a particular mutation. In the Japanese population, individuals with hypertriglyceridaemia have a higher frequency of a particular chromosome defined by the SstI and MspI RFLPs[41]. There is preliminary evidence[32] (and Kessling, unpublished) that a higher proportion than expected of individuals with Type V hyperlipidaemia, carry a chromosome with the X2S2 haplotype. If this chromosome occurs in only a small proportion of the general population, but in a significant proportion of individuals with Type V, it points the way to developing a more useful diagnostic approach.

None of the RFLPs of the apo AI-CIII-AIV cluster so far reported are in themselves genetic markers for hypertriglyceridaemia or for low levels of HDL. Thus there are healthy individuals in the population who have the particular allele of the RFLP, and patients who do not. Many of these RFLPs are, however, showing allelic population associations with variations in genes that are involved, for example, in determining the serum levels of triglyceride. Presumably, genetic variation must be altering the function, or level of expression, of a protein coded for by a gene near to the polymorphic restriction enzyme site. Of the three genes known to be within this region, the gene for apo CIII would appear to be the most likely candidate for such an alteration. Apo CIII is found on triglyceride-rich lipoproteins, and is known to inhibit the activity of lipoprotein lipase in vitro[43]. However, it is possible that important variation may also be occurring in the apo AI gene, or the apo AIV gene, or in another, unknown, neighbouring gene. To distinguish these possibilities, these genes must be isolated from a normal individual and a patient, and the sequence of the genes compared, to try to distinguish the functionally significant DNA changes. One such change, a G to A substitution in the −75bp position of the apo AI promoter has recently been found in individuals with high apo AI[44,45]. It is possible that this sequence change affects binding for a positive trans-acting protein, that increases transcription of the apo AI gene. This increases apo AI mRNA and thus apo AI protein secretion from the liver or intestine. There will, however, be many differences between two regions of DNA taken at random, since studies, for example in the globin genes, have indicated that 'neutral' DNA changes occur at the rate of roughly 1/100 to 1/200 bases[46]. Other techniques will therefore be needed to examine the functional significance of such changes detected, but in principle this can be done, and is being attempted by several research groups.

The goal of this research, as with FH, is to understand how defects in the apolipoprotein genes cause the development of dyslipidaemia and CAD. Taken overall, the major conclusion that can be made from these studies, is that genes near or within the apo AI/CIII/AIV gene cluster are important in apolipoprotein and lipid metabolism. Different studies, both in patients and the normal population, show that genetic variation in this region is involved in the determination of serum triglyceride, apo AI and HDL levels. At the present time, these RFLPs are not useful for diagnosis. They do, however, give strong clues that detailed studies of the apo AI/CIII/AIV genes will enable the identification of the DNA changes that are causing the different phenotypes. This information can be used to develop tests that will be 'mutation specific' and that may be useful for early diagnosis of individuals with a predisposition to hyperlipidaemia.

POPULATION ASSOCIATION IN THE NORMAL POPULATION.
THE APO B GENE AS AN EXAMPLE

Several studies have shown that there is a roughly linear relationship between serum cholesterol levels and the risk of developing coronary artery disease. Individuals with serum cholesterol levels in the first or second quintile of the distribution are, therefore, at significantly lower risk of developing arterial disease than those in the fourth or fifth quintile. One of the important topics of research is thus to analyse the genetic component of the determination of lipid levels within the normolipidaemic population. Individuals who are predisposed for example to developing both LDL-cholesterol levels in the top quintile, and HDL-cholesterol levels in the lowest quintile, may be at particular risk, and it would be useful to identify these individuals at an early age, particularly if they have a positive family history of arterial disease. This approach will clearly require analysis of genetic variation in a number of different genes, since in the general population, elevated lipid levels are not caused by a single gene defect, like FH, but are the result of polygenic interaction.

Recently, several groups have isolated DNA probes for the apolipoprotein apo B[47,48]. As with the apo AI-CIII-AIV gene RFLPs, studies have detected differences in allele frequency between cases and controls in some but not all populations[49-51], indicating that variation in the apo B gene determines CAD risk by some mechanism. It is now known that apo B, which is the major protein component of LDL, is a protein of 4536 amino acids, with a molecular weight of 512 kd. The gene for apo B is on chromosome 2, and several DNA polymorphisms of the gene have been reported. For any one of these polymorphisms, for example the XbaI RFLP of apo B, individuals can be divided by genotype into three classes, and the mean serum total cholesterol, LDL-cholesterol, or apo B level estimated for each group. Several reports[52-55] have shown that in the normolipidaemic population, individuals with a particular apo B XbaI genotype, designated *X1X1* in Figure 11.6, have a lower mean serum cholesterol level than individuals with the genotype *X2X2*, while individuals heterozygous for the polymorphism have intermediate mean serum cholesterol levels. Similar variation with XbaI genotype of the level of LDL-cholesterol and serum apo B, have been reported[54]. In the London study, two other apo B polymorphisms, detected with the enzymes Eco RI and MspI, were not associated with any significant differences in serum cholesterol levels[53]. Using statistical methods, the average effect in this study sample of the two alleles of the XbaI RFLP can be calculated. The allele *X1* has an average effect of reducing mean serum cholesterol by 0.23 mmol l^{-1} and *X2* of increasing it by a similar amount.

The XbaI polymorphism is, therefore, detecting genetic variation, in or around the apo B gene that is involved in determining serum cholesterol levels. The DNA change that creates or destroys the XbaI site occurs within the coding region of the gene, but the base change is in the third (wobble) position of a codon, and does not alter the amino acid sequence. Presumably, by a model similar to that proposed earlier, there is a population association, due to evolutionary history, between the XbaI site and a DNA sequence change elsewhere in or around the apo B gene. This change may alter the amino acid sequence, which may change the functional properties of the protein and perhaps alter its affinity for the LDL-receptor. Support for the hypothesis has come from LDL turnover studies, where individuals with the *X2* allele have a lower fractional catabolic rate (clearance) of LDL and thus a higher plasma LDL-cholesterol level, than individuals with the *X1* allele[56,57]. Alternatively, the DNA change may affect the level of transcription of the gene, and therefore alter the amount of apo B protein produced by the liver. The next stage in the analysis would be to isolate and sequence the apo B gene from individuals with different apo B genotypes, to determine the DNA change that is causing the altered levels of serum cholesterol.

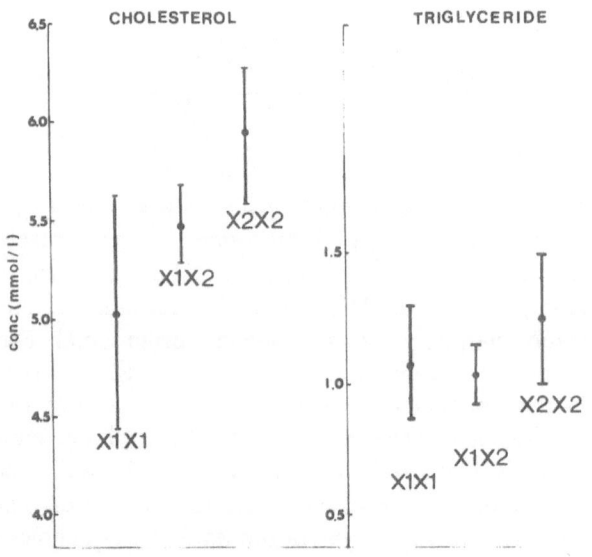

Figure 11.6 Lipid levels in normolipidaemic individuals with different XbaI genotypes. The mean plus 95% confidence limits are shown for serum cholesterol and triglyceride levels for individuals with the genotype *X1X1, X1X2* and *X2X2*.
The respective means and standard deviations of cholesterol levels (mmol/l) for the three genotypes were: 5.03 (±0.945), 5.48 (±0.65), 5.96 (±0.52). (Data from ref. 53)

Plasma levels of LDL-cholesterol are determined largely by the activity of LDL-receptors, which interact with a specific region of the apolipoprotein B-100 (apo B-100) protein moiety of LDL-particles[58] and remove LDL from the circulation. Reduced removal of LDL could either be caused by defects in the

LDL-receptor, as in FH[3], or by defects in the ligand (apo B-100). Familial defective apolipoprotein B-100 (FDB) is a recently identified, dominantly inherited genetic disorder, which leads to increased serum concentration of LDL-cholesterol with reduced affinity for the LDL receptor[59-62]. This disorder is associated with a G to A mutation in exon 26 of the apo B gene (in the putative receptor binding region of the protein) which results in a substitution of the amino acid glutamine for arginine in codon 3500. This mutation has been detected in the USA[59-62], in the UK and Denmark[63], and in the FRG[64]. So far all individuals identified have been heterozygous for the apo B($arg_{3500} \rightarrow gln$) mutation. A crude estimate of the frequency in the general population in the UK is 1/600, or similar to the frequency of FH[63] although this estimate needs to be confirmed in larger studies. The most striking feature of this disorder is that plasma lipid levels and clinical characteristics are similar to those reported for heterozygous FH[63,64]. Thus, FDB is associated with moderate to severe hypercholesterolaemia with frequencies of coronary artery disease (CAD), of tendon xanthomas and of arcus corneae resembling those reported for FH heterozygotes. Furthermore, the cumulative frequency of CAD with age is similar in FDB and FH heterozygotes (Table 11.3). In two studies, about 3% of patients with a clinical diagnosis of FH were heterozygous for the apo B ($arg_{3500} \rightarrow gln$) mutation, and had normal LDL-receptor activity[63,64].

Table 11.3 Cumulative frequency of coronary artery disease (CAD) as a function of age in men and women heterozygous for familial defective apolipoprotein B-100 (FDB) and in men and women heterozygous for familial hypercholesterolemia (FH) (Numbers in parentheses indicate number of individuals with CAD out of total) (Data from ref. 63, Table 4)

	Males		Females	
	FDB	FH[a]	FDB[a]	FH
By age 40	20% (1/5)	20%	0% (0.0)	3%
By age 50	60% (3/5)	45%	20% (1/5)	20%
By age 60	100% (5/5)	75%	40% (2/5)	45%

[a] Data from ref.3, Table 33–4

In the patients studied in the USA, roughly 70% of LDL particles in plasma contain the mutant apo B, and bind poorly to the LDL receptor[59-62]. Drugs which act to increase the number of LDL-receptors on cells (HMG-CoA reductase inhibitors or bile acid binding resins) may therefore be of limited use in treating such patients. Alternatively, drugs such as fibrates and nicotinic acid which reduce the production of apo B containing lipoproteins by the liver, may be indicated. If so, it will be important, from a clinical point of view, to identify these individuals. With the present techniques, screening for the presence of the apo B (arg$_{3500}$→gln) mutation is relatively easy. The mutation can be identified unambiguously by using a relatively new technique, the polymerase chain reaction (PCR), developed by Saiki and coworkers[65–66], followed by oligomelting[67].

PCR is a method for the selective amplification of DNA (or RNA) segments up to 2 kb or more in length[68]. Synthetic oligonucleotides flanking the sequences of interest are used in repeated cycles of enzymatic primer extension in opposite and overlapping direction (Figure 11.7). The essential steps in each cycle are thermal denaturation of the double-stranded DNA target molecules, primer annealing to both strands and enzymatic synthesis of DNA. The use of heat-stable DNA polymerase makes the reaction amenable to automation. Since both strands of a given DNA segment are used as templates, the number of target sequences increases exponentially. The reaction is simple, fast and extremely sensitive. The DNA (or RNA) content of a single cell is sufficient to detect a specific sequence. DNA for this purpose can therefore be extracted from a blood spot[69,70], a hair follicle or saliva sample[70].

To detect the apo B(arg$_{3500}$→gln) mutation, the PCR was used to amplify a 345 base pair (bp) region of the apo B gene spanning this mutation at position 10 699 bp[72] in exon 26 (Figure 11.8). Allele specific oligos (ASOs) were used to detect the presence of the G or A base at this position. The PCR reactions were conducted in an automated thermal cycler using thermostable thermus aquaticus DNA polymerase (Taq polymerase) for 30 cycles. One fiftieth of each PCR reaction was applied to nylon filters and hybridized with radioactively labelled ASOs and the filters were autoradiographed over night (Figure 11.9). This whole procedure can thus be completed within a day.

As opposed to FH where more than 30 different mutations in the LDL receptor give rise to the same phenotype, FDB is caused by one mutation in the apo B gene and can therefore be screened for in the general population as well as in families at risk. However, this is most certainly not the only mutation in the apo B gene causing primary hypercholesterolaemia through reduced binding of LDL to receptors[60], but is at present the only disorder where the underlying mutation in the apo B gene is known.

In the next few years analyses as indicated for the apo B gene will be carried out with RFLPs of all the other apolipoproteins, and some of the enzymes, receptors and carrier proteins known to be involved in lipid metabolism. Hopefully, by this approach we will be able to quantify and assign the majority of the genetic variation responsible for determining the levels of serum LDL and HDL cholesterol. As we understand more about the genetic factors that are involved in determining serum lipid levels, the diagnostic power of the battery of tests that we develop will increase. The challenge for the next few years will be to move from the imprecise use of RFLPs, to the detection and characterization of the underlying DNA changes in the different genes, which collectively predispose to hyperlipidaemia. This will allow the development of precise tests such as that for apo B 3500 that will have a high degree of accuracy and diagnostic potential.

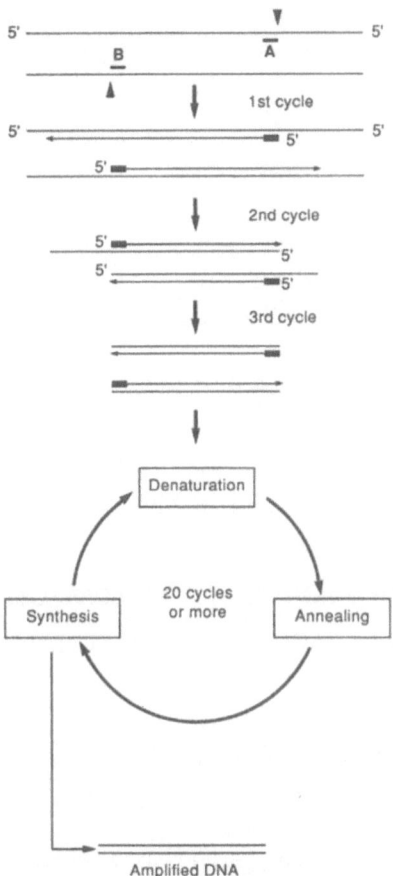

Figure 11.7 Scheme of the polymerase chain reaction (PCR) with double-stranded DNA as template. The two primers A and B serve to initiate DNA synthesis in a defined region. The arrows indicate the direction of synthesis in each cycle, which consists of template denaturation by heat, primer annealing and enzymatic synthesis. The DNA products of discrete length (defined by the distance between the 5' ends of the primers; see the arrowheads in the top two lines) are generated from the third cycle on, only these molecules are amplified exponentially.

FUTURE RESEARCH

Just as there are genes involved in determining the level of serum LDL, or HDL in a particular individual, there must be genes involved in determining the response, for example, of the cells of the artery wall, to a high level of serum cholesterol. At present, we do not know which genes are involved. One cell that has an important role in the development of the atherosclerotic lesion is the macrophage[73]. Macrophages have the ability to take up damaged or excess

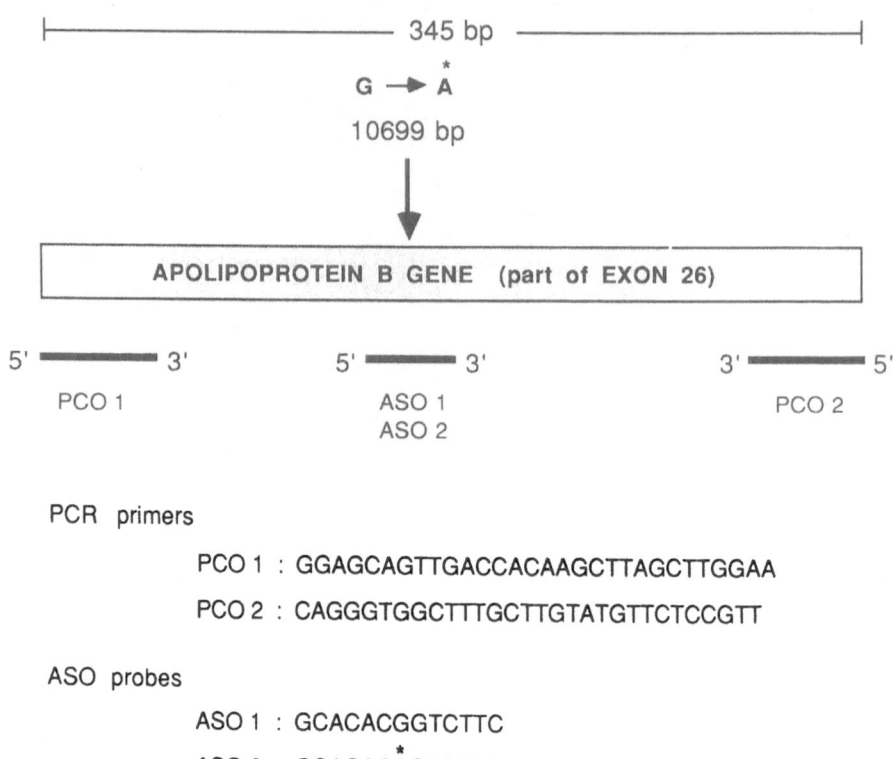

PCR primers

PCO 1 : GGAGCAGTTGACCACAAGCTTAGCTTGGAA

PCO 2 : CAGGGTGGCTTTGCTTGTATGTTCTCCGTT

ASO probes

ASO 1 : GCACACGGTCTTC

ASO 2 : GCACAC*AGTCTTC

Figure 11.8 Position of the apo B(arg$_{3500}$→gln) mutation in base pairs (bp), and sequence of polymerase chain reaction (PCR) primers and of allele specific oligonucleotide (ASO) probes, and their relation to the apo B gene[72]. The two PCR primers, PCO 1 and PCO 2, are 30 bases long and are complementary to the (−) and (+) strands respectively. The two ASO probes, ASO 1 and ASO 2, are 13 bases long and span the site of the mutation (asterisk). ASO 1 identifies the normal apo B allele, ASO 2 identifies the mutant allele. (Ref. 63, Figure 1; reproduced with permission)

lipoproteins through specific receptors. This leads to the accumulation of cholesterol esters within the cell that cause it to fill with cholesterol ester droplets, and take on a foamy appearance in the atherosclerotic tissue. These foam cells synthesize apo E, as well as specific receptors for HDL, the lipoprotein to which excess cholesterol is transferred, in the process known as reverse cholesterol transport[74]. A study of the genes for the receptors, enzymes and growth factors produced in these cells would be interesting, and might lead to further diagnostic tools.

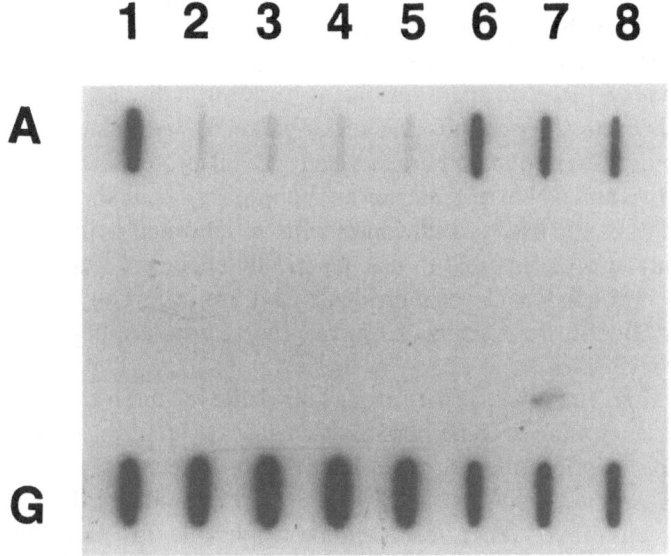

Figure 11.9 Autoradiogram of slot blot of amplified genomic DNA hybridized with ^{32}P-labelled allele specific oligonucleotide (ASO) probes. Lane G was probed with ASO 1, lane A was probed with ASO 2, detecting the normal G and the mutated A base respectively. 1, positive control; 2–5, homozygous GG; 6–8, heterozygous GA. (Ref. 63, Figure 2; reproduced with permission)

By extension of this argument, there must also be genetic control of the processes of thrombosis such as clotting, thrombolysis and platelet aggregation. For example, high levels of fibrinogen and Factor VII have both been shown by epidemiological studies to predispose an individual to ischaemic heart disease[75]. RFLP studies have shown that variation at the fibrinogen gene locus itself contributes in part to determining levels of plasma fibrinogen[76] and this opens up the way for detailed molecular studies to identify the precise molecular mechanism responsible. In addition, there may be inherited defects in some of the structural components of the heart and the blood vessel walls, which may predispose to cardiovascular disease in later life. For instance, subtle defects in a Type III collagen found in the walls of the aorta may cause some forms of abdominal aortic aneurysm (AAA), and this too would be amenable to these methods of analysis. An example of using this approach to study AAA has recently been published indicating that genes on chromosome 16 may be involved in the development of the disease[77]. The identification of the mechanism of the association at the protein and finally DNA level would be useful for diagnosis and possible methods of therapy.

Finally, genetic factors affecting the function of endothelial cells in the artery wall have been reported. Endothelial cells from individuals with a defect in the enzyme cystathionine synthase, are particularly sensitive to low levels of homocysteine in the culture medium[78]. In the general population, about 1 in 70 individuals carry a defective gene for this enzyme, but in one study of patients with arterial disease 1 in 7 of the patients had the defective enzyme. Low levels of this enzyme may, therefore, be a risk factor for arterial disease.

It is also theoretically possible that recombinant DNA techniques could, in the future, be used to produce therapeutically useful proteins. For example, if biologically active and stable enzymes or apolipoproteins could be produced, this might be of therapeutic use for individuals with an inherited deficiency of these proteins. It may also be possible to use genetically engineered apolipoproteins, to alter the lipoprotein profile of individuals who are at risk of atherosclerosis because of variation in these genes. However, these areas are beyond the scope of the present review.

Taken together, the hope is that as our knowledge of these common genetic variants increases, it may become possible to devise a battery of DNA tests that will enable us to diagnose individuals at high risk of developing arterial disease. Although this will initially be within 'high risk' families, later, as our understanding increases, these tests will be applicable to individuals in the general population. This information should make a useful contribution as part of an overall strategy to reduce the mortality from coronary artery disease.

ACKNOWLEDGEMENTS

The work in the author's laboratory was supported by the British Heart Foundation, and the Charing Cross Sunley Research Trust. Anne Tybjærg-Hansen is supported by the Danish Heart Foundation, the Danish Medical Research Council and a Wellcome–Carlsberg Travelling Research Fellowship. We thank Munksgaard International Publishers, Copenhagen, and Elsevier Publishers (Amsterdam) for permission to reproduce material from several published papers, Dr Anna Kessling for helpful comments, and Miss Helen Pritchard for assistance in preparation of the manuscript.

References

1. Humphries, S.E. (1988). DNA polymorphisms of the apolipoprotein genes; their use in the investigation of the genetic component of hyperlipidaemia and atherosclerosis. *Atherosclerosis*, **72**, 89–108
2. Lusis, A. (1988). Genetic factors affecting blood lipoproteins: the candidate gene approach. *J. Lipid Res.*, **29**, 387
3. Goldstein, J.L. and Brown, M.S. (1983). Familial hypercholesterolaemia. In Stanbury, J.B., Wyngaarden, J.B., Fredrickson, D.S., Goldstein, J.L. and Brown, M.S. (eds.). *The Metabolic Basis of Inherited Human Disease*, 5th Edn., pp. 672–712. (New York: McGraw-Hill)
4. Brown, M.S. and Goldstein, J.L. (1984). How LDL-receptors influence cholesterol and atherosclerosis. *Sci. Am.*, **251**, 52–60

5. Tolleshaug, H., Hobgood, K.K., Brown, M.S. and Goldstein, J.L. (1983). The LDL receptor locus in familial hypercholesterolaemia – Multiple mutations disrupt transport and processing of membrane receptor. *Cell*, 32, 941–51

6. Yamamoto, T., Davis, L.G., Brown, M.S. Schneider, W.J., Casey, M.L., Goldstein, J.L. and Russell, D.W. (1984). The human LDL receptor: a cysteine-rich protein with multiple Alu sequences in its mRNA. *Cell*, 39, 27–38

7. Lehrman, M.A., Schneider, W.J., Südhof, T.C. Brown M.S., Goldstein, J.L. and Russell, D.W. (1985). Mutations in the LDL receptor. Alu-Alu recombination deletes exons encoding transmembrane and cytoplasmic domains. *Science*, 227, 140–6

8. Horsthemke, B., Kessling, A.M., Seed, M., Wynn, V., Williamson, R. and Humphries, S.E. (1985). Identification of a deletion in the low density lipoprotein (LDL) receptor gene in a patient with familial hypercholesterolaemia. *Hum. Genet.*, 71, 75–8

9. Humphries, S.E., Kessling, A.M., Horsthemke, B., Donald, J.A., Seed, M., Jowett, N.I., Holm, M., Galton, D.J., Wynn, V. and Williamson, R. (1985). A common DNA polymorphism of the low density lipoprotein (LDL) receptor gene and its use in diagnosis. *Lancet*, 1, 1003–5

10. Southern, E. (1975). Detection of specific sequences among DNA sequences separated by gel electrophoresis. *J. Mol. Biol.*, 98, 503–17

11. Humphries, S.E. and Williamson, R. (1983). Recombinant DNA technology in prenatal diagnosis. *Br. Med. Bull.*, 39, 343–7

12. Humphries, S.E. (1986). Familial hypercholesterolaemia as an example of early diagnosis of coronary artery disease risk by DNA techniques. *Br. Heart J.*, 56, 1–5

13. Malcolm, A.D.B. (1981). The use of restriction enzymes in genetic engineering. In Williamson, R. (ed.). *Genetic Engineering*. Vol. 2., pp. 129–73. (London: Academic Press)

14. Leitersdorf, E., Chakravarti, A. and Hobbs, S. (1989). Polymorphic DNA haplotypes at the LDL receptor locus. *Am. J. Hum. Genet.*, 44, 409–21

15. Taylor, R., Jeenah, M., Seed, M. and Humphries S. (1988). Four DNA polymorphisms in the LDL receptor gene: their genetic relationship and use in the study of variation at the LDL receptor locus. *J. Med. Genet.*, 25, 653–9

16. Hobbs, H.H., Lehrman, M.A., Yamamoto, T. and Russell, D.W. (1985). Polymorphism and evolution of Alu sequences in the human low density lipoprotein receptor gene. *Proc. Natl. Acad. Sci. USA*, 82, 7651–5

17. Antonarakis, S.E., Kazazian, H.H. and Orkin, S.H. (1985). DNA polymorphism and molecular pathology of the human globin gene clusters. *Hum. Genet.*, 69, 1–14

18. Seftel, H.C., Baker, S.G., Sandler, M.P., Forman, M.B., Joffe, B.I., Mendelsohn, D., Jenkins, T. and Mieny, C.J. (1980). A host of hypercholesterolaemic homozygotes in South Africa. *Br. Med. J.*, 281, 633–6

19. Henderson, H., Kotze, M.J. and Berger, G.M.B. (1989). Multiple mutations underlying familial hypercholesterolemia in the South African population. *Hum. Genet.*, 83, 67–70

20. Horsthemke, B., Dunning, A. and Humphries, S. (1987). Identification of deletions in the human low-density lipoprotein (LDL) receptor gene. *J. Med. Genet.*, 24, 144–7

21. Hobbs, H.H., Brown, M.S., Russell, D.W., Davignon, J. and Goldstein, J.L. (1987). Deletion in the gene for the LDL receptor in majority of French Canadians with familial hypercholesterolemia. *N. Engl. J. Med.*, 317, 734–7

22. Ma, Y., Betard, C., Roy, M., Davignon, J. and Kessling, A. (1989). Identification of a second 'French Canadian' LDL receptor gene deletion and development of a rapid method to detect both deletions. *Clin. Genet.*, 36, 219–28

23. Leitersdorf, E., Van der Westhuyzen D.R., Coetzee, G.A. and Hobbs, H.H. (1989). Two common low density lipoprotein receptor gene mutations cause familial hypercholesterolemia in Afrikaaners. *J. Clin. Invest.*, 84, 954–61

24. Humphries, S., Taylor, R. and Munroe, A. (1988). Resolution by DNA probes of uncertain diagnosis of inheritance of hypercholesterolaemia. *Lancet*, 10, 794–5

25. Kessling, A.M., Rajput-Williams, J., Bainton, D., Scott, J., Miller, N.E., Baker, I. and Humphries, S.E. (1987). DNA polymorphisms of the apolipoprotein AII and AI-CIII-AIV genes: a study in men selected for differences in high density lipoprotein cholesterol concentration. *Am. J. Hum. Genet.*, 42, 458–67

26. Ordovas, J.M., Schaefer, E.J., Salem, D., Ward, R.H., Glueck, C.J., Vergani, C., Wilson, P.W.F. and Karathanasis, S.K. (1986). Apolipoprotein A-I gene polymorphism associated with premature coronary artery disease and familial hypoalphalipoproteinaemia. *N. Engl. J. Med.*, **314**, 671–7

27. Wile, D.B., Barbir, M., Gallagher, J., Myant, N.B., Ritchie, C.D., Thompson, G.R. and Humphries, S.E. (1989). Apolipoprotein A-I gene polymorphisms: frequency in patients with coronary artery disease and healthy controls and association with serum apo A-I and HDL-cholesterol concentration. *Atherosclerosis*, **78**, 9–18

28. Paulweber, B., Friedl, W., Krempler, F., Humphries, S.E., Sandhofer, F. (1988). Genetic variation in the apolipoprotein AI-CIII-AIV gene cluster and coronary heart disease. *Atherosclerosis*, **73**, 125–33

29. Sidoli, A., Giudici, G., Soria, M. and Vergani, C. (1986). Restriction-fragment-length polymorphisms in the AI-CIII gene complex occurring in a family with hypoalphalipoproteinaemia. *Atherosclerosis*, **62**, 81–7

30. Rees, A., Stocks, J., Shoulders, C.C., Galton, D.J. and Baralle, F.E. (1983). DNA polymorphism adjacent to human apoprotein AI gene: relation to hypertriglyceridaemia. *Lancet*, **1**, 444–6

31. Rees, A., Stocks, J., Sharpe, C.R., Vella, M.A., Shoulders, C.C., Katz, J., Jowett, N.I., Baralle, F.E. and Galton, D.J. (1985). DNA polymorphism in the apo AI-CIII gene cluster: association with hypertriglyceridaemia. *J. Clin. Invest.*, **76**, 1090–5

32. Hayden, M.R., Kirk, H., Clark, C., Frohlich, J., Rabkin, S., Kirby, L., McLeod, R. and Hewitt, J. (1986). DNA polymorphisms in and around the apo AI-CIII genes and genetic hyperlipidaemias. *Am. J. Hum. Genet.* (Submitted)

33. Shoulders, C.C., Ball, J.M. and Baralle, F.E. (1989). Variation in the apo AI/CIII/AIV gene complex: its association with hyperlipidaemia. *Atherosclerosis*, **80**, 111–18

34. Kessling, A., Taylor, R., Temple, A., Hidalgo, A. and Humphries, S.E. (1988). A PvuII polymorphism in the 5' flanking region of the apolipoprotein AIV gene: its use to study genetic variation determining serum lipid and apolipoprotein concentration. *Hum. Genet.*, **78**, 237–9

35. Karathanasis, S.K. (1985). Apolipoprotein multigene family: tandem organisation of apolipoprotein AIV, AI and CIII genes. *Proc. Natl. Acad. Sci. USA*, **82**, 6374–8

36. Karathanasis, S.K., Zannis, V.I. and Breslow, J.L. (1985). Isolation and characterisation of cDNA clones corresponding to two different human apoC-III alleles. *J. Lipid Res.*, **26**, 451–6

37. Vella, M., Kessling, A., Jowett, N., Rees, A., Stocks, J., Wallis, S. and Galton, D. (1985). DNA polymorphisms flanking the apo A-1 and insulin genes and type III hyperlipidaemia. *Hum. Genet.*, **69**, 275–6

38. Utermann, G. (1985). Genetic polymorphism of apolipoprotein E – impact on plasma lipoprotein metabolism. In Crepaldi, G. (ed.). *Diabetes, Obesity and Hyperlipidaemia – III.* pp. 1–27. (Amsterdam: Elsevier Science Publishers)

39. Kessling, A.M., Berg, K., Mockleby, E. and Humphries, S.E. (1986). DNA polymorphisms around the apo AI gene in normal and hyperlipidaemic individuals selected for a twin study. *Clin. Genet.*, **29**, 485–90

40. Cole, S.A., Szathmary, E.J.E. and Ferell, R.E. (1989). Gene and gene-product variation in the apolipoprotein A-I/C-III/A-IV cluster in the Dogrib Indians of the Northwest territories. *Am. J. Hum. Genet.*, **44**, 835–43

41. Rees, A., Stocks, J., Paul, H., Ohuchi, Y. and Galton, D. (1986). Haplotypes identified by DNA polymorphisms at the apo A-1 and C-III loci and hypertriglyceridaemia. A study in a Japanese population. *Hum. Genet.*, **72**, 168–71

42. Utermann G., Vogelberg, K.H., Steinmetz, A., Schoenborn, W., Pruin, N., Jaeshcke, M., Hees, M. and Canzler, H. (1979). Polymorphism of apolipoprotein E. II. Genetics of hyperlipoproteinaemia type III. *Clin. Genet.*, **15**, 37–62

43. Brown, W.V. and Baginsky, M.L. (1972). Inhibition of lipoprotein lipase by an apoprotein of human very low density lipoprotein. *Biochem. Biophys. Res. Commun.*, **46**, 375–81

44. Pagani, F., Sidoli, A., Giudici, G.A., Vergani, A. and Baralle, F.E. (1989). Association of a polymorphism in the apo AI gene promoter with hyperalphalipoproteinemia. In Miller N. (ed.). *High Density Lipoproteins and Atherosclerosis.* (Amsterdam: Elsevier Science Publishers)

45. Jeenah, M., Kessling, A., Miller, N. and Humphries, S. (1990). A G to A substitution in the promoter region of the apolipoprotein AI gene is associated with elevated serum apolipoprotein AI and high density lipoprotein cholesterol concentrations. *Mol. Biol. Med.* (Submitted)

46. Jeffreys, A.J. (1979). DNA sequence variants in the Gy- Ay-d- and B-globin genes of man. *Cell*, **18**, 1–10

47. Knott, T.J., Pease, R.J., Powell, L.M., Wallis, S. C., Rall Jr, S.C., Innerarity, T.L., Blackhart, B., Taylor, W.R., Lusis, A.J., McCarthy, B.J., Mahley, R.W., Levy-Wilson, B. and Scott, J. (1986). Complete protein sequence and identification of structural domains of the human apolipoprotein B. *Nature*, **323**, 734–8

48. Yang, C-Y, Chen, S-H., Sparrow, J.T., Gianturco, S.H., Bradley, W.A. *et al.* (1986). Sequence, structure, receptor-binding domains and internal repeats of human apolipoprotein B-100. *Nature*, **323**, 738

49. Hegele, R.A., Huang, S-S., Herbert, P.N., Blum, C.B., Buring, J.E., Hennekens, C.H. and Breslow, J.L. (1986). Apolipoprotein B-gene DNA polymorphisms associated with myocardial infarction. *New Engl. J. Med.*, **515**, 1509–15

50. Myant, N.B., Gallagher, J., Barbir, M., Thompson, G.R., Wile, D. and Humphries, S.E. (1989). Restriction fragment length polymorphisms in the apo B gene in relation to coronary artery disease. *Atherosclerosis*, **77**, 193–201

51. Paulweber, B., Friedl, W., Krempler, F., Humphries, S.E. and Sandhofer, F. (1990). Association of DNA polymorphism at the apolipoprotein B gene locus with coronary heart disease and serum very low density lipoprotein levels. *Atherosclerosis*, **10**, 117–24

52. Law, A., Powell, L.M., Brunt, H. *et al.* (1986). Common DNA polymorphism within coding sequence of apolipoprotein B gene associated with altered lipid levels. *Lancet*, **1**, 1301–3

53. Talmud, P.J., Barni, N., Kessling, A.M., Carlsson, P., Darnfors, C., Bjursell, G., Galton, D.J., Wynn, V. and Humphries, S.E. (1987). Apolipoprotein B gene variants are involved in the determination of serum cholesterol levels: a study in normo- and hyperlipidaemic individuals. *Atherosclerosis*, **67**, 81–9

54. Berg, K. (1986). DNA polymorphism at the apolipoprotein B locus is associated with lipoprotein level. *Clin. Genet.*, **30**, 515–20

55. Rajput-Williams J., Knott, T.J., Wallis, S.C., Sweetnam, P., Yarnell, J., Bell, G.I., Cox, N., Miller, N.E. and Scott, J. (1988). Variation of apolipoprotein-B gene is associated with obesity, high blood cholesterol levels, and increased risk of coronary heart disease. *Lancet*, **24**, 1442–6

56. Demant, T., Houlston, R., Caslake, M.J., Series, J.J., Shepherd, J., Packard, C.J. and Humphries. S.E. (1988). Catabolic rate of low density lipoprotein is influenced by variation in the apolipoprotein B gene. *J. Clin. Invest.*, **82**, 797–802

57. Houlston, R.S., Turner, P.R., Revill, J., Lewis, B. and Humphries, S.E. (1988). The fractional catabolic rate of low density lipoprotein in normal individuals is influenced by variation in the apolipoprotein B gene: a preliminary study. *Atherosclerosis*, **71**, 81–5

58. Brown, M.S. and Goldstein, J.L. (1986). A receptor-mediated pathway for cholesterol homeostasis. *Science*, **232**, 34–47

59. Vega, G.L. and Grundy, S.M. (1986). In vivo evidence for reduced binding of low density lipoproteins to receptors as a cause of primary moderate hypercholesterolaemia. *J. Clin. Invest.*, **78**, 1410–14

60. Innerarity, T.L., Weisgraber, K.H., Arnold, K.S. *et al.* (1987). Familial defective apolipoprotein B-100: low density lipoproteins with abnormal receptor binding. *Proc. Natl. Acad. Sci. USA*, **84**, 6419–923

61. Weisgraber, H., Innerarity, T.L., Newhouse, Y.E. *et al.* (1988). Familial defective apolipoprotein B-100: enhanced binding of monoclonal antibody MB47 to abnormal low density lipoproteins. *Proc. Natl. Acad. Sci. USA*, **86**, 587–91

62. Soria, L.F., Ludwig, E.H., Clarke, H.R.G., Vega, G.L., Grundy, S.M. and McCarthay, B.J. (1989). Association between a specific apolipoprotein B mutation and familial defective apolipoprotein B-100. *Proc. Natl. Acad. Sci. USA*, **86**, 587–91

63. Tybjærg-Hansen, A., Gallagher, J., Vincent, J. *et al.* (1990). Familial defective apolipoprotein B-100: detection in the United Kingdom and Scandinavia, and clinical characteristics of ten cases. *Atherosclerosis*, **80**, 235–241

64. Schuster, H, Rauh, G., Kormann, B. *et al.* Familial defective apolipoprotein B-100: 18 cases detected in Germany (submitted)

65. Saiki, R.K., Scharf, S., Faloona, F. *et al.* (1985). Enzymatic amplification of β-globin genomic sequences and restriction site analysis for diagnosis of sickle cell anemia. *Science*, **230**, 1350–4

66. Saiki, R.K., Bugawan, T.L., Horn, G.T., Mullis, K.B. and Erlich, H.A. (1986). Analysis of enzymatically amplified β-globin and HLA-DQ α DNA with allele specific oligonucleotide probes. *Nature*, **324**, 162–6

67. Saiki, R.K., Gelfand, D.H., Stoffel, S. *et al.* (1988). Primer-directed enzymatic amplification of DNA with a thermostable DNA polymerase. *Science*, **239**, 487–94

68. Vosberg, H-P. (1989). The polymerase chain reaction: an improved method for the analysis of nucleic acids (review article). *Hum. Genet.*, **83**, 1–15

69. Witt, M. and Erickson, R.P. (1989). A rapid method for detection of Y-chromosomal DNA from dried blood specimens by the polymerase chain reaction. *Hum. Genet.*, **82**, 271–74

70. Rubin, E.M., Andrews, K.A. and Kan, Y.W. (1989). Newborn screening by DNA analysis of dried blood spots. *Hum. Genet.*, **82**, 134–6

71. Lench, N., Stainer, P. and Williamson, R. (1988). Simple non-invasive method to obtain DNA for gene analysis. *Lancet*, **1**, 1356–8

72. Cladaras, C., Hadzoupoulou-Cladaras, M., Nolte, R.T., Atkinson, D. and Zannis, V.I. (1986). The complete sequence and structural analysis of human apolipoprotein B-100: relationship between apo B-100 and apo B-48 forms. *E.M.B.O. J.*, **5**, 3495–507

73. Brown, M.S. and Goldstein, J.L. (1983). Lipoprotein metabolism in the macrophage: implications for cholesterol deposition in atherosclerosis. *Ann. Rev. Biochem.*, **52**, 223–61

74. Reichl, D. and Miller, N.E. (1989). Pathophysiology of reverse cholesterol transport. Insights from inherited disorders of lipoprotein metabolism. *Arteriosclerosis*, **9**, 785–97

75. Meade, T.W., Mellows, S., Brozovic, M. *et al.* (1986). Haemostatic function and ischaemic heart disease: principal results of the Northwick Park Study. *Lancet*, **2**, 533–7

76. Humphries, S.E., Dubowitz, M., Cook, M., Stirling, Y. and Meade, T.W. (1987). Role of genetic variation at the fibrinogen locus in determination of plasma fibrinogen concentrations. *Lancet*, 1451–5

77. Powell, J., Bashir, A., Dawson, S., Vinde, N., Henney, A.M., Humphries, S.E. and Greenhalgh, R.M. (1990). Genetic variation on chromosome 16 is associated with abdominal aortic aneurysm. *Clin. Sci.*, **78**, 13–16

78. Boers, G.H.J., Smals, A.G.H., Trijbels, F.J.M., Fowler, B., Bakkeren, J.A.J.M., Schoonderwaldt, H.C., Kleijer, W.J. and Kloppenborg, P.W.C. (1985). Heterozygosity for homocystinuria in premature peripheral and cerebral occlusive arterial disease. *N. Engl. J. Med.*, **313**, 709–15

Index